Mental Disorders in Primary Care
A Guide to their Evaluation and Management

Mental Disorders in Primary Care
A Guide to their Evaluation and Management

Edited by

André F. Carvalho
Associate Professor, Department of Clinical Medicine, Head,
Translational Psychiatry Research Group, Faculty of Medicine,
Federal University of Ceará, Fortaleza, Brazil

Roger S. McIntyre, M.D., FRCPC
Professor of Psychiatry and Pharmacology,
University of Toronto

Executive Director, Brain and Cognition
Discovery Foundation (BCDF)

Head, Mood Disorders Psychopharmacology Unit

Toronto, Ontario Canada

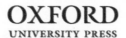

OXFORD
UNIVERSITY PRESS

OXFORD
UNIVERSITY PRESS

Great Clarendon Street, Oxford, OX2 6DP,
United Kingdom

Oxford University Press is a department of the University of Oxford.
It furthers the University's objective of excellence in research, scholarship,
and education by publishing worldwide. Oxford is a registered trade mark of
Oxford University Press in the UK and in certain other countries

© Oxford University Press 2017

The moral rights of the authors have been asserted

First Edition published in 2017

Impression: 1

Published in the United States of America by Oxford University Press
198 Madison Avenue, New York, NY 10016, United States of America

British Library Cataloguing in Publication Data

Data available

Library of Congress Control Number: 2016955730

ISBN 978-0-19-874663-8

Printed in Great Britain by
Ashford Colour Press Ltd, Gosport, Hampshire

Foreword

In the year 2016, for the first time in their history, the United Nations included the promotion of mental health and the treatment of mental disorders among its Sustainable Development Goals. This was not surprising: what is astonishing is that they have not done it earlier. The Millennium Development Goals did not mention mental health and the discussions of the United Nations about the serious problems produced by non-communicable diseases focused on diabetes, cardiovascular disease, cancer and pulmonary obstructive disease. They did not consider mental disorders – there is only one sentence about them in the report of the session acknowledging that "mental and neurological diseases and Alzheimer's disease" are also contributing to the countries' burden of disease, although by then it was well known that a significant proportion – at least a third of years lost to disability because of the disease worldwide – were caused by mental disorders.

The delay in pointing at mental disorders as one of the major public health problems may have been caused by the doubt that present knowledge about the treatment and prevention of mental disorders does not allow an effective action. It might have also been a reflection of the statistics showing that the numbers of mental health professionals are far too small to provide mental health care to five hundred million people with mental disorders across the world. However, the latter fact should not have stopped the United Nations to urge their member states to act; in 1973 a World Health Organization's Expert Committee report already spoke about the extension of mental health care by task-shifting and enabling primary health care staff to take on a major part of the burden of care for the mentally ills. Somewhat later, in 1978, the members of the World Health Organization (WHO) adopted the Declaration of Alma Ata and the Report of the Alma Ata Conference on Primary health care which included the promotion of mental health among the essential elements of primary health care. The studies on extension of mental health care carried out by the WHO demonstrated that the primary health care staff, given some training, can deal with a significant proportion of mental disorders in a competent way; since then numerous other studies have confirmed these findings.

The reluctance of the United Nations was probably, at least in part, caused by the stigma of mental disorders which is still widely spread and presents a major obstacle to the provision of care to people with mental illness and other progress in this field. To dispel this and make mental health care an obvious and important priority for the worlds' health systems, we need additional evidence that it is possible to manage mental disorders in primary health care, which in turn calls for tireless action to enable primary health care staff to take on a significant part of the responsibility for the treatment of mental illness. Such action depends on the willingness and capacity of the general practitioners, nurses and other general health care workers to deal with mental disorders which they encounter in their work. An essential requirement to achieve this is to offer primary care workers knowledge about the management of mental disorders in a clear and pragmatic way. The book which André Carvalho and Roger McIntyre constructed does this by its chapters based on evidence and presented in a manner that makes it easy to understand and use the knowledge necessary for a competent treatment and care for people with mental illness.

The editors of this volume made the wise decision to complement the chapters dealing with the management of different groups of disorders by a chapter summarizing the knowledge about the neurobiology of mental illness, and by chapters presenting two major modern trends in the organization of services – those of collaborative care and patient centredness. They have also allowed the contributing authors to support their chapters by comprehensive and rich sets of references to work on which their chapter was based: this makes the book not only a teaching tool but also a well-documented source of indications about the relevant evidence.

It is to be hoped that the Carvalho and McIntyre's Mental Disorders in Primary Care will be widely read and used, enabling primary care workers to deal with mental disorders, thus providing the evidence which supports the thesis that the scarcity of highly trained mental health personnel must not be taken as a reason to neglect mental health care and that well-trained primary care workers can play a significant role in dealing with mental disorders thus offering people who suffer from them and their families a new hope and a chance to live a life of quality while reducing the enormous burden of disease which these disorders may represent for both the rich and the poor countries of the world.

Norman Sartorius, MD, PhD, FRC Psych

Contents

Abbreviations

5-HIAA	5-hydroxyindoleacetic acid
5-HT	serotonin
5-HTT	5HT transporter
5HTTPR	serotonin transporter promoter locus
ACC	anterior cingulate cortex
ACTH	adrenocorticotropin
AD	anxiety disorder
ADH	anti-diuretic hormone
ADHD	attention-deficit hyperactivity disorder
ADL	activities of daily living
ADORA2A	adenosine 2A receptor gene
AHRQ	Agency for Healthcare Research and Quality
AIDS	acquired immune deficiency syndrome
ALT	alanine aminotransferase
APA	American Psychiatric Association
ASAM PPC	American Society of Addiction Medicine Patient Placement Criteria
ASD	acute stress disorder
ASRS	Adult Self-Report ADHD Scale
AUD	alcohol use disorder
AUDIT	Alcohol Use Disorders Identification Test
AWS	alcohol withdrawal syndrome
BAI	Beck Anxiety Inventory
BDI	Beck Depression Inventory
BDNF	brain-derived neurotrophic factor
BPD	borderline personality disorder
BSDS	bipolar spectrum disorders scale
BUD	benzodiazepine use disorder
CADDRA	Canadian ADHD Resource Alliance
CAGE	Cut Down, Annoyed, Guilty and Eye Opener
CAM	complementary and alternative medicine
CBT	Cognitive-Behavioural Therapy

CBTp	Cognitive-Behavioural Therapy for Psychosis
CD	conduct disorder
CDC	Centers for Disease Control
CEA	cost effectiveness analysis
CEN	cognitive-executive network
CHD	coronary heart disease
CIDI	Composite International Diagnostic Interview
CIWA-Ar	Clinical Institute Withdrawal Assessment for Alcohol
CL	psychiatric consultant
CM	care manager
CMD	common mental disorders
CNS	central nervous system
COMBINE	The COMbined pharmacotherapies and Behavioral INtErventions for alcohol dependence study
COMT	catechol-O-methyl transferase
COPD	chronic obstructive pulmonary disease
CRF	corticotropin-releasing factor
CRH	corticotrophin-releasing hormone
CRP	C-reactive protein
CSF	cerebrospinal fluid
CSFs	colony stimulating factors
CVD	cardiovascular disease
CYP	a group of approximately 50 oxidative heterogeneous isoenzymes classified into families by numbers (e.g., CYP1, CYP2 and CYP3)
DA	dopamine
dACC	dorsal ACC
DALY	disability-adjusted life-years
DAT	dopamine transporter
DCPR	Diagnostic Criteria for Psychosomatic Research
DDI	drug-drug interaction
DILI	drug-induced liver injury
DLPFC	dorsolateral PFC
DMDD	disruptive mood dysregulation disorder
DMN	default mode network
DMPFC	dorsomedial PFC
DSM-5	Diagnostic and Statistical Manual of Mental Disorders, Fifth Edition

DSM-IV	Diagnostic and Statistical Manual of Mental Disorders, Fourth Edition
DST	dexamethasone test
EAAD	European Alliance Against Depression
EAGG	European ADHD Guidelines Group
ECT	electro-convulsive therapy
EF	executive functioning
EMDR	eye movement desensitisation and reprocessing
EPS	extrapyramidal side effects
FDA	Food and Drug Administration
GABA	gamma-amino-butyric acid
GAD	generalized anxiety disorder
GAD-7	Generalized Anxiety Disorder 7-item survey
GDNF	glia-derived neurotrophic factor
GDS	geriatric depression scale
GFR	glomerular filtration rate
GI	gastrointestinal
GP	general practitioner
GR	glucocorticoid receptors
GWAS	genome-wide association studies
HAM-D	Hamilton Depression Scale
HARS	Hamilton Anxiety Rating Scale
HAV	Hepatitis A
HBV	Hepatitis B
HCL-32	hypomania check-list-32 items
HCV	Hepatitis C
HDRS	Hamilton Depression Rating Scale
HIC	high-income countries
HIV	human immunodeficiency virus
HPA	hypothalamic pituitary adrenal axis
HRV	heart rate variability
HVA	homovanillic acid
IAPT	improved access to psychological treatments
ICD	International Classification of Mental and Behavioral Disorders
ICPE	International Consortium in Psychiatric Epidemiology
IDO	indoleamine 2,3- dioxygenase
IED	intermittent explosive disorder

IPT	inter-personal therapy
KA	kynurenic acid
LLD	late-life depression
LMIC	low- and middle-income countries
LOPFC	lateral orbital PFC
LTC	lateral temporal cortex
MAO	monoamine oxidase
MAOI	monoamine oxidase inhibitors
MDD	major depressive disorder
MDQ	mood disorder questionnaire
MHPG	3-methoxy-4-hydroxyphenylglycol
MI	Motivational interviewing
MI	myocardial infarction
MITI	Motivational Interviewing Treatment Integrity
MMSE	Mini-Mental State Examination
MRS	magnetic resonance spectroscopy
MTL	medial temporal lobe
MUS	medically unexplained symptoms
NAcc	nucleus accumbens
nAChR	nicotinic acetylcholine receptor
NAPQI	N-acetyl-p-benzoquinone imine
NaSSA	Noradrenergic and specific serotonergic anti-depressant
NCS-R	National Comorbidity Survey Replication
NDRI	norepinephrine-dopamine reuptake inhibitor
NE	norepinephrine
NET	norepinephrine transporter
NMDA	N-Methyl-D-aspartate
NRAMP	National Register of Antipsychotic Medication in Pregnancy
NRI	norepinephrine reuptake inhibitor
NRT	nicotine replacement therapy
NSSI	non-suicidal self-injury
OARS	Open questions, Affirmations, Reflective listening, and Summarizing
ODD	oppositional defiant disorder
OFC	olanzapine-fluoxetine combination
OROS	oral release osmotic system
OTC	over-the-counter

OUD	opioid use disorder
PARC	Prevention and Recovery Centres
PCC	posterior cingulate cortex
PCMH	patient-centred medical home
PCP	primary care practitioner/primary care physician
PD	personality disorder
PD	panic disorder
PET	positron emission tomography
PFC	prefrontal cortex
P-gp	P-glycoprotein
PHQ-15	15 item Patient Health Questionnaire
PHQ-9	Patient Health Questionnaire-9
PMDD	pre-menstrual dysphoric disorder
PNS	parasympathetic nervous system
PST	problem-solving therapy
PTSD	post-traumatic stress disorder
QUIN	quinolinic acid
RCT	randomized controlled trial
RDoC	Research Domain Criteria
RNS	reactive nitrogen species
ROS	reactive oxygen species
SAIB	Scale for the Assessment of Illness Behavior
SAMSHA	Substance Abuse and Mental Health Services Administration
SARI	serotonin antagonist-reuptake inhibitor
SBIRT	Screening, Brief Intervention, Referral and Treatment
SCUD	stimulant and cannabis use disorder
SDM	shared decision making
SERM	selective estrogen receptor modulators
SERT	type of monoamine transporter protein that transports serotonin from the synaptic cleft to the presynaptic neuron
sgACC	subgenual anterior cingulate cortex
SHIP	Survey of High Impact Psychosis
SIADH	syndrome of inappropriate antidiuretic hormone
SJS	Steven Johnson's Syndrome
SMI	severe mental illness
SN	salience network

SNP	single nucleotide polymorphism
SNRI	serotonin norepinephrine reuptake inhibitors
SNS	sympathetic nervous system
SODAS	spheroidal oral drug absorption system
SSD	somatic symptom and related disorders
SSRI	selective serotonin reuptake inhibitor
STAR-D	Sequential Treatment Alternative to Relieve Depression
SUD	substance use disorder
T2DM	type 2 diabetes mellitus
TAU	treatment as usual
TCA	tricyclic antidepressants
TdP	torsades de pointes
TEN	toxic epidermal necrolysis
TMS	transcranial magnetic stimulation
TPH2	tryptophan hydroxylase-2
TRH	thyrotropin releasing hormone
TSH	thyroid stimulating hormone
TUD	tobacco use disorder
UGT	5'-diphosphate glucuronosyltransferase
VEGF	vascular endothelial growth factor
VLPFC	ventrolateral PFC
vmPFC	ventromedial PFC
WBC	white blood count
WFSBP	World Federation of Societies of Biological Psychiatry
WHO	World Health Organization
WMH	World Mental Health Surveys
WML	white matter lesions
WONCA	World Organization of Family Doctors
YLD	years lived with disability
YMRS	Young Mania Rating Scale

Contributors

Giovanni Amodeo
Associate Professor of Psychiatry,
Department of Molecular Medicine,
University of Siena, Italy

Michael Berk
Professor and Alfred Deakin
Chair of Psychiatry,
Deakin University,
Victoria, Australia

Lea Bouché
student, Ulm University,
Günzburg, Germany

Kathleen Broad
Fifth year resident in psychiatry,
Department of Psychiatry,
University of Toronto,
Toronto Canada

André F. Carvalho
Associate Professor,
Department of Clinical Medicine Head,
Translational Psychiatry Research
Group,
Faculty of Medicine,
Federal University of Ceará,
Fortaleza, Brazil

Fiammetta Cosci
Associate Professor of Clinical
Psychology,
Department of Health Sciences,
University of Florence,
Florence, Italy

Bernadette DeMuri
Clinical Instructor,
Department of Psychiatry and
Behavioral Medicine,
Medical College of Wisconsin,
Wisconsin, USA

Elizabeth A. Dinapoli
Postdoctoral Fellow,
Department of Psychiatry,
University of Pittsburgh,
Pittsburgh, USA

Markus Dold
Department of Psychiatry and
Psychotherapy,
Medical University of Vienna,
Vienna, Austria

Andrea Fagiolini
Professor of Psychiatry,
Department of Molecular Medicine,
University of Siena, Italy

Giovanni Andrea Fava
Professor, Department of Clinical
Psychology,
University of Bologna,
Bologna, Italy

Deborah S. Finnell
Associate Professor,
Director of the Masters and Doctor of
Nursing Practice Programs,
Johns Hopkins School of Nursing,
Baltimore, USA

John Furler
Associate Professor,
Department of General Practice,
University of Melbourne,
Melbourne, Australia

Fabian Fußer
Consultant Psychiatrist,
Department of Psychiatry,
Psychosomatic Medicine and
Psychotherapy,
University Hospital Frankfurt,
Frankfurt am Main, Germany

Emorfia Gavrilidis
Women's Mental Health Team
Coordinator,
Monash Alfred Psychiatry Research
Centre,
Melbourne, Australia

Tony P. George
Professor of Psychiatry,
Department of Psychiatry,
University of Toronto,
Toronto, Canada

David W. Goodman
Director,
Adult Attention Deficit Disorder
Center of Maryland,
Lutherville, USA

Adam J. Gordon
Department of Medicine,
School of Medicine,
University of Pittsburgh,
Pittsburgh, USA

Jasmin Grigg
Post Doctorate Researcher,
Monash Alfred Psychiatry Research
Centre,
Melbourne, Australia

Jane Gunn
Professor,
Department of General
Practice,
University of Melbourne,
Australia

Jeffrey P. Haibach
Health Services Research and
Development Service,
US Department of Veterans
Affairs,
Washington, DC, USA

Erkki Isometsä
Professor of Psychiatry,
University of Helsinki,
Helsinki, Finland

Tarik Karakaya
Department of Psychiatry,
Psychosomatic Medicine and
Psychotherapy,
University Hospital Frankfurt,
Frankfurt am Main, Germany

John W. Kasckow
VA Pittsburgh Healthcare System,
US Department of Veterans Affairs;
Pittsburgh, PA, USA;
Department of Psychiatry,
School of Medicine,
University of Pittsburgh,
Pittsburgh, USA

Siegfried Kasper
Department of Psychiatry and
Psychotherapy,
Medical University of Vienna,
Vienna, Austria

Cristiano A. Köhler
Researcher,
Translational Psychiatry Research Group
and Department of Clinical Medicine,
Federal University of Ceará,
Fortaleza, Brazil

Markus Kösters
Research Associate,
Ulm University,
Günzburg, Germany

Jayashri Kulkarni
Director,
Monash Alfred Psychiatry Research
Centre,
Melbourne, Australia

Bernd Löwe
Director,
Department of Psychosomatic Medicine,
University Medical Center Hamburg-
Eppendorf & Head Physician,
University Clinic for Psychosomatic
Medicine and Psychotherapy,
Schön Klinik Hamburg Eilbek,
Hamburg, Germany

Subramoniam Madhusoodanan
Associate Chairman,
Department of Psychiatry,
St John's Episcopal Hospital,
Far Rockaway, USA;
Clinical Professor of Psychiatry,
SUNY Downstate Medical
Center,
Brooklyn, USA

Giuseppe Maina
Associate Professor of Psychiatry,
Department of Neuroscience,
University of Turin,
Turin, Italy

Vladimir Maletic
Clinical Professor of Neuropsychiatry
and Behavioral Science,
University of South Carolina School of
Medicine,
Greenville, USA

Andrea Feijó Mello
Psychiatrist,
Violence and Stress Research and
Treatment Program,
Department of Psychiatry,
Federal University of São Paulo,
São Paulo, Brazil

Alexandra M. Murray
Post-Doctoral Researcher,
Department of Psychosomatic
Medicine,
University Medical Center Hamburg-
Eppendorf & University Clinic
for Psychosomatic Medicine and
Psychotherapy,
Schön Klinik Hamburg Eilbek,
Hamburg, Germany

Shainal Nathoo
Medical Officer,
Monash Alfred Psychiatry Research
Centre,
Melbourne, Australia

Paulo R. Nunes Neto
Translational Psychiatry Research Group
and Department of Clinical Medicine,
Federal University of Ceará,
Fortaleza, Brazil

Chi-Un Pae
Assistant Professor,
Department of Psychiatry,
The Catholic University of Korea College
of Medicine, Seoul, Republic of Korea;
Department of Psychiatry and
Behavioral Sciences,
Duke University Medical Center,
Durham, USA

Victoria J. Palmer
Senior Research Fellow,
Mental Health Department of General
Practice,
Melbourne Medical School,
The University of Melbourne,
Melbourne, Australia

Johannes Pantel
Head of Geriatric Medicine,
Institute of General Practice,
Geriatric Medicine,
Goethe-University Frankfurt am Main,
Frankfurt am Main, Germany

Joel Paris
Professor of Psychiatry,
McGill University,
Institute of Community and Family
Psychiatry,
Montreal, Canada

Ives Cavalcante Passos
UT Center of Excellence on Mood
Disorder,
Department of Psychiatry and
Behavioral Sciences,
The University of Texas Science Center
at Houston,
Houston, USA

Bernd Puschner
Senior Researcher,
Ulm University,
Günzburg, Germany

Leona Hakkaart-van Roijen
Associate Professor,
Erasmus University Rotterdam,
Rotterdam, Netherlands

Manu S. Sharma
Second Year Resident,
University of Texas Health Science
Center at Houston,
Department of Psychiatry and
Behavioral Sciences,
The University of Texas Science
Center at Houston,
Houston, USA

Leah R. Steinberg
Resident PGY-1,
Department of Psychiatry,
St John's Episcopal Hospital,
Far Rockaway, USA

Nitin Tandan
MD Candidate,
Medical University of Lublin,
Lublin, Poland

Anne Toussaint
Post-Doctoral Researcher,
Department of Psychosomatic
Medicine,
University Medical Center Hamburg-
Eppendorf & University Clinic
for Psychosomatic Medicine
and Psychotherapy,
Schön Klinik Hamburg Eilbek,
Hamburg, Germany

Marina Tsoy-Podosenin
Resident PGY-1,
Department of Psychiatry,
StJohn's Episcopal Hospital,
Far Rockaway, USA

Christina van der Feltz-Cornelis
Professor of Social Psychiatry,
Tilburg University,
Tillburg, Netherlands

Harm van Marwijk
Clinical Chair in Primary Care Research,
University of Manchester,
Manchester, UK

Sheng-Min Wang
Professor,
Department of Psychiatry,
The Catholic University of Korea College
of Medicine,
Seoul, Republic of Korea

Stefan Weinmann
Consultant Psychiatrist,
Psychiatric University Hospital Basel,
Basel, Switzerland

Rob Whitley
Assistant Professor Psychiatry,
Department of Psychiatry,
Douglas Mental Health University
Institute,
McGill University,
Montreal, Canada

Mary Sau Ling Yeh
Psychiatrist,
Violence and Stress Research and
Treatment Program,
Department of Psychiatry,
Federal University of São Paulo,
São Paulo, Brazil

Chapter 1

The epidemiology, burden and treatment of mental disorders in primary care

Bernd Puschner, Markus Kösters, Lea Bouché, and Stefan Weinmann

Introduction to epidemiology, burden, and treatment of mental disorders in primary care

Mental disorders are highly prevalent in the community, but poorly detected and treated in primary care (Bijl et al., 2003; King et al., 2008; Goldberg, 1995). This high unmet need entails a range of negative consequences, including reduced quality of life, high risk of chronicity, a detrimental bidirectional effect on various comorbid communicable and non-communicable diseases and injuries, and unnecessary diagnostic and therapeutic procedures which do not address the main mental health condition, which commonly goes unrecognized.

There are a variety of health conditions which increase the risk of developing mental disorders or impact on their long-term course and prognosis, while there are relatively few studies distinguishing independent somatic diseases and somatic symptoms preceding the diagnosis of mental disorders (Kroenke et al., 1994). These complex interactions illustrate the importance of the comorbidity concept and put into question the artificial separation of somatic and mental health and disease (Iacovides and Siamouli, 2008; Feltz-Cornelis et al., 2014).

In this chapter, we will:

1. report important findings on the epidemiology of treated and untreated mental disorders in the community and primary care systems in different regions of the world, including an elaboration on factors that could influence incidence and prevalence rates as well as health care utilization;

2. describe measures and results of studies on the burden of mental health as well as disease-related and societal costs;

3. discuss main challenges for the correct detection of mental disorders in primary care;

4. describe evidence-based treatment approaches; in order to;

5. draw conclusions and identify future clinical and research implications.

Epidemiology

General population

In order to obtain precise estimates of the prevalence of mental disorders, community surveys need to investigate representative samples of the general population, with the proper use of standard diagnostic criteria (WHO International Consortium in Psychiatric Epidemiology, 2000). However, methodological differences across studies limit comparability. An early review of epidemiological studies on selected psychiatric disorders in the general population published until 1997 did not identify any cross-national studies among the 43 surveys (Kohn et al., 2000). The authors found substantial variations in the prevalence rates. However, sample sizes in many studies were low, and the external validity of the estimates was questionable. Kohn and colleagues (2000) report on an inverse relation between socioeconomic status and the prevalence of mental disorders, balanced overall rates of disorders among men and women, but higher rates of depression and anxiety disorders among women. Conversely, substance use disorders and antisocial personality disorder are more prevalent among men.

Since then a number of community epidemiological studies have been published (Girolamo and Bassi, 2003). In addition, in 1998, the WHO established the International Consortium in Psychiatric Epidemiology (ICPE) to enable joint analysis of community surveys and to refine survey and data collection tools such as the Composite International Diagnostic Interview (CIDI) (Kessler and Ustün, 2004). ICPE analyses have shown that 12-month prevalence rates of common mental disorders vary widely (between a high 40% rate in the Netherlands and a low 12% rate in Turkey). ICPE has also confirmed delays in proper treatment as well as high under-treatment rates in general (WHO International Consortium in Psychiatric Epidemiology, 2000). The World Mental Health Surveys (WMH) were established in 1998, and involved 24 countries (Demyttenaere et al., 2004). This largest cross-national study used uniform diagnostic criteria which assessed prevalence rates, severity of common mental disorders, healthcare utilization, and adequacy of treatment, as well as socioeconomic predictor variables (Kessler and Ustün, 2008). The authors found widely varying prevalence rates ranging from 4.3% in Shanghai to 26.4% in the United States for any WMH-CIDI/*DSM-IV* disorder in the 12 months preceding interviews (Demyttenaere et al., 2004). In Europe, Wittchen and Jacobi (2005) identified and synthesized 27 community studies with variable designs and methods including over 150,000 subjects from 16 European countries, showing that 27% of the adult European population was affected by at least one mental disorder in the past 12 months. Only 26% of all cases had any consultation with a GP or a mental health care provider.

Steel and colleagues (2014) recently undertook a comprehensive review and meta-analysis of psychiatric epidemiological population surveys published between 1980 and 2013 which reported data on common mental disorders (CMD), i.e., mood, anxiety, and alcohol use disorders. The review included 174 surveys across 63 countries. Twenty-six studies reported data from high income countries (HIC), and 37 from low and middle income countries (LMIC), respectively. This meta-analysis estimated an overall period prevalence (an integration of point and period estimates, with preferences for one-year prevalence) of 17.6% and a lifetime prevalence of 29.2% for CMD. Heterogeneity of estimates was considerable (e.g. lifetime prevalence rate ranging from 2.9% to 81.8% across different surveys). Bearing this in mind, no differences between HIC and LMIC were found for the period prevalence estimates, while the lifetime prevalence estimates were significantly higher in HIC (32.2% vs. 22.7%). However, it seems that regional differences were more distinct than income differences: regardless of country income levels, prevalence rates in Asian regions and sub-Saharan Africa were relatively low, whereas these estimates were higher in Latin America. Furthermore, consistent gender-related differences were observed: women had substantially higher rates of lifetime and period prevalence for mood (7.3% vs. 4%) and anxiety disorders (8.7% vs. 4.3%), whereas men presented considerably higher prevalence of substance use disorders (2.0% vs. 7.5%). For Europe, Steel and colleagues (2014) have found significantly lower one-year prevalence rates than figures from the foregoing study by Wittchen and Jacobi (2005) which may be partly explained by a number of methodological differences between included studies, e.g. the inclusion of phobia and somatoform disorders by Wittchen and Jacobi (2005).

Only very few prospective studies are available. During a 30-year follow-up period, the Zurich study (Angst et al., 2015) reported rates of mental disorders ranging from 32.5% for major depressive disorder to 1.2% for Bipolar I disorder. The cumulative probability of experiencing any of mental disorder assessed by the age of 50 was 73.9%. Thus, Angst and colleagues (2015) confirm results of cross-sectional studies showing an almost universal distribution of mental disorders fulfilling current diagnostic criteria during the lifetime.

Primary care

Prevalence rates for mental disorders in primary care settings vary considerably across different studies. Table 1.1 provides a non-systematic overview of studies published after 2005, which estimated prevalence rates for affective and anxiety disorders among primary care users.

Prevalence rates range from 10% to 39% for affective disorders, from 7.2% to 37.6% for any anxiety disorder, and from 6.3% to 27.2% for major depressive disorder in these studies. Notwithstanding the substantial variability in estimates, these studies illustrate that CMDs are highly prevalent in primary care settings. Furthermore, comorbid illnesses are frequent, with concurrent chronic somatic illnesses reported for more than 50% of patients with depression (Menear et al., 2015), while multi-morbidity, i.e. more than two chronic conditions, is also very common (Gunn et al., 2012).

Burden of mental disorders in primary care

Since the publication of the World Bank Study 'Investing in health' (World Bank, 1993), which heavily relied on the Global Burden of Disease project, the disability-adjusted life-years (DALYs) metric has been increasingly employed to rate the aggregated impact of diagnostic entities in populations. By measuring the quality of life when living with a disease including valuation of health states, this instrument goes beyond estimations of incidence, prevalence, and mortality rates. Mental disorders are

Table 1.1 Prevalence rates of mental disorder in primary care settings

	Publication	Country	N	Estimated Prevalence (%)
Affective Disorders	Roca et al., 2009	Spain	7,936	35.8 (point)
	Grandes et al., 2011	Spain	2,539	10 (12 month)
	Aillon et al., 2014	Kenya	300	39.0 (point)
Anxiety	Ansseau et al., 2004	Belgium & Luxemburg	13,677	19 (point)
	Mergl et al., 2007	Germany	394	15.7 (point)
	Kroenke et al., 2007	USA	965	19.5 (point)
	Löwe et al., 2008	USA	2,091	8.0 (point)
	Roca et al., 2009	Spain	7,936	25.6 (point)
	Martín-Merino et al., 2010	UK	40,873	7.2 (point)
	Serrano-Blanco et al., 2010	Spain	3,815	18.49 (12 month)
	Grandes et al., 2011	Spain	2,539	9 (point)
	Aillon et al., 2014	Kenya	301	31.3 (point)
	Gonçalves et al., 2014	Brazil	1,857	37.6 (point)
	Bunevicius et al., 2014	Lithuania	998	21 (point)
Depression	Ansseau et al., 2004	Belgium & Luxemburg	13,677	6.3 (point)
	Mergl et al., 2007	Germany	394	22.8 (point)
	Löwe et al., 2008	USA	2,091	6.6 (point)
	Mitchell et al., 2009	Worldwide	50,371	19.5 (average from 118 studies)
	Serrano-Blanco et al., 2010	Spain	3,815	9.6 (12 month)
	Vermani et al., 2011	Canada	840	27.2 (point)
	Chin et al., 2014	Hong Kong	10,179	10.7 (point)
	Gonçalves et al., 2014	Brazil	1,466	25.1 (point)
	Bunevicius et al., 2014	Lithuania	998	15 (point)

leading sources of DALYs and have continuously moved up in the health priority lists over the last years (Wahlberg and Rose, 2015).

In 1990, depression was the most disabling disorder worldwide measured in years lived with disability (Vos et al., 2013), and the fourth leading cause of overall disease burden measured in DALYs (Global Burden of Disease Study 2013 Collaborators, 2015; Murray et al., 2013). The Global Burden of Disease 2010 estimates rank unipolar depression second in the priority list (Whiteford et al., 2013a), with mental disorders accounting for more than 7% of the DALYs, for 23% of the total years lived with disability, and only for 0.5% of lost life years. These figures are highly dependent on how disabilities are weighted. It is indisputable that CMDs substantially contribute to disease burden and costs, especially to direct health care costs in HIC, as well as to indirect costs (e.g. reduced labour productivity, absenteeism and loss of income) in all countries (Jack et al., 2014).

Detection

A variety of studies showed that a significant proportion of mental disorders in primary care go undetected. Two decades ago, a ground-breaking large international WHO study found that, overall, GPs recognize half of the common mental disorders according to ICD-10 diagnostic criteria verified by the Composite Diagnostic Interview (Üstün and Sartorius, 1995). There was a high variation across primary care centres. More recently, a meta-analysis also reported poor rates of depression detection (sensitivity = 36.4%; specificity = 83.7%) in primary care (Cepoiu et al., 2008). In Australia, GPs without any training detected 51% of patients with depression, and the specificity of the depression diagnosis was 81% (Carey et al., 2014). Another meta-analysis pooling 41 studies reported similar detection rates (sensitivity = 50.1%; specificity = 81.3%; Mitchell et al., 2009). Findings suggest that among 100 unselected patients seen in primary care, there are more false positives (n = 15) than either missed (n = 10) or identified cases (n = 10). This means that 15% of patients received a diagnosis of a mental disorder although they had none according to standard diagnostic criteria (verified through gold-standard structured diagnostic interviews). The consequences of overdiagnosis depend on the steps taken by the GP—with the improper use of psychopharmacological agents posing the highest risk.

In the case of depression, an under-diagnosis of patients with major depressive disorder (MDD) seems to be due to errors of clinical judgment regarding the severity of symptoms (Mitchell et al., 2009). That is, the physician recognizes depressive symptoms, but considers these manifestations as subthreshold (i.e. clinically insignificant), most likely due to time constraints and the erroneous attribution of psychopathological manifestations as resulting from physical symptoms. However, GPs may also be reluctant to grant a definitive diagnosis of depression and may fear a 'labelling effect' on patients due to the stigma associated with this diagnosis. For example, non-depressed primary care patients who labelled themselves as depressive were twice as likely to develop a depressive disorder in the following year compared to those who were not diagnosed as clinically depressive (Barkow et al., 2002). Furthermore, GPs may be reluctant to make a diagnosis of depression if they face a limited availability of specialized services to refer the patients who may be difficult to manage (Burroughs et al., 2006).

Even when depression or other CMDs are properly recognized, they often go untreated indefinitely or for a prolonged period of time following a correct diagnosis. Data from the National Comorbidity Survey Replication (NCS-R) study, which enrolled more than 9,000 participants, found that in the vast majority of cases with lifetime major depression treatment is eventually initiated, but delays may be excessive, which often leads to a chronic relapsing course (Pence et al., 2012; Wang et al., 2005).

Consequently, efforts have been implemented worldwide to increase GPs' detection rates for CMDs, especially MDD. Use of scales modestly increases diagnostic accuracy (Gilbody et al., 2008). However, screening alone and increasing diagnostic accuracy does not itself result in better outcomes.

Treatment and outcomes

Most individuals with mental illnesses are primarily treated in primary care settings (Bijl and Ravelli, 2000; Patel et al., 2013). Up to 90% of people with CMDs are treated solely in primary care (National Institute for Health and Care Excellence, 2011). There is some evidence showing that illness severity and chronicity is lower among individuals with mental illnesses receiving primary care treatment (Schwenk et al., 1996). However, GPs also provide treatment for a large number of people with severe and long-standing mental illnesses of whom only a small proportion are referred to specialist care (Bijl and Ravelli, 2000; Kessler et al., 2005). Over the last decade, a number of meta-analyses have summarized the results from many randomized controlled trials which examined the effectiveness of treatments offered to people with mental illness in primary care. Interventions tested have included psychosocial and pharmacological treatments, as well as treatments incorporating some form of collaboration between GPs and other health professionals (collaborative care, liaison). Table 1.2 gives an overview of the results of these meta-analyses.

First, there is compelling evidence from a large number of meta-analyses showing that psychosocial treatments such as cognitive-behavioural therapy (CBT), psychodynamic therapies (including interpersonal therapy, IPT) and problem-solving therapy (PST) considerably improve outcomes, which in most instances have been measured with standardized measures, such as the Beck Depression Inventory (BDI) or the Hamilton Depression Rating Scale (HDRS). In the vast majority of studies, participants included individuals with depression, and the most solid evidence base has been established for CBT, also backed by a systematic review without meta-analysis (Høifødt et al., 2011). The evidence for PST and IPT is also convincing, while effect sizes for counselling approaches are comparably small, with questionable long-term benefits. Notably, brief treatments also yield impressive effects which are in agreement with findings that treatment length does not seem to influence outcomes (Linde et al., 2015b). Furthermore, over the last years, an ever-increasing number of RCTs have tested the effectiveness of minimal-contact and/or computerized psychotherapies, and there is emerging evidence that these approaches are not necessarily less effective than psychotherapy delivered face to face.

Second, solid evidence has also been accumulated showing that pharmacological treatment of CMDs with tricyclic antidepressants (TCAs) and selective serotonin reuptake inhibitors (SSRIs) is effective in treating depression in primary care, with a higher rate of adverse effects for TCAs (Arroll et al., 2009). Some positive results not justifying a clear recommendation have been shown for other agents (Linde et al., 2015a). SSRIs have become the most prescribed antidepressant class in most parts of the world. Despite profiles of untoward side-effects differing among agents, there is no

Table 1.2 Effectiveness of interventions for the treatment of mental illness in primary care (meta-analyses)

Reference (year)	$N_{included\ studies}$ Year of publication (range)	Diagnoses	Intervention(s)	Control	N_{total} N_{mean} N_{SD} N_{range}	Effect	Summary of results
Psychosocial interventions							
Bortolotti et al., 2008	10 1995–2005	Depression	CBT (f:f and computerized), PST (f:f and by phone), IPT, counselling, PD	TAU	1,579 157.90 82.84 48–276	$d = -0.42$ (short term, £6 months); −0.30 (long-term, >6 months)	Psychological interventions are significantly linked to clinical improvement.
Cape et al., 2010	34 1982–2007	Anxiety, depression, or mixed common mental health problems	Brief (£ 10 sessions) CBT, PST, or counselling	TAU	4,024 118.35 92.20 20–429	$d = -0.17$–1.06	Brief psychological interventions are effective treatments.
Bower et al., 2011	9 1994–2001	Anxiety, stress, depression, emotional difficulties, somatoform disorder	Counselling (non-directive, psychodynamic, cognitive-behavioural), 6–24 sessions	TAU, CBT, acupuncture	1384 152.33 87.86 40–327	$d = -0.28$ (short-term); −0.09 (long-term)	Counselling is associated with significantly greater clinical effectiveness in short-term mental health outcomes, but provides no additional advantages in the long-term.
Huntley et al., 2012	19 1983–2010	Depression	Group CBT	TAU	1,365 71.84 78.92 16–322	$d = -0.55$ (immediate), −0,47 (short- and long-term)	CBT-based psychotherapy compared to TAU is effective. Individual delivery CBT is more effective immediately post-treatment, but no longer at 3-month follow-up.

(continued)

Table 1.2 Continued

Reference (year)	$N_{included\ studies}$ Year of publication (range)	Diagnoses	Intervention(s)	Control	N_{total} N_{mean} N_{SD} N_{range}	Effect	Summary of results
Psychosocial interventions							
Linde et al., 2015b	30 1984–2013	Depression	CBT, PST, IPT, guided self-help	TAU	5,190 173.00 113.37 29–453	$d = -0.30$ (−0.14–0.69)	Psychological treatments are effective. Minimal contact or computerized CBT are as effective as treatment delivered face-to-face.
Pharmacological interventions							
Arroll et al., 2005	10 1979–2002	Depression (MDD and heterogenous)	TCA, SSRI	Placebo	1,685 168.50 113.78 36 380	RR = 1.26 (TCS vs. placebo), 1.37 (SSRI vs. placebo)	TCAs and SSRIs are effective.
Arroll et al., 2009	14 1979–2002	Range of depressive disorders	TCA, SSRI	Placebo	3,046 217.57 137.17 52–469	$d = -0.49$ (TCA vs. placebo), 1.28 (SSRI vs. placebo)	Both TCAs and SSRIs are effective.
Linde et al., 2015a	66 1971–2012	Depression	TCA, SSRI, SNRI, NRI, SARI, NaSSA, rMAO-A, Hypericum	Placebo or head-to-head	15,161 229.71 221.47 21–1385	OR (response) mean = 1.46, range 0.83–3.83)	Antidepressants are significantly more effective than placebo. Antidepressants have higher short-term effects when compared with placebo.

Collaborative care

Study	k	Years	Condition	Intervention	Comparator	Data	Effect size	Conclusion
Bower et al., 2006	37	1993–2004	Depression	Collaborative care[a]	TAU	12,294 / 361.59 / 350.77 / 61–1801	$d = 0.24$ (depressive outcomes), OR = 1.92 (antidepressant use)	Collaborative care significantly increases the use of antidepressants and reduces depressive symptoms.
Gilbody et al., 2006a	37	1993–2004	Depression	Collaborative care[b]	TAU	12,355 / - / - / -	$d = 0.25/0.15$ (short-/long-term)	Collaborative care is more effective than standard care in improving depression outcomes in the short and longer terms.
Feltz-Cornelis et al., 2010	10	1986–2006	Depression, somatoform disorders	Psychiatric consultation	TAU	5,209 / 520.90 / 684.83 / 38–1,801	$d = 0.313$ (0.210–0.614)	Psychiatric consultation is effective, especially in people with somatoform disorder, and when a consultation letter has been provided.
Archer et al., 2012	84	1993–2011	Depression, anxiety	Collaborative care[c]	TAU or other intervention	28,047 / 332.35 / 418.79 / 34–2,796	$d = -0.34/0.35$ (depression short-/long-term); $d = -0.30/-0.20$ (anxiety short-/long-term);	Collaborative care is associated with significant improvement in depression and anxiety outcomes compared with usual care.
Thota et al., 2012	32	2004–2009	Depression	Collaborative care[d]	TAU or other intervention		$d = 0.34$ (depression); OR = 2.22 (adherence); OR = 1.74 (remission)	Collaborative care models are effective in achieving clinically meaningful improvements in depression outcomes and public health benefits in a wide range of populations, settings, and organizations.

(continued)

Table 1.2 Continued

Reference (year)	$N_{included\ studies}$ Year of publication (range)	Diagnoses	Intervention(s)	Control	N_{total} N_{mean} N_{SD} N_{range}	Effect	Summary of results
Collaborative care							
Woltmann et al., 2012	57 (39 in primary care)	Depression, bipolar disorder, anxiety disorder, mixed disorders	Collaborative care[e]	TAU	22,037 386.61 446.06 55–2796	d = 0.31 (depression), 0.20 (mental QoL), 0.33 (physical QoL), 0.20 (overall QoL), 0.09 (global mental health), 0.23 (social role function)	Significant small-to-medium effects of CCMs across multiple disorders with regard to clinical symptoms, mental and physical QoL, and social role function, with no net increase in total health care costs.
Miller et al., 2013	15 2001–2010	Depression, bipolar disorder, anxiety disorder, mixed disorders	Collaborative care[e]	TAU	4,976 331.73 432.59 58 1801	d = 0.31 (depression), 0.20 (mental QoL), 0.33 (physical QoL)	CCM effect sizes for depression and mental and physical QoL have achieved statistical significance. QoL outcomes attained this status more recently than depression outcomes.

Author, year	N	Years	Condition	Intervention	Comparator	Data	Effect size	Conclusion
Coventry et al., 2014	70	1995–2011	Depression	Collaborative care[c]	TAU	23,834 380.71 422.23 38–2796	d = −0.28 (depressive outcomes) OR = 1.53 (antidepressant use)	Collaborative care successfully improves both patient outcomes and the process of care for depression.
Sighinolfi et al., 2014	15		Depression	Collaborative care[f]	TAU	3,696 246.40 188.61 62–626	d = −0.19/−0.24/ −0.21 (short-/ medium-/ long-term)	Collaborative care is more effective than treatment as usual in improving depression outcomes in European countries.

CBT: cognitive-behavioural therapy; CT: cognitive therapy; d = Cohens' d effect size (standardized mean difference); ftf: face-to-face; Hypericum: extracts from Hypericum perforatum L. (St. John's wort); IPT: interpersonal therapy; MAO: reversible inhibitors of monoaminoxidase A; NaSSA: noradrenergic and specific serotonergic antidepressive agents; NRI: noradrenaline reuptake inhibitor; OR = odds ratio; PD: psychodynamic therapy; PST: Problem solving therapy; RR: relative risk; SARI: serotonin (5-HT2) antagonists and reuptake inhibitor; SMD: standardized mean difference; SNRI, serotonin–noradrenaline reuptake inhibitor; SSRI: selective serotonin reuptake inhibitors; TAU: treatment as usual; TCA: tricyclic and tetracyclic antidepressants.

[a] (i) The introduction of a new role (case manager) into primary care; (ii) the introduction of mechanisms to foster closer liaison between primary care clinicians and mental health specialists (including case managers); (iii) the introduction of mechanisms to collect and share information on the progress of individual patients.

[b] A multifaceted intervention involving combinations of 3 distinct professionals working collaboratively within the primary care setting: a case manager, a primary care practitioner, and a mental health specialist. To be included, studies had to involve 2 of these 3 components.

[c] Meeting the 4 criteria: (i) a multi-professional approach to patient care; (ii) a structured management plan; (iii) scheduled patient follow-ups; (iv) enhanced inter-professional communication.

[d] Included at least a case manager, primary care provider, and mental health specialist with collaboration among these roles.

[e] At least three of six elements: (i) self-management support; (ii) clinical information systems; (iii) delivery system redesign; (iv) decision support; (v) healthcare organization; (vi) linkages to community resources.

[f] According to Katon et al. (1995; 2001): A multi-professional approach involving a primary care provider and at least one other health professional or paraprofessional such as a mental health specialist or case manager.

reliable evidence to guide GPs in choosing the best antidepressant for a given patient (Staudigl et al., 2014).

Third, a growing number of studies have evaluated the effectiveness of collaborative care models. Collaborative care is a multicomponent system–level intervention where case managers link primary care providers, patients, and mental health specialists in order to improve the follow-up of patients, assessing patient adherence, monitoring patient progress, and delivering psychological support (Archer et al., 2012; Korff and Goldberg, 2001; Thota et al., 2012). Psychiatric consultation, a very basic form of collaborative care, is effective (Feltz-Cornelis et al., 2010). Further meta-analytic findings drawing on a large number of RCTs show robust effects of more comprehensive collaborative (chronic) care models across mental disorders and outcome domains. Meta-regressions aiming at identifying moderators and mechanisms of effect have yielded unequivocal results, with different components predicting effects on certain outcomes only (Bower et al., 2006; Coventry et al., 2014), or components being entirely unrelated to outcome (Miller et al., 2013). It is still unclear which or how many components are necessary (Woltmann et al., 2012). However, is has been repeatedly shown that people with more severe mental illnesses might benefit more from collaborative care (Woltmann et al., 2012).

Preferences and costs

For a very long time, pharmacotherapy has been the first-line treatment of mental disorders in primary care, while psychotherapy is seldom used (Robinson et al., 2005). This is in sharp contrast to a three-fold service user preference for psychological treatment relative to medication, which is even higher among women and younger people (McHugh et al., 2013). Given the overall similar effectiveness of these treatments for CMDs (Huhn et al., 2014; Bortolotti et al., 2008; Wolf and Hopko, 2008, also see Table 1.2), and picking up on recent initiatives (Clark et al., 2009), we recommend a combined effort across care pathways to improve access to psychological therapies while increasing research into to the reasons and consequences of neglecting patient preferences.

One of the reasons for the dominance of pharmacological treatment may be higher costs for psychotherapy when compared to drug treatment. Notwithstanding flaws in cost studies in the field, especially pertaining to the proper assessment of total costs, there is some evidence suggesting that while psychotherapy is indeed more expensive than usual care, it is not more expensive than antidepressant treatment (Bosmans et al., 2008). Furthermore, it has been shown that the overall costs of counselling and usual care are similar (Bower et al., 2011). It has also been shown that the introduction of collaborative care models is associated with increased costs, with costs per additional depression-free day ranging from US$13–$24 (Gilbody et al., 2006b), and per additional quality-adjusted life year ranging from US$21,478–$49,500 (Steenbergen-Weijenburg et al., 2010). The question remains how much health insurers and society as a whole are able and willing to pay for the provision of better collaborative care models for CMDs.

Conclusion

Primary care providers are the first contact point for most people seeking treatment because of a mental illness (Goldberg, 2003). The low detection rates of mental illnesses by GPs are an ongoing concern, indicating that the awareness of mental illnesses and training in the correct application of diagnostic procedures deserve improvements. However, while a valid diagnosis does not necessarily mean that a specific treatment is required, neither does it guarantee the provision of the right evidence-based treatment. While CMDs bear a risk of a chronic disease course, there are also high rates of spontaneous remission (Chin et al., 2015; Whiteford et al., 2013b), suggesting that sometimes watchful waiting may be a viable option.

A wide range of interventions (psychosocial, pharmacological, collaborative care) are effective for the treatment of CMDs in primary care. However, it is highly questionable whether primary care interventions for depression are really able to substantially reduce the current burden of this illness (Chisholm et al., 2004). Notwithstanding some evidence of the efficacy of specific treatments for mental disorders in low- and middle-income countries (Hyman et al., 2006), these numbers disregard many socioeconomic risk factors for depression, which creates an illusion that treatments are equally effective in different sociocultural contexts. Even in the most affluent regions of the world, while medical interventions may have contributed to reductions in psychological stress and suicide rates (Isacsson et al., 2009; Rihmer, 2001), they have so far failed to bring about substantial reductions in depression-related burden. To further suppress undue optimism, it has been estimated that even when providing the best treatment, about 60% of the burden of mental disorders is unavertable (Andrews et al., 2004).

Reasons for this sobering situation are manifold, including lack of or flawed implementation of effective treatments and undue distribution of treatment resources. Common measures to increase treatment effectiveness have included GP training that focuses on diagnosis and referral procedures, and the implementation of treatment guidelines. However, effects of these measures are doubtful (Barbui et al., 2014; Gilbody et al., 2008; Thompson et al., 2000; Weinmann et al., 2007). While tackling the research-practice gap and GPs' lack of guideline adherence is important, researchers should move beyond global efficacy testing towards providing answers to the classic question, 'What treatment, by whom is most effective for this individual, with that specific problem, and under what specific set of circumstances'? (Paul, 1967: 111). A first step in this direction are studies aiming at identifying active ingredients of collaborative care (Coventry et al., 2014; Bower et al., 2006; Miller et al., 2013), taking into consideration that the treatment in a primary care setting of people with mental illness is a complex intervention (Moore et al., 2015). A major research challenge is the development of feasible and effective stepped care models balancing patient preferences and availability of treatment resources. Recent progress in delivering interventions using modern information and communication technologies (internet, smartphone), with a special focus on resource-limited settings, offers promising perspectives (Gureje et al., 2015; Joska and Sorsdahl, 2012; Patel et al., 2008).

References

Aillon J-L, Ndetei DM, Khasakhala L, Ngari WN, Achola HO, Akinyi S, and Ribero S. (2014). Prevalence, types and comorbidity of mental disorders in a Kenyan primary health centre. *Social Psychiatry and Psychiatric Epidemiology*, 49/8: 1257–68.

Andrews G, Issakidis C, Sanderson K, Corry J, and Lapsley H. (2004). Utilising survey data to inform public policy: comparison of the cost-effectiveness of treatment of ten mental disorders, *British Journal of Psychiatry*, 184/6: 526–33.

Angst J, Paksarian D, Cui L, Merikangas KR, Hengartner MP, Ajdacic-Gross V, and Rössler W. (2015). The epidemiology of common mental disorders from age 20 to 50: results from the prospective Zurich cohort Study. *Epidemiology and Psychiatric Sciences*, first view: 1–9.

Ansseau M, Dierick M, Buntinkx F, Cnockaert P, Smedt J. de, Van Den Haute M, and Vander Mijnsbrugge D. (2004). High prevalence of mental disorders in primary care. *Journal of Affective Disorders*, 78/1: 49–55.

Archer J, Bower PJ, Gilbody S, Lovell K, Richards D, Gask L, Dickens, C, and Coventry P. (2012). Collaborative care for depression and anxiety problems in primary care. *Cochrane Database of Systematic Reviews*, 2: CD006525.

Arroll B, Elley C, Fishman T, Goodyear-Smith F, Kenealy T, Blashki G, Kerse N, and MacGillivray S. (2009). Antidepressants versus placebo for depression in primary care. *Cochrane Database of Systematic Reviews*, 3: CD007954.

Arroll B, Macgillivray S, Ogston S, Reid I, Sullivan F, Williams B, and Crombie I. (2005). Efficacy and tolerability of tricyclic antidepressants and SSRIs compared with placebo for treatment of depression in primary care: a meta-analysis. *Annals of Family Medicine*, 3/5: 449–56.

Barbui C, Girlanda F, Ay, E, Cipriani A, Becker T, and Koesters M. (2014). Implementation of treatment guidelines for specialist mental health care. *Cochrane Database of Systematic Reviews*, 1: CD009780.

Barkow K, Heun R, Maier W, Wittchen HU, and Ustün TB. (2002). Risk factors for new depressive episodes in primary health care: an international prospective 12-month follow-up study. *Psychological Medicine*, 32/4: 595–607.

Bijl RV, Graaf, R. de, Hiripi E, Kessler RC, Kohn R, Offord DR, Ustün TB, Vicente B, Vollebergh Wilma AM, Walters EE, and Wittchen HU. (2003). The prevalence of treated and untreated mental disorders in five countries. *Health Affairs*, 22/3: 122–33.

Bijl RV and Ravelli A. (2000). Psychiatric morbidity, service use, and need for care in the general population: results of The Netherlands Mental Health Survey and Incidence Study. *American Journal of Public Health*, 90/4: 602–7.

Bortolotti B, Menchetti M, Bellini F, Montaguti MB, and Berardi D. (2008). Psychological interventions for major depression in primary care: a meta-analytic review of randomized controlled trials. *General Hospital Psychiatry*, 30/4: 293–302.

Bosmans JE, van Schaik DJ, de Bruijne MC, van Hout HP, van Marwijk HW, van Tulder MW, and Stalman WA. (2008). Are psychological treatments for depression in primary care cost-effective?. *Journal of Mental Health Policy and Economics*, 11/1: 3–15.

Bower P, Gilbody S, Richards D, Fletcher J, and Sutton A. (2006). Collaborative care for depression in primary care. Making sense of a complex intervention: systematic review and meta-regression. *British Journal of Psychiatry*, 189/6: 484–93.

Bower P, Knowles S, Coventry PA, and Rowland N. (2011). Counselling for mental health and psychosocial problems in primary care. *Cochrane Database of Systematic Reviews*, 9: CD001025.

Bunevicius R, Liaugaudaite V, Peceliuniene J, Raskauskiene N, Bunevicius A, and Mickuviene N. (2014). Factors affecting the presence of depression, anxiety disorders, and suicidal ideation in patients attending primary health care service in Lithuania. *Scandinavian Journal of Primary Health Care*, 32/1: 24–9.

Burroughs H, Lovell K, Morley M, Baldwin R, Burns A, and Chew-Graham C. (2006). Justifiable depression: how primary care professionals and patients view late-life depression? A qualitative study. *Family Practice*, 23/3: 369–77.

Cape J, Whittington C, Buszewicz M, Wallace P, and Underwood L. (2010). Brief psychological therapies for anxiety and depression in primary care: meta-analysis and meta-regression. *BMC Medicine*, 8/1: 38.

Carey M, Jones K, Meadows G, Sanson-Fisher R, D'Este C, Inder K, Yoong SL, and Russell G. (2014). Accuracy of general practitioner unassisted detection of depression. *Australian and New Zealand Journal of Psychiatry*, 48/6: 571–8.

Cepoiu M, McCusker J, Cole MG, Sewitch M, Belzile E, and Ciampi A. (2008). Recognition of depression by non-psychiatric physicians—a systematic literature review and meta-analysis. *Journal of General Internal Medicine*, 23/1: 25–36.

Chin WY, Chan KTY, Lam, CLK, Wan EYF, and Lam TP. (2015). 12-Month naturalistic outcomes of depressive disorders in Hong Kong's primary care. *Family Practice*, 32/3: 288–96.

Chin WY, Chan KTY, Lam CLK, Wong SYS, Fong DYT, Lo YYC, Lam TP, and Chiu BCF. (2014). Detection and management of depression in adult primary care patients in Hong Kong: a cross-sectional survey conducted by a primary care practice-based research network. *BMC Family Practice*, 15: 30.

Chisholm D, Sanderson K, Ayuso-Mateos JL, and Saxena S. (2004). Reducing the global burden of depression: population-level analysis of intervention cost-effectiveness in 14 world regions. *British Journal of Psychiatry*, 184/5: 393–403.

Clark DM, Layard R, Smithies R, Richards DA, Suckling R, and Wright B. (2009). Improving access to psychological therapy: Initial evaluation of two UK demonstration sites. *Behaviour Research and Therapy*, 47/11: 910–920.

Coventry PA, Hudson JL, Kontopantelis E, Archer J, Richards DA, Gilbody S, Lovell K, Dickens C, Gask L, Waheed W, and Bower P. (2014). Characteristics of effective collaborative care for treatment of depression: a systematic review and meta-regression of 74 randomised controlled trials. *PLoS One*, 9/9: e108114. doi: 10.1371/journal. pone.0108114

De Girolamo G and Bassi M. (2003). Community surveys of mental disorders: recent achievements and works in progress. *Current Opinion in Psychiatry*, 16/4: 403–11.

Demyttenaere K, Bruffaerts R, Posada-Villa J, Gasquet I, Kovess V, Lepine JP, Angermeyer MC, Bernert S, Girolamo, G de, Morosini P, Polidori G, Kikkawa T, Kawakami N, Ono Y, Takeshima T, Uda H, Karam EG, Fayyad JA, Karam AN, Mneimneh ZN, Medina-Mora ME, Borges G, Lara C, Graaf R de, Ormel J, Gureje O, Shen Y, Huang Y, Zhang M, Alonso J, Haro JM, Vilagut G, Bromet EJ, Gluzman S, Webb, C, Kessler RC, Merikangas KR, Anthony JC, Von Korff Michael R, Wang PS, Brugha TS, Aguilar-Gaxiola S, Lee S, Heeringa S, Pennell B-E, Zaslavsky AM, Ustun TB, and Chatterji S. (2004). Prevalence, severity, and unmet need for treatment of mental disorders in the World Health Organization World Mental Health Surveys. *JAMA*, 291/21: 2581–90.

van der Feltz-Cornelis CM, van Os J, Knappe S, Schumann G, Vieta E, Wittchen HU, Lewis SW, Elfeddali I, Wahlbeck K, Linszen D, Obradors-Tarragó C, and Haro JM. (2014). Towards Horizon 2020: challenges and advances for clinical mental health research—outcome of an expert survey. *Neuropsychiatric Disease and Treatment,* 10: 1057–68.

van der Feltz-Cornelis CM, van Os TW, van Marwijk HW, and Leentjens AFG. (2010). Effect of psychiatric consultation models in primary care. A systematic review and meta-analysis of randomized clinical trials. *Journal of Psychosomatic Research,* 68/6: 521–33.

Gilbody S, Bower P, Fletcher J, Richards D, and Sutton AJ. (2006a). Collaborative care for depression: a cumulative meta-analysis and review of longer-term outcomes. *Archives of Internal Medicine,* 166/21: 2314–21.

Gilbody S, Bower P, and Whitty P. (2006b). Costs and consequences of enhanced primary care for depression. *British Journal of Psychiatry,* 189/4: 297–308.

Gilbody S, Sheldon T, and House A. (2008). Screening and case-finding instruments for depression: a meta-analysis. *Canadian Medical Association Journal,* 178/8: 997–1003.

Global Burden of Disease Study 2013 Collaborators. (2015). Global, regional, and national incidence, prevalence, and years lived with disability for 301 acute and chronic diseases and injuries in 188 countries, 1990–2013: a systematic analysis for the Global Burden of Disease Study 2013. *Lancet,* 386/9995: 743–800.

Goldberg D. (1995). Epidemiology of mental disorders in primary care settings. *Epidemiologic Reviews,* 17/1: 182–90.

Goldberg D. (2003). Psychiatry and primary care. *World Psychiatry,* 2/3: 153–7.

Gonçalves DA, Mari Jair de Jesus, Bower P, Gask L, Dowrick C, Tófoli LF, Campos M, Portugal FB, Ballester D, and Fortes S. (2014). Brazilian multicentre study of common mental disorders in primary care: rates and related social and demographic factors. *Cadernos de Saúde Pública,* 30/3: 623–32.

Grandes G, Montoya I, Arietaleanizbeaskoa MS, Arce V, and Sanchez A. (2011). The burden of mental disorders in primary care. *European Psychiatry,* 26/7: 428–35.

Gunn JM, Ayton DR, Densley K, Pallant JF, Chondros P, Herrman HE, and Dowrick CF. (2012). The association between chronic illness, multimorbidity and depressive symptoms in an Australian primary care cohort. *Social Psychiatry and Psychiatric Epidemiology,* 47/2: 175–84.

Gureje O, Oladeji BD, Araya R, and Montgomery AA. (2015). A cluster randomized clinical trial of a stepped care intervention for depression in primary care (STEPCARE)- study protocol. *BMC Psychiatry,* 15: 148.

Høifødt RS, Strøm C, Kolstrup N, Eisemann M, and Waterloo K. (2011). Effectiveness of cognitive behavioural therapy in primary health care: a review. *Family Practice,* 28/5: 489–504.

Huhn M, Tardy M, Spineli L, Leucht C, Samara M, Dold M, Davis JM, and Leucht S. (2014). Efficacy of pharmacotherapy and psychotherapy for adult psychiatric disorders: a systematic overview of meta-analyses. *JAMA Psychiatry,* 71/6: 706–15.

Huntley AL, Araya R, and Salisbury C. (2012). Group psychological therapies for depression in the community: systematic review and meta-analysis. *British Journal of Psychiatry,* 200/3: 184–90.

Hyman S, Chisholm D, Kessler RC, Patel V, and Whiteford HA. (2006), Mental Disorders. In DT Jamison, JG Breman, AR Measham, G Alleyne, M. Claeson, DB Evans, P Jha, A Mills, and P Musgrove, eds. *Disease control priorities in developing countries,* 2nd edn, New York: Oxford University Press, 605–26.

Iacovides A and Siamouli M. (2008). Comorbid mental and somatic disorders: an epidemiological perspective. *Current Opinion in Psychiatry,* 21/4: 417–21.

Isacsson G, Holmgren A, Ösby U, and Ahlner J. (2009). Decrease in suicide among the individuals treated with antidepressants: a controlled study of antidepressants in suicide, Sweden 1995–2005. *Acta Psychiatrica Scandinavica*, 120/1: 37–44.

Jack H, Wagner RG, Petersen I, Thom R, Newton CR, Stein A, Kahn K, Tollman S, and Hofman KJ. (2014). Closing the mental health treatment gap in South Africa: a review of costs and cost-effectiveness. *Global Health Action*, 7, doi: 10.3402/gha.v7.23431

Joska JA and Sorsdahl KR. (2012). Integrating mental health into general health care: lessons from HIV. *African Journal of Psychiatry*, 15/6: 420–3.

Katon W, Korff M von, Lin E, and Simon G. (2001). Rethinking practitioner roles in chronic illness: the specialist, primary care physician, and the practice nurse. *General Hospital Psychiatry*, 23/3: 138–44.

Katon W, Korff M von, Lin E, Walker E, Simon GE, Bush T, Robinson P, and Russo J. (1995). Collaborative management to achieve treatment guidelines: impact on depression in primary care. *JAMA*, 273/13: 1026–31.

Kessler RC, Lane M, Olfson M, Pincus HA, Wang PS, and Wells KB. (2005). Twelve-month use of mental health services in the United States: results from the national comorbidity survey replication. *Archives of General Psychiatry*, 62/6: 629–40.

Kessler RC and Ustün TB. (2004). The World Mental Health (WMH) Survey Initiative Version of the World Health Organization (WHO) Composite International Diagnostic Interview (CIDI). *International Journal of Methods in Psychiatric Research*, 13: 93–121.

Kessler RC and Ustün TB. (2008). *The WHO World Mental Health Surveys: Global perspectives on the epidemiology of mental disorders*. Published in collaboration with the World Health Organization, Cambridge, New York, Geneva, Cambridge University Press.

King M, Nazareth I, Levy G, Walker C, Morris R, Weich S, Bellón-Saameño JÁ, Moreno B, Švab I, Rotar D, Rifel J, Maaroos H-I, Aluoja A, Kalda R, Neeleman J, Geerlings MI, Xavier M, Caldas de Almeida Manuel, Correa B, and Torres-Gonzalez F. (2008). Prevalence of common mental disorders in general practice attendees across Europe. *British Journal of Psychiatry*, 192/5: 362–7.

Kohn R, Dohrenwend BP, and Mirotznik J. (2000). Epidemiological findings on selected psychiatric disorders. In BP Dohrenwend, ed. *Adversity, stress and psychopathology*. Cambridge, Cambridge University Press, 235–84.

Korff M von and Goldberg D. (2001). Improving outcomes in depression. The whole process of care needs to be enhanced. *British Medical Journal*, 323/7319: 948–9.

Kroenke K, Spitzer RL, Williams Janet BW, Linzer M, Hahn SR, deGruy III Frank V, and Brody D. (1994). Physical symptoms in primary care: predictors of psychiatric disorders and functional impairment. *Archives of Family Medicine*, 3/9: 774–9.

Kroenke K, Spitzer RL, Williams Janet BW, Monahan PO, and Löwe B. (2007). Anxiety disorders in primary care: prevalence, impairment, comorbidity, and detection. *Annals of Internal Medicine*, 146/5: 317–25.

Linde K, Kriston L, Rücker G, Jamil S, Schumann I, Meissner K, Sigterman K, and Schneider A. (2015a). Efficacy and acceptability of pharmacological treatments for depressive disorders in primary care: systematic review and network meta-analysis. *Annals of Family Medicine*, 13/1: 69–79.

Linde K, Sigterman K, Kriston L, Rücker G, Jamil S, Meissner K, and Schneider A. (2015b). Effectiveness of psychological treatments for depressive disorders in primary care: systematic review and meta-analysis. *Annals of Family Medicine*, 13/1: 56–68.

Löwe B, Spitzer RL, Williams Janet BW, Mussell M, Schellberg D, and Kroenke K. (2008). Depression, anxiety and somatization in primary care: syndrome overlap and functional impairment. *General Hospital Psychiatry*, 30/3: 191–9.

Martín-Merino E, Ruigómez A, Wallander M-A, Johansson S, and García-Rodríguez LA. (2010). Prevalence, incidence, morbidity and treatment patterns in a cohort of patients diagnosed with anxiety in UK primary care. *Family Practice*, 27/1: 9–16.

McHugh RK, Whitton SW, Peckham AD, Welge JA, and Otto MW. (2013). Patient preference for psychological vs. pharmacological treatment of psychiatric disorders: a meta-analytic review. *The Journal of Clinical Psychiatry*, 74/6: 595–602.

Menear M, Doré I, Cloutier A-M, Perrier L, Roberge P, Duhoux A, Houle J, and Fournier L. (2015). The influence of comorbid chronic physical conditions on depression recognition in primary care: a systematic review. *Journal of Psychosomatic Research*, 78/4: 304–13.

Mergl R, Seidscheck I, Allgaier A-K, Möller H-J, Hegerl U, and Henkel V. (2007). Depressive, anxiety, and somatoform disorders in primary care: prevalence and recognition. *Depression and Anxiety*, 24/3: 185–95.

Miller CJ, Grogan-Kaylor A, Perron BE, Kilbourne AM, Woltmann E, and Bauer MS. (2013). Collaborative chronic care models for mental health conditions: cumulative meta-analysis and meta-regression to guide future research and implementation. *Medical Care*, 51/10: 922–30.

Mitchell AJ, Vaze A, and Rao S. (2009). Clinical diagnosis of depression in primary care: a meta-analysis. *Lancet*, 374/9690: 609–19.

Moore GF, Audrey S, Barker M, Bond L, Bonell C, Hardeman W, Moore L, O'Cathain A, Tinati T, Wight D, and Baird J. (2015). Process evaluation of complex interventions: Medical Research Council guidance. *British Medical Journal*, 350, doi: 10.1136/bmj.h1258.

Murray CJL, Vos T, Lozano R, Naghavi M, Flaxman AD, Michaud C, Ezzati M, Shibuya K, Salomon JA, and Abdalla S. (2013). Disability-adjusted life years (DALYs) for 291 diseases and injuries in 21 regions, 1990–2010: a systematic analysis for the Global Burden of Disease Study 2010. *Lancet*, 380/9859: 2197–23.

National Institute for Health and Care Excellence (NICE). (2011). Common mental health disorders: Identification and pathways to care. Available at: https://www.nice.org.uk/guidance/cg123 (accessed 20 July 2015).

Patel V, Belkin GS, Chockalingam A, Cooper J, Saxena S, and Unützer J. (2013). Grand challenges: integrating mental health services into priority health care platforms. *PLoS Med*, 10/5: doi: 10.1371/journal.pmed.1001448

Patel VH, Kirkwood BR, Pednekar S, Araya R, King M, Chisholm D, Simon G, and Weiss H. (2008). Improving the outcomes of primary care attenders with common mental disorders in developing countries: a cluster randomized controlled trial of a collaborative stepped care intervention in Goa, India. *Trials*, 9: 4.

Paul GL. (1967). Strategy of outcome research in psychotherapy. *Journal of Consulting Psychology*, 31/2: 109–18.

Pence BW, O'Donnell JK, and Gaynes BN. (2012). The depression treatment cascade in primary care: a public health perspective. *Current Psychiatry Reports*, 14/4: 328–35.

Rihmer Z. (2001). Can better recognition and treatment of depression reduce suicide rates? A brief review. *European Psychiatry*, 16/7: 406–9.

Robinson WD, Geske JA, Prest LA, and Barnacle R. (2005). Depression treatment in primary care. *The Journal of the American Board of Family Practice*, 18/2: 79–86.

Roca M, Gili M, Garcia-Garcia M, Salva J, Vives M, Garcia Campayo J, and Comas A. (2009). Prevalence and comorbidity of common mental disorders in primary care. *Journal of Affective Disorders*, 119/1–3: 52–8.

Schwenk TL, Coyne JC, and Fechner-Bates S. (1996). Differences between detected and undetected patients in primary care and depressed psychiatric patients. *General Hospital Psychiatry*, 18/6: 407–15.

Serrano-Blanco A, Palao DJ, Luciano JV, Pinto-Meza A, Luján L, Fernández A, Roura P, Bertsch J, Mercader M, and Haro JM. (2010). Prevalence of mental disorders in primary care: results from the diagnosis and treatment of mental disorders in primary care study (DASMAP). *Social Psychiatry and Psychiatric Epidemiology*, 45/2: 201–10.

Sighinolfi C, Nespeca C, Menchetti M, Levantesi P, Belvederi Murri M, and Berardi D. (2014). Collaborative care for depression in European countries: a systematic review and meta-analysis. *Journal of Psychosomatic Research*, 77/4: 247–63.

Staudigl L, Becker T, and Kösters M. (2014). Wenn sich der Hausarzt entscheiden muss: as sagt die Evidenz zur Auswahl von Antidepressiva? [If the general practitioner has to decide: What is the evidence for the selection of antidepressants?]. *Deutsche Medizinische Wochenschrift*, 139/34–35: 1727–30.

Steel Z, Marnane C, Iranpour C, Chey T, Jackson JW, Patel V, and Silove D. (2014). The global prevalence of common mental disorders: a systematic review and meta-analysis 1980–2013. *International Journal of Epidemiology*, 43/2: 476–93.

van Steenbergen-Weijenburg KM, van der Feltz-Cornelis CM, Horn EK, van Marwijk HWJ, Beekman ATF, Rutten FFH, and Hakkaart-van Roijen L. (2010). Cost-effectiveness of collaborative care for the treatment of major depressive disorder in primary care. A systematic review. *BMC Health Services Research*, 10/1: 19.

Thompson C, Kinmonth AL, Stevens L, Pevele RC, Stevens A, Ostler KJ, Pickering RM, Baker NG, Henson A, and Preece J. (2000). Effects of a clinical-practice guideline and practice-based education on detection and outcome of depression in primary care: Hampshire Depression Project randomised controlled trial. *Lancet*, 355/9199: 185–91.

Thota AB, Sipe TA, Byard GJ, Zometa CS, Hahn RA, McKnight-Eily LR, Chapman DP, Abraido-Lanza AF, Pearson JL, Anderson CW, Gelenberg AJ, Hennessy KD, Duffy FF, Vernon-Smiley ME, Nease Donald E Jr, Williams SP, and Community Preventive Services Task Force. (2012). Collaborative care to improve the management of depressive disorders. *American Journal of Preventive Medicine*, 42/5: 525–38.

Ustün TB and Sartorius N. (1995). *Mental illness in general health care: an international study*. Chichester, John Wiley & Sons.

Vermani M, Marcus M, and Katzman MA. (2011). Rates of detection of mood and anxiety disorders in primary care: a descriptive, cross-sectional study. *The Primary Care Companion for CNS Disorders*, 13/2: doi: 10.4088/PCC.10m01013.

Vos T, Flaxman AD, Naghavi M, Lozano R, Michaud C, Ezzati M, Shibuya K, Salomon JA, Abdalla S, and Aboyans V. (2013). Years lived with disability (YLDs) for 1160 sequelae of 289 diseases and injuries 1990–2010: a systematic analysis for the Global Burden of Disease Study 2010. *Lancet*, 380/9859: 2163–96.

Wahlberg A and Rose N. (2015). The governmentalization of living: calculating global health', *Economy and Society*, 44/1: 60–90.

Wang PS, Berglund P, Olfson M, Pincus HA, Wells KB, and Kessler RC. (2005). Failure and delay in initial treatment contact after first onset of mental disorders in the National Comorbidity Survey Replication. *Archives of General Psychiatry*, 62/6: 603–13.

Weinmann S, Koesters M, and Becker T. (2007). Effects of implementation of psychiatric guidelines on provider performance and patient outcome: systematic review. *Acta Psychiatrica Scandinavica*, 115/6: 420–33.

Whiteford HA, Degenhardt L, Rehm J, Baxter AJ, Ferrari AJ, Erskine HE, Charlson FJ, Norman RE, Flaxman AD, Johns N, Burstein R, Murray CJL, and Vos T. (2013a). Global burden of disease attributable to mental and substance use disorders: findings from the Global Burden of Disease Study 2010. *Lancet*, 382/9904: 1575–86.

Whiteford HA, Harris MG, McKeon G, Baxter A, Pennell C, Barendregt JJ, and Wang J. (2013b). Estimating remission from untreated major depression: a systematic review and meta-analysis. *Psychological Medicine*, 43/08: 1569–85.

WHO International Consortium in Psychiatric Epidemiology. (2000). Cross-national comparisons of the prevalences and correlates of mental disorders. *Bulletin of the World Health Organization*, 78/4: 413–26.

Wittchen H-U and Jacobi F. (2005). Size and burden of mental disorders in Europe--a critical review and appraisal of 27 studies. *European Neuropsychopharmacology the Journal of the European College of Neuropsychopharmacology*, 15/4: 357–76.

Wolf NJ and Hopko DR. (2008). Psychosocial and pharmacological interventions for depressed adults in primary care: a critical review. *Clinical Psychology Review*, 28/1: 131–61.

Woltmann E, Grogan-Kaylor A, Perron B, Georges H, Kilbourne AM, and Bauer MS. (2012). Comparative effectiveness of collaborative chronic care models for mental health conditions across primary, specialty, and behavioral health care settings: systematic review and meta-analysis. *American Journal of Psychiatry*, 169/8: 790–804.

World Bank. (1993). *World Development Report 1993: Investing in Health*. New York, Oxford University Press).

Chapter 2

Across the spectrum: Strategies to improve recognition and treatment of mental disorders in primary care

Victoria J. Palmer and Rob Whitley

Introduction

The year 2016 marks 50 years since the important role that primary care plays in the recognition, treatment, and management of mental disorders began to be more widely acknowledged in the published literature. It began with the findings of a large British study which showed that patients at risk of a mental disorder had consulted with their general practitioner (GP) at least once in the past 12 months (Sheperd, Cooper et al. 1966). The GP role in mental health care continued to be identified across international research, and seminal work by Goldberg and Blackwell (1970) raised the profile of the problem with the phrase 'hidden psychiatric morbidity', which was used to refer to unrecognized mental illness in primary care (Higgens 1994). In the early 1970s a European working group of the World Health Organization (WHO) then asked, 'How could GPs be better integrated within the mental health team'? The question prompted further recognition by the United States Institute of Medicine (IoM) and the National Institutes of Mental Health (NIMH) of the need to integrate primary care in the treatment of mental disorders (Shepherd 1987). Since then, the arguments have continued to vacillate between how primary care clinicians under-recognize, misdiagnose or now over-treat mental disorders like depression and bipolar disorder (Culpepper 2010). Early research suggested that not only were GPs poor at recognizing mental disorders, but that where disorders were identified, treatment was inappropriate (Mechanic 2001). Recent evidence indicates that misidentification of cases outweighs the numbers of missed cases (Mitchell, Vaze et al. 2009). The evidence varies considerably depending on whether recognition is defined by diagnosis via the Diagnostic Statistical Manual, Fifth Edition (DSM-5), via the International Statistical Classification of Diseases and Related Health Problems, Tenth Revision (ICD-10) or via other types of documented treatment and support for emotional disorders in case records (Higgens, 1994; APA, 2013; Stein et al., 2013). There has also been a misconception that primary care only provides treatment and support for mild to moderate mental disorders like anxiety and depression (Pirl et al., 2001).

Given these debates, numerous attempts have been made using various research strategies in order to improve the recognition and treatment of mental disorders in primary care; these have been mostly levelled at depression and other related disorders (Chew-Graham et al., 2002). Depression has received the most attention due to its higher prevalence in the primary care setting compared to the general population (Dowrick 2009). Estimates from the US indicates that one in four patients in primary care may have a mental disorder, which is equivalent to a prevalence rate between 23–29% of the primary care population (Kessler et al., 2005). To date, research-driven attempts to improve the recognition, treatment, and management of mental disorders in primary care have been through randomized controlled trials (RCTs) of collaborative care, stepped care, and tailored care models. UK and US studies of these models have shown improved patient outcomes but they nonetheless remain difficult to routinely implement in different international contexts (Lee et al., 2007; Gask et al., 2010; Reilly et al., 2013). Other research has examined how to best organize primary care for depression, and has had a particular focus on understanding what patient and community expectations of ideal treatment and support might be (Gunn et al., 2010). Other trials have been conducted to improve GP education and training on prevalent mental disorders with ultimate goals of increasing their recognition and treatment (Kroenke et al., 2000, Gask et al., 2004).

Mental disorders at the more severe end of the spectrum and (e.g. schizophrenia, bipolar disorder, and psychosis) are referred to as severe mental illness (SMI), and have not received the same attention in primary care. This may be explained by the assumption that SMIs are more appropriately managed in secondary and tertiary settings. Yet, de-institutionalization in the 1980s increased community-based care (Crews et al., 1998), and because of this, for many people primary care is their only contact with the health care system (Phelanet al., 2001). Those who recommend specialist or psychiatric management for SMIs suggest that GPs do not have adequate skills, training, or interest to manage them (Lester et al., 2005). However, early research findings have indicated that mental disorders treated in primary care resolve almost as quickly as those treated by mental health specialists (Scott, 1992). Other studies have highlighted that greater acknowledgement is needed of the fact that GPs and nurses could be skilled in both recognizing and treating mental disorders (Oud et al., 2009).

Conversely, Crews et al. (1998) argue that mental disorders are better managed by GPs because of the multiple physical morbidities associated with mental illnesses. Prevalence rates for mental disorders and mortality due to poor physical health and other lifestyle factors continue to grow exponentially (Morgan et al., 2014). Primary care is essential to improving physical health care, and the 2010 Survey of High Impact Psychosis (SHIP) conducted in Australia found that 88.2% of 1,825 people living with psychotic illnesses aged 18–64 years old had visited a GP in the last 12 months. Of these visits, 76.3% were for physical health problems and 49.3% were for mental health problems (Morgan et al., 2011). The five most common reasons reported for GP visits were for a new/repeat prescription (68.8%), followed by blood tests (52.8%), reviewing psychotic symptoms (42.0%), a general check-up (35.3%), and a blood pressure and or cardiovascular check (35.0%). The SHIP also identified that people living with SMIs had nearly twice the amount of contact with a GP annually for co-morbid physical health conditions (nine visits/year compared to the five for the general population) (Morgan et al., 2014). As the rate of co-morbidities rises in this population, the role of the GP and the primary care setting will also increase (Mercer et al., 2011). These trends indicate that it is paramount that integrated, multi-disciplinary team models are implemented to recognize, treat, and manage mental disorders. Cross-collaboration across the spectrum of clinical, non-clinical, specialist, government, and non-government agencies will be required (Lee et al., 2013).

The importance of recognizing and treating both common mental disorders (CMDs) and SMIs in primary care hinges on four interrelated factors. The first is that primary care is the first (and sometimes the only) point of access for the majority of people to many healthcare systems. Combined with having first contact, it is now accepted that new treatments for mental disorders are also better suited to delivery via the primary care setting (Wittchen et al., 2003). These new treatments include pharmacological and non-pharmacological interventions and are well suited to primary care coordination. The second factor is that improved recognition and treatment of mental disorders may reduce the economic costs of avoidable emergency and hospital admissions. For some people, if mental disorders (and any associated physical conditions) can be treated early in the primary care setting, their severity may be greatly reduced. The third, and perhaps newest, factor is the philosophical fit between the person-centred, bio-psycho-social approach of GP care and facilitating psychosocial recovery (Whitley et al., 2015). Psychosocial recovery is now a central tenet in all mental health policies and at the heart of recovery-oriented treatment. This approach recognizes the subjective nature of recovery and the importance of both the individual's identity in and ownership of recovery. The final factor is that there is greater acceptance of those seeking help via primary care, which has resulted in fewer barriers for many in how, and when, to access support and treatment (Wittchen et al., 2003).

That being said, barriers to recognition and treatment of mental illness remain. For example, some primary health care professionals view severe mental illness as a lifelong, chronic, and disabling condition (Lester et al., 2005). This is in opposition to the psychosocial recovery focus in mental health policy, practice, and theory (Slade, 2015). Previous research undertaken by Thielke et al. (2007) has also identified an additional four overlapping barriers: disease processes (the broad range of conditions, the undifferentiated symptoms, and the limited success of treatments), the patient/person (stigma associated with mental illness, negative beliefs about treatment, symptoms affecting help-seeking and management), the provider (trained in a medical model, competing demands, and knowledge overload) and the system (financial incentives, time constraints, systems for follow up, limited access to mental health specialists for referral, and a limited ability to provide psychosocial interventions). Galon and Graor (2012) found that people with more severe mental illness had a greater reluctance to seek help via primary care due to their fears of detention because of psychiatric symptoms, lack of insurance (specifically in the US context), co-occurrence of substance use, severe infectious illnesses like hepatitis and tuberculosis, and severe depression. Galon and Graor's research certainly indicates that there are areas for improvement.

Improvements at the clinical/practice level to recognize and treat mental disorders in primary care are well documented and well known. Indeed, many have challenged the misconception that primary care ought to focus on the mild to moderate or common disorders such as depression and anxiety, and have proposed it has a role to play across the mental illness spectrum (Dowrick 2009). Such authors advocate for less focus on the diagnostic categorization of the illnesses identified in primary care and a greater focus on enabling narratives that facilitate people to flourish, live well, and engage in their communities while still having their mental and physical health issues attended to (Dowrick 2009). This approach is based on treatment of the whole individual and their needs, rather than the implementation of routine screening programs to identify new and undetected cases of depression and other mental disorders (Thombs et al., 2012).

Published literature supports a re-direction of government funding in order to implement and support new primary care-led models of treatment to facilitate the person-centred, narrative-based, and holistic care of the patient. The critical issue is that successful strategies are not only dependent on re-directed and increased funding from governments but also the development of appropriate policy to guide said funding. Additionally, success also requires overcoming the implementation challenges that come with turning evidence into practice. For example, having a team of professionals available in the primary care setting with mixed skill sets is important for the delivery of holistic and integrated care. This can be difficult, however, if there are technological barriers that limit inter-professional communication and data collection and sharing, as well as physical space limitations to house teams. Additionally, there can be paradigm differences in professional approaches to the treatment of mental disorders. The rest of this chapter focuses on the strategies that could currently be implemented to improve recognition and treatment of mental disorders in primary care.

Fig. 2.1 depicts four levels of the health care system where strategies can be directed. The fig moves from the outer level (funding, infrastructure and policy) to the inner level (engaged, whole person/integrated person-centred care). We outline the strategies to achieve this in turn.

Purpose built environments

The physical environment of any health service is critical to the care process and how it shapes an individuals' experience of care and their engagement. Qualitative studies have found that the nature of waiting rooms and reception areas influences the experience of primary health care (Lester et al., 2005). Cramped, dark, and windowless waiting rooms may be particularly stressful for those with anxiety and schizophrenia. Additionally, paying attention to average waiting times and how staff, including receptionists, interact with patients is important (Lester et al., 2005). While evidence exists regarding the important part the physical environment plays in patient engagement and experience, it is not known how well existing primary care environments have been designed with this in mind. The physical environment of all treatment settings needs to be welcoming and carefully designed to accommodate people's specific needs.

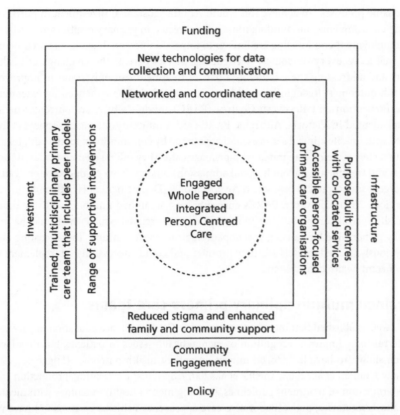

Fig. 2.1 Primary care strategies to improve recognition and treatment of mental disorders

Some innovative mental health services have made strident efforts to ensure that their internal physical environments are welcoming (e.g. Headspace in Australia, a prevention service provided to young people (18–24 y/o) (Rickwood et al., 2015). There have also been indications that co-located services are successful for supporting people with SMIs. Earlier models developed and implemented in the US included specific primary care clinics only for people with SMIs in order that the mental and physical health needs of these individuals could be appropriately addressed with continuity of care at the fore (Crews et al., 1998). In Australia a trial care model between GPs, non-government services, public mental health services, and a mobile primary care service using peer support workers was used successfully to improve the treatment of physical health problems for people living with SMIs (Lee et al., 2013). The contemporary manifestation of this type of model could be a 'one stop shop' service where the physical, mental and social needs of patients are met in a safe and supportive environment. This service might be housed in a building with a healthcare facility at the top and a shared café/social space at the bottom. Combined professional support options to address employment, housing, and other needs could also be available on the same premises. To achieve this would require substantial investment in purpose-built environments, and funding must be re-directed to primary health care.

Employment and housing are known to impact on personal health and well-being as well as recovery outcomes. Recognizing this as part of the challenge of health care and addressing these issues as a part of treatment can only result in improved health outcomes. Recognition and treatment could also be enhanced by extending the Prevention and Recovery Centres (PARC) models which are currently being implemented in Victoria, Australia. PARCs are community-managed services delivered with on-site clinical services, and are offered by community mental health teams with a view to being integrated with primary care. They offer a step up (focused support and treatment to avoid hospital admission) or step down (support for early discharge from hospital to promote recovery) model (Department of Health and Human Services, 2010). However, PARCs currently have small bed numbers and stay times are short, so it can be difficult to address any interrelated issues which may be initially responsible for causing psychopathological manifestations. These existing and previously trialled models all show promise and could successfully be implemented in current health care systems.

Trained multidisciplinary primary care teams

It is well established that interventions aimed at GPs to increase education or increase referrals may improve recognition of mental health issues in patients, but they have been shown to have little to no impact on patient health outcomes (Higgens, 1994; Chew-Graham et al., 2002; Thielke et al., 2007). Systematic screening, production and dissemination of treatment guidelines, tracking mental health outcomes with mental health laboratories, and collaborative care approaches (Thielke et al., 2007) have all had varied results and impact. Thus, while training and education must be incorporated into a well-rounded primary care programme, they must also be accompanied by an investment in interventions known to work as well as an investment in trialling new interventions and methods that can improve detection and management. Education and training are best positioned to enable work force capacity for primary care and should be combined with sharing knowledge and understanding of how to work via contexts and models that are interdisciplinary.

Training of GPs, nurses, and the spectrum of allied health care professionals to provide technical and relational-based care is critical. However, this must be balanced with the recognition that the primary care workforce has valuable existing skill-sets that should be utilized and harnessed in the diagnosis and management of mental health disorders. Continuing education programmes, professional development programmes, and course training need to involve the emerging notion of 'recovery', and this is best delivered in partnership with people with lived experiences from across the mental health organizational spectrum, including academic institutions and professional associations. This redefinition of recovery expands the traditional definition beyond a narrow focus on recovery as symptom remission, and instead encompasses social and functional factors as much as clinical factors to emphasize the strengths and capabilities of people with SMI (Rapp, 1998; Whitley and Drake, 2010).

The emphasis on psychosocial recovery instead of clinical and functional improvements derives from evidence that SMIs are not necessarily lifelong, chronic, and disabling. Rather, people with SMIs can make an excellent recovery if given the right services and support. Governments across the world are demanding that health services for people with SMIs become more recovery-oriented (Kirby, 2008; Slade, 2009). Currently the person-centred and bio-psycho-social approach of primary care fits well with this vision. So far, most action has been focused on transforming secondary and tertiary care towards recovery with far less attention on primary care (Drake and Whitley, 2014). While efforts exist to integrate mental health care into primary care and psychiatry, there has been little attempt to harness primary care as an agent of recovery, let alone assess the impact of any transformations. As such, the time is ripe for new approaches and initiatives, and training and education will play a fundamental role here.

Education about the models of care which are necessary for whole person support will require involvement of a wide range of people involved in the recognition and treatment of mental disorders. GPs continue to provide first-contact care at the community level, but nurses, social workers, occupational therapists, physiotherapists, exercise physiologists, and psychologists all have a role to play in the strategies to increase recognition and treatment of mental disorders in primary care. Service models that encourage and facilitate professional collaboration (rather than a silo service system) are clearly more conducive to better treatment. A variety of peer-support models also exist that could be incorporated into primary care-led models for recognition and treatment of mental disorders.

Technologies for data collection and communication

A critical way forward is to appreciate that, while fundamental, the treatment of mental health disorders goes beyond therapeutic and pharmacological management. As discussed, there is a need for a balance between a technical and relational approach. The technical side of care is all about continuing to increase skill sets, and having the available tools at hand to complement diagnosis and recognition, and to develop treatment and management plans that can be used for goal setting and to coordinate care. The relational side is about positive relationships where individuals feel noticed, have attention paid to them, feel important because someone is concerned or cares for them, feel a sense of purpose and social obligation, and feel that others have an interest in them. These have been identified as some of the main factors for accessing primary care support (Galon and Graor, 2012). The idea is that the technical and relational aspects of care are interrelated concepts which must be given equal attention.

In Australia the opportunity exists for GPs to develop a number of care plans that are billable through Medicare, the universal health care system. Under these plans people can access a range of mental health or chronic disease treatments and support either through further access to psychologists, or to podiatry, exercise physiology, and dental care, respectively, under a chronic disease plan. including nurse review and coordination of treatment and management plans. Treatment plans include needs assessment, establishing goals, and referrals to other providers. Currently, there is criticism regarding how feedback is given across the providers, and improvements could be made to coordinate the use of such treatment plans. Ensuring that plans have a focus on holistic patient treatment to include both physical and mental health needs assessments with goal setting and shared decision-making would be a good first step. Additionally, particular primary care teams could be involved in the development and implementation of recovery plans that are being used in the community mental health setting in Australia and other countries. To achieve this, investment is needed in data sharing systems and technologies by which different health care providers across settings can communicate with each other, and therefore plans can be tailored to individual needs. Person-centred approaches that facilitate connection between referral and social supports are important in the recovery-oriented mental health care approach.

There are also a range of low-intensity interventions available that are suited to CMDs in primary care. These must involve stretching the traditional notion of 'treatment' to ensure that GPs are aware of the full range of recovery-oriented interventions that differ for specific illnesses. For example, in treating schizophrenia, evidence-based recovery-oriented interventions include supported employment and housing, illness self-management programmes, and integrated dual-diagnosis treatment (Corrigan et al., 2008). GPs, nurses, and social workers can be educated about the availability and impact of such interventions, and can be encouraged to make referrals to such services. However, this must be coupled with active communication so that the coordination and continuity of care of people with SMIs remains at the forefront. In jurisdictions where GPs have power over purchasing (e.g. the UK), they can also consider providing such services (housing or employment support) in house in larger practices.

Additionally, it is becoming increasingly important to involve members of the family and other carers in treatment. Currently, while policy incorporates the role of carers and families, the tools and models for doing this work are limited. Part of the family/carer role is clearly necessary when advance planning takes place. Advance planning for people living with SMIs should be part of all recognition and treatment approaches for mental disorders for where there are shared care arrangements between both primary and specialist care providers. Having an advance plan means setting out a patient's treatment wishes in advance for during a period of illness where decision-making capacity might be impaired. A shared decision-making framework needs to underpin this and be implemented widely in practice settings (Puschner et al., 2015). Again, all primary care providers must be educated and trained in how to facilitate shared decision-making for their patients.

Rates of treatment discontinuation in primary care for people with mental illness are high, with some studies suggesting that over 70% of patients are non-adherent to treatment plans three months after the initial visit (Olfson et al., 2006; O'Connor et al., 2009). The early work of Puschner et al. (2015) in shared decision making has identified that adherence rates can increase with a shared model of decision making in place. This indicates that more can be done to monitor the follow-up phases of treatment. Bipolar disorder is one example where symptoms fluctuate cyclically and there is scope to better develop follow-up and monitoring procedures (Culpepper, 2010). These procedures could be managed in the primary care setting by practice nurses, mental health nurses, or social workers. A growing and popular intervention is the use of mental health peer support workers (people with a lived experience of mental illness who work collaboratively within the team) to enhance recovery, treatment adherence, and general well-being. Peer support workers are traditionally located within secondary or tertiary settings, or work from dedicated mental health support organizations (Perez and Kidd 2015). The integration of mental health peer support workers into primary care settings would be a bold and visionary advance that may go some way to improving service engagement among people with mental illness.

Community Engagement

Stigma is a pervasive problem for people with mental illness. Goffman (1963) defined stigma as 'an attribute that is deeply discrediting … turning a whole and usual person to a tainted and discounted one'. In western societies, the possible or actual presence of a mental illness is generally considered a highly discrediting attribute (Stuart et al., 2014). Additionally, so is the use of health services for such a problem, especially mental health services. Stigma is considered one of the main factors behind the low rates of service engagement for people with mental illness, with surveys regularly showing that approximately 50–60% of people with mental illness do not voluntarily engage with health services (Wang et al., 2007). An active focus on reducing stigma and engaging people in primary care is needed. Routine measurement and feedback from service users and carers about how well care is working for them is essential. Participant-led studies are growing and could provide another model to augment the peer support models of team care currently in place (Pelletier et al., 2015). To achieve this, mechanisms for community engagement are required at a range of levels and across sectors.

Some studies indicate that primary care is a favoured location for services for people with mental illnesses. As discussed, this may be due to various factors, including the familiarity of primary care clinics and clinicians, less association with stigma than secondary and tertiary care, and the possibility to treat multi-morbidity using a multi-dimensional framework and approach. Because primary care clinics are also located in neighbourhood settings, visits are easier to integrate into everyday routines, and also cheaper as they may not involve long trips across town on public transport. Therefore, identifying ways to implement primary care-led models that are localized and can skilfully provide a range of services is a good use of existing and available resources.

Conclusion

There is currently a unique opportunity to think about ways to innovate the existing community and health services to improve recognition and treatment of mental disorders. It has been well established that just implementing screening for mental disorders does not improve recognition and health outcomes, and that there need to be other system elements put into place (Thombs et al., 2012; Deneke et al., 2014). Screening for new cases needs to be coupled with the appropriate treatment and management for particular conditions, which signals a greater need for tailored models of primary care for mental disorders. The strategies that have been outlined point to this need. Efforts to improve recognition and treatment through improved infrastructure should result in accessible, person-focused primary care organizations. Funding new technologies for data collection and communication will make building a networked and coordinated system of care possible. Investment in trained, multidisciplinary teams and inclusion of successful peer models of support will enable people to have a range of supportive interventions tailored to their individual needs. All of this needs to be underpinned by focused policy development that will facilitate community engagement to reduce both individual and public stigma and enhance family and community support. The ideal outcome of these strategies is thus an engaged individual who receives holistic, integrated, person-centred care. This highlights the substantive opportunities to expand primary care and its role in the care of people living with mental disorders.

References

APA. (2013). *Diagnostic and Statistical Manual of Mental Disorders* (*DSM-5®*). Washington, DC: American Psychiatric Publishing.

Chew-Graham CA, Mullin, S, May CR, Hedley S, and Cole H. (2002). Managing depression in primary care: another example of the inverse care law? *Fam Pract*, 19/6: 632–7.

Corrigan P, Mueser K, Bond G, Drake R, and Solomon P, *Principles and Practice of Psychiatric Rehabilitation*. New York: Guilford Press.

Crews C, Batal H, Elasy T, Casper E, and Mehler P. (1998). Primary care for those with severe and persistent mental illness. *Western Journal of Medicine*, 169/4: 245–50.

Culpepper L. (2010). The Role of Primary Care Clinicians in Diagnosing and Treating Bipolar Disorder. *Primary Care Companion to The Journal of Clinical Psychiatry*, 12/Suppl 1: 4–9.

Deneke DE, Schultz H, and Fluent TE. (2014). Screening for Depression in the Primary Care Population. *Primary Care: Clinics in Office Practice*, 41: 399–420.

Department of Health and Human Services. *Adult prevention and recovery services framework and operational guidelines*. Victoria, Department of Health and Human Services.

Dowrick C. (2009). *Beyond Depression: A New Approach to understanding and management*. Oxford: Oxford University Press.

Drake R and Whitley R. (2014). Recovery and severe mental illness: description and analysis. *Canadian Journal of Psychiatry*, 59/5: 236–42.

Galon P and Graor, CH. (2012). Engagement in Primary Care Treatment by Persons With Severe and Persistent Mental Illness. *Archives of Psychiatric Nursing*, 26: 272–84.

Gask L, Bower P, Lovell K, Escott D, Archer J, Gilbody S, Lankshear AJ, Simpson AE, and Richards, DA. (2010). What work has to be done to implement collaborative care for depression? Process evaluation of a trial utilizing the Normalization Process Model. *Implement Sci*, 5: 15.

Gask L, Dowrick C, Dixon C, Sutton C, Perry R, Torgerson D, and Usherwood T. (2004). A pragmatic cluster randomized controlled trial of an educational intervention for GPs in the assessment and management of depression. *Psychological Medicine*, 34: 63–72.

Goffman E. (1963). *Stigma: notes on the management of spoiled identity*. New York: Simon and Schuster.

Gunn J, Palmer V, Dowrick C, Herrman H, Griffiths F, Kokanovic R, Blashki G, Hegarty K, Johnson C, Potiriadis M, and May C. (2010). Embedding effective depression care: using theory for primary care organisational and systems change. *Implementation Science*, 5/1): 62.

Higgens E. (1994). A review of unrecognised mental illness in primary care: prevalence, natural history, and efforts to change the course. *Archives of Family Medicine*, 3: 908–17.

Kessler RC, Demler O, Frank RG, Olfson M, Pincus HA, Walters EE, Wang P, Wells KB, and Zaslavsky AM. (2005). Prevalence and Treatment of Mental Disorders, 1990 to 2003. *New England Journal of Medicine*, 352/24: 2515–23.

Kirby M. (2008). Mental health in Canada: out of the shadows forever. *Canadian Medical Association Journal*, 178/10: 1320–2.

Kroenke K, Taylor-Vaisey A, Dietrich AJ, and Oxman TE. (2000). Interventions to Improve Provider Diagnosis and Treatment of Mental Disorders in Primary Care: A Critical Review of the Literature. *Psychosomatics*, 41/1: 39–52.

Lee PW, Dietrich AJ, Oxman TE, Williams JW, and Barry SL. (2007). Sustainable Impact of a Primary Care Depression Intervention. *The Journal of the American Board of Family Medicine*, 20/5: 427–33.

Lee SJ, Crowther E, Keating C, and Kulkarni J. (2013). What is needed to deliver collaborative care to address comorbidity more effectively for adults with a severe mental illness? *Australian and New Zealand Journal of Psychiatry*, 47/4: 333–46.

Lester H, Tritter JQ, and Sorohan H. (2005). Patients' and health professionals' views on primary care for people with serious mental illness: focus group study. *BMJ*, 330/7500: 1122.

Mechanic D. (2001). Closing gaps in mental health care for persons with serious mental illness. *Health Services Research*, 36/6: 1009–17.

Mercer SW, Gunn J, and Wyke S. (2011). Improving the health of people with multimorbidity: the need for prospective cohort studies. *Journal of Comorbidity*, 1/1: 4–7.

Mitchell AJ, Vaze A, and Rao A. (2009). Clinical diagnosis of depression in primary care: a meta-analysis. *Lancet*, 374/9690: 609–19.

Morgan V, Waterreus A, Jablensky A, Mackinnon A, McGrath J, Carr V, Bush R, Castle D, Cohen M, Harvey C, Galletly C, Stain H, Neil A, McGorry P, Hocking B, Shah S, and Saw S. (2011). *People living with psychotic illness 2010: report on the second national survey*. Canberra, Commonwealth of Australia.

Morgan VA, McGrath JJ, Jablensky A, Badcock JC, Waterreus A, Bush R, Carr V, Castle D, Cohen M, Galletly C, Harvey C, Hocking B, McGorry P, Neil AL, Saw S, Shah S, Stain HJ, and Mackinnon A. (2014). Psychosis prevalence and physical, metabolic and cognitive co-morbidity: data from the second Australian national survey of psychosis. *Psychological Medicine*, 44/10: 2163–76.

O'Connor EA, Whitlock EP, Beil TL, and Gaynes BN. (2009). Screening for depression in adult patients in primary care settings: a systematic evidence review. *Annals of Internal Medicine*, 151/11: 793–803.

Olfson M, Marcus SC, Tedeschi M, and Wan GJ. (2006). Continuity of Antidepressant Treatment for Adults with Depression in the United States. *American Journal of Psychiatry*, 163/1: 101–8.

Oud M, Schuling J, Slooff C, Groenier K, Dekker J, and Meyboom-de Jong B. (2009). Care for patients with severe mental illness: the general practitioner's role perspective. *BMC Family Practice*, 10/Suppl:1–8.

Pelletier JF, Lesage A, Boisvert C, Denis F, Bonin JP, and Kisely A. (2015). Feasibility and acceptability of patient partnership to improve access to primary care for the physical health of patients with severe mental illnesses: an interactive guide. *International Journal for Equity in Health*, 14: 78.

Perez J and Kidd J, Peer support workers: an untapped resource in primary mental health care, *Journal of Primary Health Care*, 7/1 (2015), 84.

Phelan M, Stradins L, and Morrison S. (2001). Physical health of people with severe mental illness: Can be improved if primary care and mental health professionals pay attention to it. *BMJ*, 322/7284: 443–4.

Pirl WF, Beck BJ, Safren SA, and Kim H. (2001). A Descriptive Study of Psychiatric Consultations in a Community Primary Care Center. *Primary Care Companion to The Journal of Clinical Psychiatry*, 3/5: 190–4.

Puschner B, Becker T, Mayer B, Jordan H, Maj M, Fiorillo A, Égerházi A,Ivánka T, Munk-Jørgensen P, Krogsgaard Bording M, Rössler W, Kawohl W, and Slade M. (2015). Clinical decision making and outcome in the routine care of people with severe mental illness across Europe (CEDAR). *Epidemiology and Psychiatric Sciences*, 25/1: 69–79.

Rapp CA. (1998). *The strengths model: case management for people suffering from severe and persistent mental illness*. New York: Oxford University Press.

Reilly S, Planner C, Gask L, Hann M, Knowles S, Druss B, and Lester H. (2013). Collaborative care approaches for people with severe mental illness. Cochrane Database of Systematic Reviews, 11/CD009531, doi: 10.1002/14651858.CD009531.pub2

Rickwood D, Van Dyke N, and Telford N. (2015). Innovation in youth mental health services in Australia: common characteristics across the first headspace centres. *Early Intervention in Psychiatry*, 91/1: 29–37.

Scott AI and Freeman CP. (1992). Edinburgh primary care depression study: treatment outcome, patient satisfaction, and cost after 16 weeks. *BMJ*, 304/6831: 883–7.

Sheperd M, Cooper B, Brown A, and Kalton G. (1966). *Psychiatric Illness in General Practice*. Oxford: Oxford University Press.

Shepherd M. (1987). Mental illness and primary care. *American Journal of Public Health*, 77/1: 12–13.

Slade M. (2009). *Personal Recovery and Mental Illness*. Cambridge, UK: Cambridge University Press.

Slade M and Longden E. (2015). *The empirical evidence about mental health and recovery: how likely, how long, what helps?* Victoria: Mental Illness Fellowship.

Stein DJ, Lund C, and Nesse R. (2013). Classification systems in psychiatry: diagnosis and global mental health in the era of DSM-5 and ICD-11. *Current Opinion in Psychiatry*, 26/5: 493–95.

Stuart H, Chen, SP, Christie R, Dobson K, Kirsh B, Knaak S, and Whitley R. (2014). Opening Minds: The Mental Health Commission of Canada's Anti-Stigma Initiative: Opening Minds in Canada: Background and Rationale. *Canadian Journal of Psychiatry*, 59/10, Suppl 1: S8.

Thielke, S, Vannoy S, and Unützer J. (2007). Integrating Mental Health and Primary Care. *Primary Care: Clinics in Office Practice*, 34/3: 571–92.

Thombs BD, Coyne JC, Cuijpers, de Jonge P, Gilbody S, Ioannidis JP, Johnson BT, Patten SB, Turner EH, and Ziegelstein RC. (2012). Rethinking recommendations for screening for depression in primary care. CMAJ: *Canadian Medical Association Journal*, 184/4: 413–8.

Wang PS, Aguilar-Gaxiola S, Alonso J, Angermeyer MC, Borges G, Bromet EJ, Bruffaerts R, Girolamo G, Graaf R, Gureje O, Haro JM, Karam EG, Kessler RC, Kovess V, Lane MC, Lee SJ, Levsion D, Ono Y, Petukhova M, Posada-Villa J, Seedat S, and Wells JE. (2007). Use of mental health services for anxiety, mood, and substance disorders in 17 countries in the WHO world mental health surveys. *Lancet* 370/9590): 841–50.

Whitley R and Drake R. (2010). Recovery: a dimensional approach. *Psychiatric Services*, 61/12: 1248–50.

Whitley R, Palmer V, and Gunn J. (2015). Recovery from severe mental illness. *CMAJ*, 187/13: 951–2.

Wittchen HU, Mühlig S, and Beesdo K. (2003). Mental disorders in primary care. *Dialogues in Clinical Neuroscience*, 5/2: 115–28.

Chapter 3

Collaborative care models for the management of mental disorders in primary care

Christina van der Feltz-Cornelis,
Harm van Marwijk,
and Leona Hakkaart-van Roijen

Mental health care in general practice

This chapter aims to provide a critical overview of collaborative care models and their clinical effectiveness, cost effectiveness, and applicability in the general practice setting with GPs as the primary target audience. For decades, it has been suggested that timely diagnosis and care might be improved for patients presenting with various forms of distress, anxiety, somatoform disorders, and depression in the general practice setting (Rollman et al., 2006). The delivery and uptake of antidepressant medication and evidence-based psychotherapies is often suboptimal (Simon, 2002; Bijl et al., 2003; National Institute for Health and Clinical Excellence, 2011; Piek et al., 2011, 2012). Improvement of care for patients with various forms of distress, anxiety, somatoform disorders and depression is more likely to come from changes in the way care is provided than from adding new treatment options at the interface between primary and secondary care (Katon & Unutzer, 2006).

Currently, the standard treatment approach for mental disorder in general practice is called matched care, i.e. the treatment does not follow a general approach but rather should match the patient's needs at an individual level. In this way, the patient is usually coached in the general practice setting using some form of short-term psychotherapy or self-management in combination with antidepressant medication. However, if symptoms are severe, if the patient feels seriously invalidated, or if there is a high risk of suicide, the referral to specialty mental health care is recommended. The therapy choice is based on severity but also matched with the patient's characteristics and preferences. As a result, the treatment varies. Available treatment options are watchful waiting, antidepressants, or different types of psychological interventions, and these options depend on patient preferences as well as on differences in setting and provider (e.g. GP, nurse, psychological wellbeing practitioner, psychologist, or consultant psychiatrist). GPs are known to vary in how they diagnose mental illness, either as more context-dependent symptoms, or as an 'illness' or disorder in its own right, and therefore treatment options can vary greatly between practices.

The problem with such matched care is that the current high variations of treatment in management are undesirable in terms of equity of access, safety, and quality, and that is if the treatment is provided at all. Variation between practices exists and some groups (e.g. the elderly, and people from different cultural backgrounds) have less access. This is the case in the Netherlands, a country deemed to have a well-developed health care system. Research shows that patients with depressive symptoms who present themselves in a general practice setting and ask for treatment receive guideline based treatment in less than 50% of the cases (Prins, 2010). It is likely that similar percentages exist in other countries as well.

A second problem with current matched care model is that it is less suitable for chronic care as it allows too many patients to 'fall through the cracks'. Central coordination and monitoring are already difficult in current fragmented health care systems, but mental health issues tend to increase such fragmentation. Mental illnesses are increasingly conceptualized as long-term conditions. Those with the more socially disruptive forms of psychopathology or those who are more vocal in their need for care may receive more care, but others with more avoidant, more long-term symptoms, and equally large major invalidating mental illnesses may receive less appropriate or less immediate care.

Although tailoring matched care to the preferences of the patient corresponds naturally to the 'regular' care received in a primary care setting, a third problem is that it lacks clear prognostic determinants with which to match patients to available treatments. It has been argued that some patients who are perhaps suffering temporarily with problems are being 'overdiagnosed' as depressed and in need of antidepressants, and perhaps receive antidepressant treatment too early (Van Marwijk et al., 2003). Others who are truly in need of thorough diagnosis and perhaps also pharmacological treatment may receive too little, or even none.

Collaborative care

We suggest that collaborative care may provide a pathway toward answering these problems. Collaborative care includes a broad range of interventions, settings, and providers, and its defining characteristics are that a team of healthcare professionals are responsible for providing the 'right' care at the 'right' time. This treatment model was developed originally as a chronic care model (Wagner et al, 1996) for the treatment of depressive disorder in general practice (Wagner et al., 1996; Katon et al., 1995; Katon et al., 1999) in the US. It was found to be effective in the US, especially when psychiatric consultation and nurse supervision of patients were a systematic part of the intervention (Bower et al., 2006; Gilbody et al., 2006). The collaborative care model has also been found effective in several other countries, such as Chile, the Netherlands, Germany, and Italy (Araya et al., 2003; Huijbregts et al., 2013). It has also been evaluated for mental disorders other than depression, such as anxiety disorders (Roy-Byrne et al., 2001; Muntingh et al., 2014), personality disorders (Stringer et al., 2011; Stringer et al., 2015a; Stringer et al., 2015b), somatoform disorders (Van der Feltz-Cornelis et al., 2006), and bipolar disorder (van der Voort, 2011). The model has also been used for treatment of comorbid depressive disorder and somatic illnesses such as diabetes mellitus (Katon et al., 2004b), cancer (Strong et al., 2008), and arthritis (Lin et al., 2006). Furthermore, it has been evaluated in other settings than general practice, such as the general hospital setting for patients with depression and comorbid chronic illness (van Steenbergen-Weijenburg et al., 2015).

The model

Collaborative care has been operationalized in different ways. Collaboration between a general practitioner (GP), a nurse that takes the role of care manager (CM), and a psychiatric consultant (CL) is the most frequent combination of health care professionals. Collaborative care has been defined as at least two of these three collaborating in treatment of a patient for a mental disorder (Katon et al., 1999), with or without comorbid medical illness (see Fig. 3.1).

A structured management plan that includes scheduled patient follow-ups and close CM supervision by a psychiatrist (Bower et al., 2006; Gunn et al., 2006) along with the participation of a central CM are key parts of the model. However, it is important to note that, depending on the country and the medical system, the roles may differ somewhat. In Europe, the nurse CM may monitor treatment by phone, as in the US model use by Kaiser Permanente, or in the oncology trial mentioned in the previous paragraph. In the UK and the Netherlands, the nurse CM may monitor symptoms with instruments like the Patient Health Questionnaire 9 according to validated cut scores (Kroenke et al., 2001). The CM will then contact the GP or CL within a few weeks if there is lack of progress, but may also provide a form of psychotherapeutic treatment. The most commonly used psychotherapeutic treatment is Problem Solving Therapy (PST), which is a directive treatment used in the general practice setting and was found to be effective for depression (Mynors-Wallis et al., 1997). Whereas in the USA, she may also provide medication after consultation with the psychiatric consultant (Unützer et al., 2002), in mainland Europe the GP provides medication according to a guideline for depression (Schulberg et al., 1999), or to a more closely described

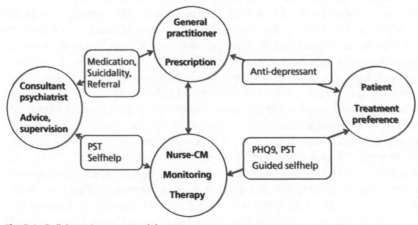

Fig. 3.1 Collaborative care model

medication algorithm (Huijbregts et al., 2013). In general, the use of detailed algorithms improves treatment outcome in collaborative care (Adli et al., 2006).

The first successful example of collaborative (stepped) care is the IMPACT model that used PST and antidepressants for major depression in later life (Unützer J et al., 1999). The IMPACT model incorporates a dedicated team that works together to provide optimal care, and patients are evaluated at predetermined time intervals according to defined improvement criteria. Care is adjusted or augmented if the patient does not improve sufficiently. Treatment is provided according to patients' needs and preferences. In all seven existing IMPACT depression studies as well as one other involving both psychological treatment (psycho-education) and antidepressants, there was no prescribed progression of increasing therapeutic intensity based on the monitoring.

Stepped Care

In later collaborative care studies, stepped care was incorporated into the monitoring approach. Stepped care has been recommended in order to increase access and efficiency of mental health care (Andrews, 2006; NICE, 2009). The patient is first evaluated via an evidence-based psychological treatment. Progress is monitored systematically and those patients who do not respond adequately are then moved into a psychological treatment of higher intensity. Nowadays, this kind of stepped care approach is always part of the collaborative care intervention with an emphasis on monitoring patient progress and acting upon lack of it.

Two concepts of stepped care have been suggested in the literature. Firstly, the key assumption of stepped care is that low-intensity treatment will suffice for many, and that only a few will need a higher-intensity treatment. This thereby makes better use of scarce and/or expensive resources, such as therapist time. Self-help treatments (through books, apps, or the Internet) are often used as a first step in this model of care. Additionally, meta-analyses of this model have shown that it may be the most effective compared to more intensive treatments of depression in stepped care (Gellatly et al., 2007; Andrews and Titov, 2010; Cuijpers et al., 2010; Richards, 2012). Thus, there is no evidence that a rigid stepped care approach for treatment of depressive disorder is the most effective (van Straten et al., 2015). Often, the patient is already following some kind of treatment that is considered to be of higher intensity than this first step in the stepped care approach model; additionally, this kind of model does not take patient preferences or physician considerations into account. For example, Muntingh et al. (2009) evaluated a collaborative stepped care approach for anxiety disorders in general practice. The model began with a recommendation of self-help in all cases, then progressing to CBT as the next step, and only in the third step were antidepressants provided. Although in general the results were favourable, it transpired that the indicated procedure was not followed, as there were patients involved in the stepped care treatment who were already on antidepressant medication (Muntingh et al., 2014).

The term 'stepped care' is also used to refer to models where at each 'step' patients switch or add treatments of different modalities (e.g. pharmacological, psychological) but here patients may start at any level, depending on the severity of symptoms or preference, e.g. with intensive psychological therapy (Araya et al., 2003; Katon, 2004a; Ell et al., 2008). This approach is currently used in collaborative care models (van Straten et al., 2015). In this model the patient may choose to start with PST alone or in conjunction with antidepressant medication (Ijff et al., 2007); interestingly, this patient preference model resulted in above-average outcomes compared to the original IMPACT model (Huijbregts et al., 2013). With this in mind, the collaborative care model may be optimal if combining a stepped care approach with patient preference for where to enter treatment.

Another aspect in the application of the model is supervision of the nurse CM if they are providing a form of psychotherapy, such as PST. PST is a directive approach and many, if trained in other mental health treatments as well, might find it difficult to adhere to the directive approach. A systematic review showed that regular supervision of the nurse CM by a psychiatrist was associated with better treatment effect (Bower et al., 2006). This suggests that providing a liaison in the consultation between general practice and specialty mental health care is important in the collaborative care model.

Treatment effect

Better outcomes are reached in collaborative care compared to care as usual. Several systematic reviews showed effect sizes ranging between 0.3 and 1.2 for collaborative care compared to care as usual in the general practice setting (Coventry et al., 2014). These differences depended on the form of collaboration between GP, CM and CL, and on the kind of mental disorder under treatment (Van der Feltz-Cornelis et al., 2010). It turns out that collaborative care models in which the CL actually sees the patient and provides written consultation advice to one professional (i.e., either GP or nurse CM) (Hoedeman et al., 2010) is the most effective model. Furthermore, the model is more effective in somatoform disorder and anxiety disorder than in depressive disorder (Van der Feltz-Cornelis et al., 2010), suggesting that depressive disorder may need a more sustained treatment effort and that anxiety disorders and somatoform disorders may be more reactive to short-term treatment in the general practice setting.

Implementation of collaborative care

According to Richards, et al. (2012), there is considerable variety in the implementation of collaborative care, especially in the number and duration of treatment steps, the types of treatments offered, the professionals involved, and the criteria used to move between treatment steps. A tracking system integrated into an electronic support system, now possible due to rapid ICT advances, makes the model more effective (Huijbregts et al., 2013; de Jong et al., 2009). Future developments will certainly take such requirements into account. The presence of nurses that can act as CMs, CLs, as well as reimbursement of patient treatments are factors needed to make wide implementation of this model possible. In many countries it may take a significant amount of time to be implemented at a national level.

For example, since 2014, the circumstances and reimbursement for collaborative care have been optimized in the basic mental health care model for general practice in the

Netherlands, and the model is widely implemented now with practice nurses. A guideline exists for psychiatric consultation in general practice (Leentjens et al., 2009) and many professionals have been trained in the application of the model. However, ten years elapsed between the initial list compiled by GPs regarding their needs to successfully collaborate with mental health organisations in the general practice setting (the first step towards collaborative care in the Netherlands) (Herbert and van der Feltz-Cornelis, 2004) and the development and full scale implementation of an effective collaborative care model including psychiatric consultation in general practice (Van der Feltz-Cornelis et al., 2006; this close collaboration also included insurance companies, governmental agencies, and professional associations (van der Feltz-Cornelis, 2011). The changes needed regarding provisions and reimbursement for GP support to successfully implement the collaborative care model took a decade to complete.

In the UK, several projects have demonstrated the difficulty in finding a central CM in general practice. With the advent of Improved Access to Psychological Treatments (IAPT), a specialized psychological service within the primary care setting was created. The coverage of IAPT is minimal, however, reaching on about 10% of the population, and there is no integrated medication provision; additionally, often the service is separate from the general practice setting, which means that if the first step of psychological treatment does not meet with success, no sequence treatment is provided. Furthermore, this is a stand-alone model, rather than a collaborative care model. For integration of care and adequate treatment of often chronic mental disorders like depression and anxiety, it would be beneficial for IAPT therapists to have the option of collaborating with a GP and a CL.

Additionally, in terms of implementation, other countries experience different problems. In Germany, reimbursement only happens if the collaborative care model is provided from a general hospital setting. This required the model to be adapted so that the hospital psychiatrist can collaborate closely with the GP. In Chile, the model is very cost effective as the salaries of the GPs providing care are very low; however, because of these low reimbursements, turnover of GPs in the community health centres is high; this 'revolving door' of GPs must be addressed promptly in order to keep the model working.

Cost effectiveness

Cost effectiveness analysis (CEA) is a tool that decision makers increasingly use to assess and potentially improve the performance of their health systems. These analyses indicate which interventions provide the highest 'value for money' to help choose the interventions and programmes that maximize health for the available resources (www.who.int). In a CEA, an intervention is compared to at least one alternative in terms of costs and (health) effects. Which costs (and effects) are to be considered depends on the perspective from which the economic evaluation is performed. If a societal perspective is adopted, all costs, including productivity/losses (e.g. absence from work) and health effects should be incorporated, regardless of who bears the costs and who experiences the health effects (Drummond et al., 2005). CEAs compare one intervention with another by calculating the difference in cost between two interventions, divided by the difference in health benefit obtained (i.e., Quality Adjusted Life Years (QALY)). The QALY takes into account both the increase in life expectancy from an intervention and any resulting change in quality of life. The QALY outcome measure is commonly used in economic evaluation as it allows comparing the cost effectiveness of different conditions.

Recently, Grochtdreis et al. (2015) updated the van Steenbergen-Weijenburg et al. (2010) review on the cost-effectiveness of collaborative care in primary care. This systematic review showed out of the 19 cost effectiveness studies, 14 showed improved effectiveness, but also higher costs. Moreover, the review showed that there was considerable uncertainty, due to inconsistent methodological quality (Grochtdreis et al., (2015). However, only a limited number of studies included productivity costs, despite the importance of including these costs in treatment of depression. Due to the recurrent nature of depressive disorders, it would be beneficial if these studies could span at least two years. Goorden et al. (2015) showed that at the intervention's finish, its effects decrease as the QOL at the end of the study also decreased for the collaborative care group. This result would support prolonging the treatment period of collaborative care beyond one or two years, which is often the maximum amount of time provided. A recent study showed that collaborative stepped care was a cost-effective intervention for panic disorder (PD) and generalized anxiety disorder (GAD) (Goorden et al., 2014). These results indicate that collaborative care is recommended as an intervention for this patient group. However, more evidence is needed to determine the cost-effectiveness of collaborative care across populations and health care insurance systems.

Conclusion

Collaborative care is an effective treatment model that can be used for providing mental health care in the general practice setting. Systematic monitoring and increasing treatment intensity according to a stepped care algorithm that incorporates the patient preference from the start improves outcomes substantially compared to usual matched care. The effectiveness of the model increases if the CM receives adequate supervision and if structural possibilities for psychiatric consultation exist. Collaborative care is cost effective depending upon willingness to pay. The implementation of collaborative care depends on the availability of nurse CMs and CLs, guidelines for psychiatric consultation, reimbursement, and adequate web-based decision aids for professionals. For implementation at a national level, long-term strategies are needed, but the results from models currently used in the Netherlands are promising as they have shown that it is possible to successfully implement this model in general practice on a large scale. In the Netherlands the model is now applied nationally applied following a period of ten years in which needs of GPs were explored, the optimal model was piloted, and its effectiveness established. This was then followed by guideline development and a national approach involving training of professionals and adapting reimbursement policies in close collaboration with the relevant professional societies, insurance companies, and the government. Other countries may need other implementation approaches depending on their specific national health and reimbursement systems.

References

Adli M, Bauer M, and Rush AJ. (2006). Algorithms and collaborative-care systems for depression: are they effective and why? A systematic review', *Biol Psychiatry*, 59/11: 1029–38.

Andrews G. (2006). Tolkein II: A needs-based, costed stepped-care model for mental health services– recommendations, executive summaries, clinical pathways, treatment flowcharts, costing structures, (Sydney: CRUFAD, University of New South Wales.

Andrews G and Titov N. (2010). Is internet treatment for depressive and anxiety disorders ready for prime time? *Med J Aust*, 192/11 Suppl: S45–S47.

Araya R, Rojas G, Fritsch R, Gaete J, Rojas M, Simon G, and Peters TJ. (2003). Treating depression in primary care in low-income women in Santiago, Chile: a randomised controlled trial. *Lancet*, 361/9362): 995–1000.

Bower P, Gilbody S, Richards D, Fletcher J, and Sutton A. (2006). Collaborative care for depression in primary care. Making sense of a complex intervention: systematic review and meta-regression. *British Journal of Psychiatry*, 189: 484–93.

Coventry PA, Hudson JL, Kontopantelis E, Archer J, Richards DA, Gilbody S, Lovell K, Dickens C, Gask L, Waheed W, and Bower P. (2014). Characteristics of effective collaborative care for treatment of depression: a systematic review and meta-regression of 74 randomised controlled trials. *PLoS One*, 9/9: doi: 10.1371/journal.pone.0108114

Cuijpers P, Donker T, van Straten A, Li J, and Andersson G. (2010). Is guided self-help as effective as face-to-face psychotherapy for depression and anxiety disorders? A systematic review and meta-analysis of comparative outcome studies. *Psychol Med*, 40/12: 1943–57.

Drummond MF, Sculpher MJ, Torrance GW, O'Brien BJ, and Stoddart GL. (2005). *Methods for the Economic Evaluation of Health Care Programmes*, Third edn, Oxford: Oxford University Press.

Ell K, Xie B, Quon B, Quinn DI, Dwight-Johnson M, and Lee PJ. (2008). Randomized controlled trial of collaborative care management of depression among low-income patients with cancer. *Journal Of Clinical Oncology: Official Journal Of The American Society Of Clinical Oncology*, 26/27: 4488–96.

Van der Feltz-Cornelis CM, van Oppen P, Adèr H, and van Dyck R. (2006). Randomised Controlled Trial of a Collaborative Care Model with Psychiatric Consultation for Persistent Medically Unexplained Symptoms in General Practice. *Psychother Psychosom*, 75/5): 282–9.

van der Feltz-Cornelis CM, Van Os TWDP, Van Marwijk HWJ, and Leentjens AF. (2010). Effect of psychiatric consultation models in primary care: a systematic review and meta-analysis of randomized clinical trials. *Journal of Psychosomatic Research*, 68: 521–33.

van der Feltz-Cornelis CM. (2011). Ten years of integrated care for mental disorders in the Netherlands', *Int J Integr Care*, 11, Spec Ed: Epub;%2011 Apr 18.:e015

Gellatly J, Bower P, Hennessy S, Richards D, Gilbody S, and Lovell K. (2007). What makes self-help interventions effective in the management of depressive symptoms? Meta-analysis and meta-regression. *Psychol Med*, 37/9: 1217–28.

Gilbody S, Bower P, Fletcher J, Richards D, and Sutton AJ. (2006). Collaborative care for depression: a cumulative meta-analysis and review of longer-term outcomes. *Arch Intern Med*, 166/21: 2314–21.

Goorden M, Muntingh A, van MH, Spinhoven P, Ader H, van Balkom A, van der Feltz-Cornelis C, and Hakkaart-van Roijen L. (2014). Cost utility analysis of a collaborative stepped care intervention for panic and generalized anxiety disorders in primary care. *J Psychosom Res,* **77**/1: 57–63.

Goorden M, Huijbregts KM, van Marwijk HW, Beekman AT, van der Feltz-Cornelis CM, and Hakkaart-van RL. (2015). Cost-utility of collaborative care for major depressive disorder in primary care in the Netherlands. *J Psychosom Res,* **79**/4: 316–23.

Grochtdreis T, Brettschneider C, Wegener A, Watzke B, Riedel-Heller S, Harter M, and König HH. (2015). Cost-effectiveness of collaborative care for the treatment of depressive disorders in primary care: a systematic review. *PLoS One,* **10**/5: e0123078.

Herbert CM and van der Feltz-Cornelis CM. (2004). Wat wil de huisarts? Inventarisatie van wensen van huisartsen ten aanzien van psychiatrische consulten in hun praktijk. (What does the GP want? Survey of psychiatric consultation needs of GPs). *Maandblad Geestelijke volksgezondheid,* **59**/3: 206–15.

Hoedeman R, Blankenstein AH, van der Feltz-Cornelis CM, Krol B, Stewart R, and Groothoff JW. (2010). Consultation letters for medically unexplained physical symptoms in primary care', *Cochrane Database Syst Rev,* **12**: CD006524.

Huijbregts KM, de Jong FJ, van Marwijk HW, Beekman AT, Adèr HJ, Hakkaart-van RL, Unützer J, and van der Feltz-Cornelis CM. (2013). A target-driven collaborative care model for Major Depressive Disorder is effective in primary care in the Netherlands. A randomized clinical trial from the depression initiative. *J Affect Disord,* **146**/3: 328–37.

Ijff MA, Huijbregts KM, van Marwijk HW, Beekman AT, Hakkaart-van Roijen L, Rutten FF, Unützer J, and van der Feltz-Cornelis CM. (2007). Cost-effectiveness of collaborative care including PST and an antidepressant treatment algorithm for the treatment of major depressive disorder in primary care; a randomised clinical trial. *BMC Health Serv Res,* **7**: 34.

de Jong FJ, van Steenbergen-Weijenburg KM, Huijbregts KM, Vlasveld MC, van Marwijk HW, Beekman AT, and Van der Feltz-Cornelis CM. (2009). The Depression Initiative. Description of a collaborative care model for depression and of the factors influencing its implementation in the primary care setting in the Netherlands. *Int J Integr Care,* **9**: e81.

Katon W, Von Korff M, Lin E, Simon GE, Bush T, Robinson P, and Russo J. (1995). Collaborative management to achieve treatment guidelines. Impact on depression in primary care. *JAMA,* **273**/13: 1026–31.

Katon W, Von Korff M, Lin E, Simon G, Walker E, Unützer J, Bush T, Russo J, and Ludman E. (1999). Stepped collaborative care for primary care patients with persistent symptoms of depression: a randomized trial. *Arch Gen Psychiatry,* **56**/12: 1109–15.

Katon W, von Korff M, Ciechanowski P, Russo J, Lin E, Simon G, Ludman E, Walker E, Bush T, and Young B. (2004a). Behavioral and clinical factors associated with depression among individuals with diabetes. *Diabetes Care,* **27**/4: 914–20.

Katon WJ, Von Korff M, Lin EH, Simon G, Ludman E, Russo J, Ciechanowski P, Walker E, and Bush T. (2004b). The Pathways Study: a randomized trial of collaborative care in patients with diabetes and depression. *Arch Gen Psychiatry,* **61**/10: 1042–9.

Kroenke K, Spitzer RL, and Williams JB. (2001). The PHQ-9: validity of a brief depression severity measure. *J Gen Intern Med,* **16**/9: 606–13.

Leentjens AF, Boenink AD, Sno HN, Strack van Schijndel RJ, van Croonenborg JJ, van Everdingen JJ, van der Feltz-Cornelis CM, van der Laan NC, van Marwijk H, van Os TW, and Netherlands Psychiatric Association. (2009). The guideline 'consultation psychiatry' of the Netherlands Psychiatric Association. *J Psychosom Res,* **66**/6: 531–5.

Lin EH, Tang L, Katon W, Hegel MT, Sullivan MD, and Unützer J. (2006). Arthritis pain and disability: response to collaborative depression care. *Gen Hosp Psychiatry,* **28**/6: 482–6.

Marwijk HWJ van , Grundmeijer HGLM, Bijl D, Van Gelderen MG, De Haan M, Van Weel-Baumgarten EM, Burgers JS, Boukes FS, Romeijnders ACM. (2003). NHG-Standaard Depressieve stoornis (depressie). *Huisarts Wet*, 46/11: 614–62.

Muntingh AD, van der Feltz-Cornelis CM, van Marwijk HW, Spinhoven P, Assendelft WJ, de Waal MW, Hakkaart-van Roijen L, Adèr HJ, and van Balkom AJ. (2009). Collaborative stepped care for anxiety disorders in primary care: aims and design of a randomized controlled trial. *BMC Health Services Research*, 9/1: 159.

Muntingh A, Feltz-Cornelis C, van Marwijk HW, Spinhoven P, Assendelft W, de Waal M, Adèr H, and van Balkom A. (2014). Effectiveness of collaborative stepped care for anxiety disorders in primary care: a pragmatic cluster randomised controlled trial. *Psychother Psychosom*, 83/1): 37–44.

Mynors-Wallis L, Davies I, Gray A, Barbour F, and Gath D. (1997). A randomised controlled trial and cost analysis of problem-solving treatment for emotional disorders given by community nurses in primary care. *Br J Psychiatry*, 170: 113–9.

National Institute for Health and Clinical Excellence. (2009). Depression in adults: recognition and management, (London, NICE).

Prins M. (2010). *Mental health care from the patient's perspective: a study of patients with anxiety and depression in general practice*; thesis. Utrecht: NIVEL, Netherlands Institute for Health Services Research.

Richards DA. (2012). Stepped care: a method to deliver increased access to psychological therapies. *Can J Psychiatry*, 57/4: 210–5.

Richards DA, Bower P, Pagel C, Weaver A, Utley M, Cape J, Pilling S, Lovell K, Gilbody S, Leibowitz J, Owens L, Paxton R, Hennessy S, Simpson A, Gallivan S, Tomson D, and Vasilakis C. (2012). Delivering stepped care: an analysis of implementation in routine practice. *Implement Sci*, 7: 3.

Rollman BL, Weinreb L, Korsen N, and Schulberg HC. (2006). Implementation of guideline-based care for depression in primary care. *Adm Policy Ment Health*, 33/1, 43–53.

Roy-Byrne PP, Katon W, Cowley DS, and Russo J. (2001). A randomized effectiveness trial of collaborative care for patients with panic disorder in primary care. *Arch Gen Psychiatry*, 58/9: 869–76.

Schulberg HC, Katon WJ, Simon GE, and Rush AJ. (1999). Best clinical practice: guidelines for managing major depression in primary medical care. *J Clin Psychiatry*, 60/Suppl 7: 19–26.

van Steenbergen-Weijenburg KM, van der Feltz-Cornelis CM, Horn EK, van Marwijk HW, Beekman AT, Rutten FF, and Hakkaart-van Roijen L. (2010). Cost-effectiveness of collaborative care for the treatment of major depressive disorder in primary care. A systematic review. *BMC Health Serv Res*, 10: 19.

van Steenbergen-Weijenburg KM, van der Feltz-Cornelis CM, van Benthem TB, Horn EK, Ploeger R, Brals JW, Leue C, Spijker J, Hakkaart-Van Roijen L, Rutten FF, and Beekman AT. (2015). [Collaborative care for comorbid major depressive disorder in chronically ill outpatients in a general hospital]. *Tijdschr Psychiatr*, 57/4: 248–57.

van Straten A, Hill J, Richards DA, and Cuijpers P. (2015). Stepped care treatment delivery for depression: a systematic review and meta-analysis. *Psychol Med*, 45/2: 231–46.

Stringer B, van Meijel B, Karman P, Koekkoek B, Kerkhof AJ, and Beekman AT. (2015a), 'Collaborative Care for Patients With Severe Personality Disorders: Analyzing the Execution Process in a Pilot Study (Part II). *Perspect Psychiatr Care*, 51/3: 220–7.

Stringer B, van Meijel B, Karman P, Koekkoek B, Hoogendoorn AW, Kerkhof AJ, and Beekman AT. (2015b). Collaborative Care for Patients With Severe Personality

Disorders: Preliminary Results and Active Ingredients From a Pilot Study (Part I); *Perspect Psychiatr Care*, 51/3: 180–9.

Stringer B, van Meijel B, Koekkoek B, Kerkhof A, and Beekman A. (2011). Collaborative Care for patients with severe borderline and NOS personality disorders: a comparative multiple case study on processes and outcomes. *BMC Psychiatry*, 11:102.

Strong V, Waters R, Hibberd C, Murray G, Wall L, Walker J, McHugh G, Walker A, and Sharpe M. Management of depression for people with cancer (SMaRT oncology 1): a randomised trial. *Lancet*, 372/9632: 40–8.

Unützer J and IMPACT Study Investigators. (1999). *Project IMPACT Intervention Manual: Improving care for depression in late life*;(Los Angeles: UCLA: NPI Center for Health Services Research).

Unützer J, Katon W, Callahan CM, Williams JW, Jr., Hunkeler E, Harpole L, Hoffing M, Della Penna RD, Noël PH, Lin EH, Areán PA, Hegel MT, Tang L, Belin TR, Oishi S, Langston C, and IMPACT Investigators (Improving Mood-Promoting Access to Collaborative Treatment). (2002). Collaborative care management of late-life depression in the primary care setting: a randomized controlled trial. *JAMA*, 288/22: 2836–45.

van der Voort TY, van Meijel B, Goossens PJ, Renes J, Beekman AT, Kupka RW. (2011). Collaborative care for patients with bipolar disorder: a randomised controlled trial. *BMC Psychiatry* 11: 133.

Wagner EH, Austin BT, and Von KM. (1996). Improving outcomes in chronic illness. *Manag Care Q*, 4/2: 12–25.

Chapter 4

Operationalizing patient-centredness to enhance recovery and primary care for mental disorders

John Furler, Victoria J. Palmer, and Jane Gunn

Introduction

Patient-centredness is not a new concept in medicine. Its roots can be traced to early twentieth-century attempts to ensure patient consent was required for medical treatments, which extended later to the notion of patient's providing informed consent. In its current manifestation, patient-centredness has become more aligned with the consumerist movement in medicine which grew out of a range of radical socio-political critiques of medical power, dominance, and hegemony in the 1970s. This focus on consumerism, and hence patient rights, has been criticized for being driven by a range of corporate, state, and economic interests that themselves shape notions of society, rather than as a sign of underlying radical shifts (McDonald et al., 2007). Currently the notion of patient-centredness has been embraced and mobilized by mainstream health institutions and organizations charged with both promoting and improving safety and quality in health care, as well as devolving accountability for these outcomes.

There is no doubt that patient-centredness has much to offer in addressing some of the challenges posed by caring for people with mental disorders. Operationalizing patient-centredness could potentially reduce stigma and thus improve access to care, help to meaningfully engage patients, families and carers in decisions about care, and thus promote adherence and retention in treatment and improve outcomes. Patient-centredness can also aid in a holistic and broad approach to managing physical health issues and to supporting recovery as a meaningful aim of delivering care for mental disorders. However, both important challenges and tensions are embedded within the practice of patient-centredness.

One challenge is that the evidence base for patient-centredness in terms of improving health outcomes is not strong. Stewart et al (2003:4) provide a rationale for the practice of a patient-centred method on the basis that not only do patients prefer it, but it also improves health outcomes and health care utilization; however, the evidence that it improves clinical outcomes is complex. Mead and Bower (2002) reviewed evidence for the effectiveness of patient-centredness, and in their review note that many individual components or dimensions of patient-centredness have in some studies been associated with better outcomes. They concluded that this evidence is suggestive of a relationship, although in their own study they found no significant association between scores of patient-centredness and patient satisfaction, and sense of enablement (Mead et al., 2002).

In a pragmatic sense, another important challenge is that patient-centred practice requires significant investment at both the level of individual encounters as well as at an organizational level. Providers need to build capacity to support patients, families, and carers to be more involved in their own care. Organizations similarly need to invest in capacity building to realize the benefits of patient-centred practice at both a community and population level. Developing clinical aids and tools to facilitate patient-centred practice is also important.

However, a focus on the technical and resource challenges needed to operationalize patient-centred practice can obscure an important tension. Like all clinical care, clinical care for mental disorders is inherently social practice, subject to variations in and implicit manifestations of power. Some see the growth of patient-centredness as an institutional 'subjectification' of the patient and as a way of reframing and limiting a new version of 'patient-hood' in the service of dominant interests (Armstrong, 2011).

In this chapter we examine how operationalizing the concept of patient-centredness could enhance recovery and primary care for mental disorders. We begin with an outline of the concept and method of patient-centredness and its applicability for the treatment of mental disorders in primary care. We draw on the current example of the patient-centred medical home (PCMH) as a model for enhancing recovery and primary care, and conclude with a discussion about the challenges and tensions for operationalizing patient-centredness in primary care.

The Concept and Method of Patient-Centredness

Patient-centred care goes by a number of related terms and concepts, including consumer-centred, person-centred, personalized care, patient empowerment, and more recently, relationship-centred care. The terms all relate to the patient or person being at the centre of their care, and being involved in making decisions about treatment and management that are informed and shared between practitioner and person. Each of these coalesces around key values and approaches to care that lie at the heart of the approach and philosophy of primary care practice, and which are key to the recovery agenda in mental health. In particular, the biopsychosocial approach of primary care practice, a focus on individuals in the context of their life stories, and a commitment to shared decision making all mean primary care can play a leading role in recovery focused care for mental disorders (Gunn et al., 2008).

There is a great deal of early work in the primary care setting that has contributed to what we understand today as patient-centredness. Michael Balint, a psychiatrist who over a period of years in the 1950s worked on a weekly basis with a group of general practitioners (GPs) in the UK, is a prime example of this early work. Balint's explored the nature of the relationship between GP and patient, particularly why the relationship was 'so often …. unsatisfactory or unhappy' (Balint, 1964:5). The group of GPs brought to their discussions stories of patients from their everyday practice. The group changed very little over the years and the patient's stories could be 'updated' and followed over time, allowing great insight into the evolving nature of the patient-GP relationship. The patients discussed in the group were most often (but not exclusively) those who presented with somatic symptoms without identifiable disease, or what is known currently as medically unexplained symptoms (MUS) (Ring et al., 2005). Balint clearly showed for the first time that the relationship between patient and doctor was important *in and of itself* in determining what happened to patients over time. This was true for patients both with and without 'physical disease'. Balint coined the term 'doctor as drug/therapy' (1964:4), and focused on the importance of GPs reaching a 'deeper diagnosis' in helping patients interpret their illness. Equally and importantly, he suggested that GPs needed to reach a deeper psychological insight and understanding of themselves if they were to understand their own contribution to the interaction. In Balint's view, the GPs in his group found this difficult.

Balint's work is an important historical antecedent to the evolution of the notion of patient-centredness in primary care. Importantly, he suggested that wider social contexts were at work, influencing both patient ('particularly as a result of urbanisation, a lot of people have lost their roots and connections') (Balint, 1964:2)) and doctor (for example, Balint suggested that the panel system of capitation payment may be influencing the behaviour and thinking of GPs). Balint suggested that a doctor's 'practice style' and limitations to the 'elasticity' with which the GP negotiates 'a great variety of relationships with various patients in his (sic) practice' (1964:217) was contingent not only on the doctors' professional milieu, but also on the social and material context in which patient and doctor live and meet.

Nevertheless, within the field of primary care practice and literature, patient-centredness retains a connection to this idea of the centrality and importance of the doctor and patient, seen as a 'meeting of experts' (Tuckett et al., 1985). This 'meeting' has also been seen as a way to recapture a sense of spontaneity and humanity in the relationship between GP and patient that has been lost in the increasingly scientific abstractions of modern technical medicine. It has been argued that this technical and abstract focus has both separated the GP and patient from each other, as well as impoverished their meeting as 'two fellow humans' (McWhinney, 1995:10). Primary care today leads the current shift to 're-centre' the patient within the clinical practice of medicine, partly driven by a desire to differentiate itself within the medical profession, and partly due to changing expectations from wider society and the growth of consumerism.

The various dimensions of patient-centredness in this sense have been brought together and described in the recent literature (Stewart and Brown, 2001; Stewart, 1995; Mead and Bower, 2000) (see Table 4.1). Stewart and Brown (2001) align the dimensions of what they refer to as the patient-centred method in a systems-type diagram (Fig. 4.1). In this model, enhancing the GP-patient relationship provides a basis for all other dimensions. Finding common ground is at the centre of the model, informed by the GP's exploration of both disease and illness, and an understanding of the whole person. Mead and Bower (2000) see the dimensions clustered at the centre of a much wider socially embedded system that is composed of external (social and societal) factors thought likely to influence patient-centred practice (Fig. 4.2).

Table 4.1 Dimensions of PCM

1	Exploring both the disease and illness experience of the patient	A 'biopsychosocial' perspective
2	Holistic understanding of the whole person	Awareness of 'patient-as-person'
3	Finding common ground and agreement on formulating the problem and management	Orientation to sharing power and responsibility
4	Attention to enhancing the GP-patient relationship	Development of a therapeutic alliance
5		Awareness of 'doctor-as-person'

Data from The *BMJ*, 322, 2001, Stewart M, 'Towards a global definition of patient-centred care', pp. 444–445; Social Science & Medicine, 51, 2000, Mead, N and Bower P., 'Patient-centredness: a conceptual framework and review of the empirical literature', pp. 1087–110.

Clearly for Mead and Bower, patient-centredness cannot be considered in isolation; social context is seen as exerting complex effects on *how* it is practised. Mead and Bower note that the term 'patient-centredness' has been 'used to refer to so many different concepts that its scientific utility may have been compromised' (Mead and Bower, 2000:1102). Nevertheless, patient-centredness as a concept continues to inform much debate about what is unique about primary care practice, and to underpin a range of research into the relationship between doctor and patient (Bower et al., 2001). One example of the way in which patient-centredness has been operationalized as a way to deliver care for people with mental disorders is the PCMH in the US, which we discuss as an example of how to enhance recovery and care for mental disorders in primary care.

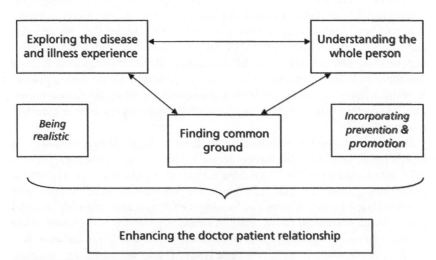

Fig. 4.1 Dimensions of the patient-centred Method
Data from Stewart M., Brown J.B., Weston W.W. et al., *Patient-centered medicine : transforming the clinical method*, second edition, 2003, Radcliffe Medical Press.

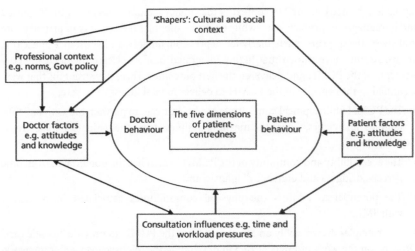

Fig. 4.2 Patient-centredness and factors influencing it
Data from *Social Science & Medicine*, 51, 2000, Mead N. and Bower P., 'Patient-centredness: a conceptual framework and review of the empirical literature', pp. 1087–110.

The patient-centred medical home: fit for purpose in enhancing care for mental disorders in primary care

Patient-centredness has played a major part in how primary care has adopted a role in the treatment and management of mental disorders, particularly in the US. In the past under managed-care and reimbursement arrangements, there has been 'carve-out' of mental health from mainstream primary care provision (Frank et al., 2003; Pincus et al., 2005) with a view that mental disorders are best treated in specialist, secondary-care settings. There is growing interest in re-connecting the two, not least because the majority of care across the spectrum of mental disorders (from common to complex) occurs in primary care (Pirl et al., 2001). Additionally there is growing recognition of the inequitable physical illness burden borne by people with mental illness, where people with severe mental illness (SMI) die up to 25 years earlier than the general population, in particular from chronic conditions like cardiovascular disease (CVD), diabetes, and respiratory disease (Shim and Rust, 2013).

The critical vehicle for this debate is the growing momentum of the PCMH movement. The PCMH is a way of organizing care delivery that is broadly consistent with elements of the Chronic Care Model (Robert Woods Johnson Foundation, 2008), and with a 'patient-centred orientation'. It is based on coordinated, comprehensive, and accessible team-based care with an embedded systems approach to safety and quality. Information technology, workforce training, and payment reforms are all important in supporting the move to a PCMH.

The Agency for Healthcare Research and Quality (AHRQ) have explicitly studied the potential for the integration of mental illness care into the PCMH model (Croghan and Brown, June 2010) and have explored the rationale, evidence base, and 'fit' for mental illness care in the PCMH, as well as how best to achieve the integration. The rationale advanced in the US context is that much mental illness goes undiagnosed and unmanaged in primary care, while evidence supports the capacity of primary care to deliver effective care, particularly for depression, anxiety, and substance abuse disorders. Results have shown that highly integrated models of care included the core elements of the PCMH and delivered the best outcomes. Three key strengths that were identified in the capacity of the PCMH to deliver mental illness care were:

- The PCMH philosophical commitment to holistic care in partnership with patients, families, and carers, where the meaning of illness from the patients' perspective is valued;
- The accessibility and continuity of the PCMH, which has the potential to overcome perceived stigma and enhance diagnosis; and
- The potential to address the physical comorbidities associated in particular with SMI.

These principles draw heavily on the potential for the PCMH to provide 'holistic care'. Drawing on the work of Engel (1977) in developing the 'biopsychosocial' framework, patient-centred models in primary care place strong emphasis on the need to understand the 'whole person', which 'may include family, work, beliefs, struggles with life's crises, ... cultural beliefs'. More recently this approach has been subsumed within the notion of generalist practice (Reeve et al., 2011; Gunn et al., 2008) with its capacity to integrate biopsychosocial care for multiple conditions. The biopsychosocial approach offers potential to contribute to a wider approach to recovery. If recovery means finding meaningful employment, building satisfying relationships, engaging in wider social activities, and securing safe and comfortable housing, as opposed to simply controlling symptoms, then generalist practice must play a leading role in supporting and facilitating recovery.

In conclusion, we explore tensions within the practice of patient-centredness, using shared decision making as an example.

Tensions in the practice of patient-centredness: shared decision making and the contingency of practice

One of the key dimensions of patient-centredness studied in mental illness care is shared decision making (SDM), and much of this work has been conducted in primary care. 'Finding common ground', (Stewart, 1995; Stewart et al., 2003) is the process through which the patient and the doctor reach a mutual understanding and agreement in three key areas: defining the problem, establishing the goals and priorities of treatment and/or management, and identifying the roles to be assumed by both the patient and the doctor. It is both process and outcome. It involves active listening, encouraging questions from the patient to elicit their ideas, concerns and expectations, and the use of plain and understandable language in exchanging information between patient and doctor. 'Sharing power and responsibility' (Mead and Bower, 2000:1089) draws on the notion of a shared, cooperative partnership between doctor and patient, based on respect for and acknowledgement of the patient's own expertise in their own illnesses. SDM is embedded within both these concepts. Clinical decision making ranges across a spectrum from paternalistic, doctor-centred styles on the one hand, to informed choice, consumer-based styles on the other, with shared decision making somewhere between the two (Elwyn, 2001). Decision support interventions and decision aids can support this style of clinical decision making. Charles et al. (1997) identified three stages to SDM: bi-directional information exchange, deliberation, and selection of treatment options consistent with the patient's preferences.

There has been considerable interest in SDM in mental illness as a strategy to improve safety and quality of care, to address the increasing complexity of treatment options, and fundamentally to empower and enhance the autonomy and quality of life of people with mental illness seeking care. Patel et al. (2008) reviewed extant literature on SDM in mental illness care and found support for the notion that people with mental illnesses across a wide spectrum that ranges from high to low prevalence disorders want information and scientific evidence about their condition. They also want to be involved in decisions about their care, particularly about medications.

Nevertheless, in practice, SDM in mental illness care is often confined to simply information sharing. It is interesting to consider the sorts of limitations that surround SDM in practice. Certainly, system levels factors such as time limitation may play a role. Cultural variations in the expectation of adopting a questioning style in an encounter with a doctor are also important. However, one of the key factors may be professional bias. Truly patient-centred SDM requires flexibility as patients and circumstances differ. While striving to encourage greater patient involvement in decisions, it is not clear to what degree the doctor-patient relationship can become genuinely symmetrical. Doctors find it difficult to explicitly discuss preferences for sharing information with patients, and instead rely on an 'intuitive feel' to determine if a patient is interested in, and capable of, participating in SDM, or not (Goossensen et al., 2007). Thus, bias and stereotype can shape the interaction between GP and patient. As the amount of information exchange is theoretically infinite, the need for flexibility, tools, and strategies to elicit patient preferences for information exchange is particularly important.

Can these tensions be overcome? Interestingly, primary care has led the way in studies of SDM interventions in mental illness care. These studies suggest positive outcomes for SDM in a range of settings. Greater involvement in decision making has been associated with more guideline-concordant care and recovery from depression (Clever et al., 2006; Swanson et al., 2007), improvement in self-efficacy (Ludman et al., 2003), and patient satisfaction without causing increased time in the consultation (Loh et al., 2007).

Written mental health plans can incorporate elements to support SDM and can provide a structure for GPs to explicitly elicit patient preferences for participation in the decisions about their care. Our own work on the use of written and negotiated care plans identified that a majority of people with depression in primary care found they were helpful in setting goals, giving direction, engaging family and friends, measuring progress, and enhancing autonomy (Palmer et al., 2013). This suggests that SDM can play a key role in recovery-oriented primary mental illness care.

Conclusion

Patient-centred practice holds great promise at both an individual encounter level and at an organizational and system level for supporting more accessible, meaningful, and recovery-focused therapeutic encounters and settings. Primary care has both the philosophical heritage and professional skill set to play a leadership role in championing and promoting such practice, in partnership with patient and user organizations. However, as we have pointed out, this is not without challenges.

Politically, patient-centred practice is at risk of simply being mobilized to serve broader powerful interests, subjecting both users of services and health professionals to a limited set of sanctioned forms of practice that serve notions of population- and individual-level accountability. Resisting this and realizing the potential of patient-centredness requires reflexivity in providers, patients, and their organizations, and a self-awareness both in and of practice. The notion of 'relationship-centred practice' (Frankel, 2004) more closely captures this liberated and emancipatory view of the encounter.

The sociologist Richard Sennett wrote of the 'art' of mutual respect as a sign of a 'character turned outward' (Sennett, 2003:227), and as the foundation of respect and equality in dealings between individuals. For Sennett, openness to change and newness—to journeying together or 'méttisage'—is the basis for mutual respect and equality between individuals. This has resonance for the ongoing project of realizing the potential of patient-centred practice in mental health care. For Sennett, 'conscious excavation is necessary for survival in a hostile world' (Sennett, 2003:235). Referring to conscious (and reflexive) excavation of the clinically routine, the known, the familiar, and the assumed, this can be simply 'a matter of curiosity' as a way of creating genuine respect and mutuality between GP and patient (Sennett, 2003:241). This can be the foundation for genuine patient-centred practice that supports recovery for people with mental disorders.

References

Armstrong, D. (2011). The invention of patient-centred medicine. *Social Theory & Health,* 9: 410–8.

Balint, M. (1964). *The doctor, his patient and the illness.* London, Pitman.

Bower, P, Gask, L, May, C, and MEAD, N. (2001). Domains of consultation research in primary care. *Patient Educ Couns,* 45: 3–11.

Charles, C, Gafni, A, and Whelan, T. (1997). Shared decision-making in the medical encounter: what does it mean? (or it takes at least two to tango). *Social Science & Medicine,* 44: 681–92.

Clever, SL, Ford, DE, Rubenstein, LV, Rost, KM, Meredith, LS, Sherbourne, CD, Wang, NY, Arbelaez, JJ, and Cooper, LA. (2006). Primary care patients' involvement in decision-making is associated with improvement in depression. *Medical Care,* 44: 398–405.

Croghan, T and Brown, J. (2010). *Integrating mental health treatment into the patient centered medical home.* Prepared for the Agency for Healthcare Research and Quality by Mathematica Policy Research under contract No. HHSA2902009000191 TO2, (Rockville, MD: Agency for Healthcare Research and Quality.

Elwyn, G. (2001). *Shared decision making: patient involvement in clinical practice.* Nijmegen: Nijmegen University.

Enge;, GL. (1977). The need for a new medical model: a challenge for biomedicine. *Science,* **196**: 129–36.

Frank, RG, Huskamp, HA, and **Pincus, HA**. (2003). Aligning incentives in the treatment of depression in primary care with evidence-based practice. *Psychiatric Services,* **54**: 682–7.

Frankel, RM. (2004). Relationship-centered care and the patient-physician relationship. *Journal of General Internal Medicine,* **19**: 1163–5.

Goossensen, A., Zijlstra, P. and Koopmanschap, M. (2007). Measuring shared decision making processes in psychiatry: skills versus patient satisfaction. *Patient Education and Counseling,* **67**: 50–6.

Gunn, JM, Palmer, VJ, Naccarella, L, Kokanovic, R, Pope, CJ, Lathlean, J, and Stange, KC. (2008). The promise and pitfalls of generalism in achieving the Alma-Ata vision of health for all. *Medical Journal of Australia,* **189**: 110–2.

Loh, A, Simon, D, Wills, CE, Kriston L, Niebling, W, and Harter, M. (2007). The effects of a shared decision-making intervention in primary care of depression: a cluster-randomized controlled trial. *Patient Education and Counseling,* **67**: 324–32.

Ludman, E, Katon, W, Bush, T, Rutter, C, Lin, E, Simon, G, Von Korff, M, and Walker, E. (2003). Behavioural factors associated with symptom outcomes in a primary care-based depression prevention intervention trial. *Psychological Medicine,* **33**: 1061–70.

McDonald, R, Mead, N Cheragi-Sohi, S, Bower, P, Whalley, D, and Roland, M. (2007). Governing the ethical consumer: identity, choice and the primary care medical encounter. *Sociology of Health & Illness,* **29**: 430–56.

McWhinney, IR. (1995). Why we need a new clinical method. *In:* A Stewart, JB Brown, WW Weston, IR McWhinney, CL McWilliam, and TR Freeman eds., *Patient-Centered Medicine: Transforming the clinical method.*London: Sage, 1–18.

Mead, N and Bower, P. (2000). Patient-centredness: a conceptual framework and review of the empirical literature. *Social Science & Medicine,* **51**: 1087–110.

Mead, N and Bower, P. (2002). Patient-centred consultations and outcomes in primary care: a review of the literature [comment]. *Patient Education & Counseling,* **48**: 51–61.

Mead, N, Bower, P, and Hann, M. (2002). The impact of general practitioners' patient-centredness on patients' post-consultation satisfaction and enablement. *Social Science & Medicine,* **55**: 283–99.

Palmer, VJ, Johnson, CL, Furler, JS, Densley, K, Potiriadis, M, and Gunn, JM. (2013). Written plans: an overlooked mechanism to develop recovery-oriented primary care for depression? *Australian Journal of Primary Health,* **20/3**: 241–9.

Patel, SR, Bakken, S, and Ruland, C. (2008). Recent advances in shared decision making for mental health. *Current Opinion in Psychiatry,* **21**: 606–12.

Pincus, HA, Houtsinger, JK, Bachman, J, and Keyser, D. (2005). Depression in primary care: bringing behavioral health care into the mainstream. *Health Affairs,* **24**: 271–6.

Pirl, WF, BECK, BJ, Safren, SA, and Kim, H. (2001). A Descriptive Study of Psychiatric Consultations in a Community Primary Care Center. *Primary Care Companion to The Journal of Clinical Psychiatry* **3**: 190–4.

Reeve, J, Irving, G, and Dowrick, CF. (2011). Can generalism help revive the primary healthcare vision? *Journal of the Royal Society of Medicine,* **104**: 395–400.

Ring, A, Dowrick, CF, Humphris, GM, Davies, J, and Salmon, P. (2005). The somatising effect of clinical consultation: what patients and doctors say and do not say when patients present medically unexplained physical symptoms. *Soc Sci Med*, **61**: 1505–15.

Robert Woods Johnson Foundation. (2008). *Improving Chronic Illness Care: The chronic care model* Available: http://www.improvingchroniccare.org/index.php?p=The_Chronic_Care_Model&s=2, Accessed 2 February 2016.

Sennett, R. (2003). *Respect in a world of inequality*. New York: W.W. Norton.

Shim, R and Rust, G. (2013). Primary Care, Behavioral Health, and Public Health: Partners in Reducing Mental Health Stigma. *American Journal of Public Health*, **103**: 774–6.

Stewart, M. (1995). *Patient-centered medicine: transforming the clinical method*. Thousand Oaks: Sage Publications.

Stewart, M. (2001). Towards a global definition of patient-centred care. *BMJ*, **322**: 444–5.

Stewart, M and Brown, J. (2001). The patient-centred clinical method. *In*: A Edwards and G Elwyn (eds.), *Evidence based patient choice: inevitable or impossible?* Oxford: Oxford University Press.

Stewart, M, Brown, JB, Weston, WW, McWhinney, IR, McWilliam, CL, and Freeman, TR., eds. (2003). *Patient-centered medicine: transforming the clinical method*. Oxford: Radcliffe Medical Press.

Swanson, KA, Bastani, R, Rubenstein, LV, Meredith, LS. and Ford, DE. (2007). Effect of mental health care and shared decision making on patient satisfaction in a community sample of patients with depression. *Medical Care Research and Review*, **64**: 416–430.

Tuckett, D, Boulton, M, Olson, C, and Williams, A. (1985). *Meetings between experts: An approach to sharing ideas in medical consultations*. London: Tavistock.

Chapter 5

Neurobiology of psychiatric disorders

Vladimir Maletic and Bernadette DeMuri

Introduction

With lifetime prevalence of approximately 16%, major depressive disorder (MDD) is amongst the most prevalent and disabling psychiatric disorders (Schosser et al., 2013). Recent estimates suggest that MDD is the second leading cause of disability worldwide (Korte et al., 2015). Despite decades of antidepressant treatment development, about 30% of patients remain without full relief, even after sequential treatment attempts (Rush et al., 2006). Our descriptive nomenclature offers little guidance in choosing the most effective treatment for a specific patient. Moreover, phenotypical presentation and biological markers of MDD (e.g. melancholy vs. atypical subtype) are generally not stable over time, and may change with episode recurrence and duration. Additionally, multiple psychiatric conditions have shared clinical manifestations, such as changes in cognition, energy levels, sleep, and appetite. Furthermore, psychiatric disorders tend not to 'breed true', as substantial genetic overlaps and similar patterns of functional and structural brain changes are more a rule, rather than exception (Goodkind et al., 2015). While we are all cognizant of the limitations of the current phenomenologically based diagnostic schema, the substantial phenotypical and biological heterogeneity of MDD–and other psychiatric disorders–has hindered our efforts to develop an alternative diagnostic system based on deeper understanding of disease etiopathogenesis. In these times of transition, better understanding of the neurobiological underpinning of MDD offers hope that individualized, integrated, multimodal treatment approaches, possibly guided by biomarkers, as well as more diverse treatments, may be developed.

Anxiety disorders, with an estimated lifetime incidence approaching 29% and 12-month prevalence of 18%, are also very common conditions and are some of the most common conditions seen by primary care physicians (Klerman et al., 1991). Like MDD, anxiety disorders are associated with substantial morbidity and suffering. Furthermore, MDD and anxiety disorders may have shared clinical symptoms, genetics, risk factors, and neurobiological underpinning, yet there are also some important physiological differences separating these conditions (Kendler et al., 2008). As many as 40% to 50% of MDD patients will also have at least one comorbid anxiety disorder (Ionescu et al., 2013). Therefore, comparison of the neurobiological basis of MDD and anxiety disorders provides a suitable context for discussion of the etiopathogenesis of psychiatric conditions and its relevance for diagnosis and treatment of these disorders.

Genetics of MDD and anxiety disorders

Estimated heritability of major depressive disorder (MDD) appears to be in the moderate range (31–42%), suggesting that environmental factors may have a dominant role in its aetiology (Sullivan et al., 2000). Furthermore, the largest mega-analysis of genome-wide association studies (GWAS), which included approximately 100 000 subjects, has failed to provide robust and replicable proof of a specific gene involvement in the aetiology of MDD (2012). As several other GWAS studies were unable to identify individual genes reaching genome-wide significance for depression, we are left with an unavoidable conclusion that MDD is so genetically and phenotypically heterogeneous, that only a small portion of its aetiology can be explained by GWAS research (Demirkan et al., 2016).

On the other hand, candidate gene research focused on finding associations between single nucleotide polymorphisms (SNPs) and depression, differentiating patient from control cohorts has identified dozens of different genes potentially implicated in a etiology of MDD. Many of these polymorphisms involve genes that regulate monoamine signalling, such as serotonin transporter promoter locus (5HTTPR), 5HT2A receptor, catechol-O-methyl transferase (COMT) and monoamine oxidase (MAO). Furthermore, genes coding for brain-derived neurotrophic factor (BDNF) and glial-derived neurotrophic factor (GDNF) may also have a role in propagating vulnerability towards MDD. More recently, genes regulating the activity of CRF, gamma-amino-butyric acid (GABA), and glutamate receptors have also been implicated in MDD a etiology (Bradley et al., 2008). Emerging theories postulate that candidate genes more likely code for 'endophenotypical traits', which increase the risk of psychiatric morbidity, rather than any specific psychiatric diagnosis (Dreher et al., 2008).

Often risk alleles, such as the short version of 5HTTLPR, interact with environmental adversity in propagating the likelihood of developing depression and suicidal ideation in individuals dealing with life stressors (Caspi et al., 2003). Moreover, gender may interact with genotype, such that women with the short 5HTTPR allele, when exposed to stress, are seven times more likely to develop depression compared to males with the long allele of the same gene (Kendler KS et al., 2005). The 's' allele of the 5HTTLPR gene has been associated with several aspects of brain function and morphology, including diminished functional and structural integrity of amygdala-ACC circuitry involved in regulation of emotional, behavioural and endocrine response to stress (Pezawas et al., 2005). Moreover, the 's' 5HTTPR allele interacts with other genes—a process known as genetic epistasis. For instance, the combination of the 5HTTPR short allele with a less competent allele of the 5HT1A receptor gene has been associated with augmented amygdala reactivity, even in medicated MDD patients, relative to controls (Dannlowski et al., 2007). Studies linking less functional 5HT2A and tryptophan hydroxylase-2 (TPH2) alleles with vulnerability for developing depression and suicidality in adverse circumstances have been equivocal (Frokjaer et al., 2008).

Other alleles regulating monoamine transmission, such as MAO-A, COMT, DAT, NAT, have also been linked with the etiology of depression, neuroendocrine homeostasis, and treatment response, albeit inconsistently (Xu et al., 2009, Lavretsky et al., 2008).

Emerging evidence has also tied the polymorphism of genes coding for subunits of glutamate and GABA receptors with the risk for developing depression in conjunction with adversity, treatment response, and antidepressant-related suicidality (Sequeira et al., 2009)

Furthermore, genes tasked with control of neurotrophic factors, cellular resilience, neuroplasticity, and neurogenesis may have diminished function in MDD patients (Manji and Duman, 2001,). Less efficient, the BDNF allele has been associated with unfavourable structural brain changes, increased risk for developing depression in adverse circumstances, and suicidality in MDD (Pezawas et al., 2004).

Additionally, polymorphisms of genes regulating HPA function and inflammation-related genes have confer susceptibility to major depression in the face of adversity and influence antidepressant response (Wong et al., 2008).

In conclusion, genes regulating monoamine, GABA, and glutamate transmission seem to individually or jointly contribute to predilection towards MDD, especially in adverse circumstances (Haavik et al., 2008). Through complex epistatic interactions, these genes and the ones modulating corticosteroid, neurotrophic, and inflammatory signalling, have a convergent impact on the structural integrity and functional connectivity of key brain structures involved in generating adaptation to stress (Manji et al., 2001).

Heritability estimates for anxiety disorders range between 35% and 50%. As was the case with MDD, large GWAS studies failed to identify specific genes reaching genome-wide significance. Instead, they indicate interactions between myriad genes with small individual contributions and significant heterogeneity (Shimada-Sugimoto et al., 2015). Several studies have implicated the adenosine 2A receptor gene (ADORA2A), genes encoding 5HT1A & 5HT2A receptors, COMT (Catechol-O-methyltransferase), an enzyme involved in the metabolism of noradrenaline and dopamine, and polymorphisms of the SCL6A4 promoter 5-HTTLPR in propagating the risk for anxiety disorders (Hohoff et al., 2010, Sumner et al., 2016).

Heritability of anxiety disorders is most pronounced in early age groups, while family environment plays an increasing etiological role from mid-childhood to puberty (Franic et al., 2010). Anxiety disorders not only share genetic risk factors with each other, but also with other stress-related disorders such as MDD (Schosser et al., 2013).

Functional and structural brain changes in MDD and anxiety disorders

Rather than describing functional and structural changes related to MDD by sequentially focusing on individual brain areas, we explain the extant information in the context of resting functional brain networks. Aberrant communication between the large functional networks, and amongst their constituent components, reflects clinical manifestations of MDD with much greater accuracy than attempts to associate depressive symptoms with dysfunction of specific brain regions.

The Salience Network (SN) is tasked with accepting and processing relevant information about changes in both the internal and external environment and conveying this information to the Cognitive-Executive Network (CEN), which then organizes and initiates an adaptive response. The chief components of the SN are the subgenual and pregenual anterior cingulate (ACC) and insula, but the SN also includes the amygdala, ventral striatum/nucleus accumbens, hypothalamus, and related subcortical areas encompassing the dorsomedial thalamus and periaqueductal grey (Menon, 2011).

Most of the functional imaging studies report increased amygdala activity in depressed patients relative to controls (Sheline et al., 2001). Furthermore, excessive amygdala activity in response to negative cues has been recognized either as a risk for a new-onset depressive episode or a prognosticator of relapse in established MDD patients (Chan et al., 2009). Findings regarding structural changes of amygdala in MDD are inconsistent (Hajek et al., 2009). It is tempting to speculate that altered amygdala activity propagated via its connections with the hypothalamus and autonomic nervous system may contribute to sympathetic and neuroendocrine disturbances, commonly encountered in MDD (Drevets et al., 2002).

Intensity of anhedonia in depressed patients may be related to reduced nucleus accumbens (NAcc) volume and its attenuated response to rewards (Wacker et al., 2009). Additionally, it appears that the ventral striatum/NAcc is selectively unresponsive only to positive cues in MDD patients, since there was no difference between depressed patients and controls in their responses to negative or neutral cues (Epstein et al., 2006).

The insula-ACC unit acts as the central switch regulating communication between the SN, default mode network (DMN) and CEN. While depressed patients manifested diminished insula activity in response to positive visual cues, negative images elicited an exaggerated insular response, and this response correlated with the severity of MDD symptomatology (Lee et al., 2007). Furthermore, both current and remitted MDD patients had reductions in insular volume compared to healthy individuals (Takahashi et al., 2010). Moreover, main depressive symptoms, such as diminished capacity to experience pleasure, are inversely correlated with insular and ACC grey matter volumes (Sprengelmeyer et al., 2011).

While some authors refer to ACC as a DMN component, its more conventional designation is in the SN (Pizzagalli, 2011). For the most part, functional imaging studies report increased sgACC activity in MDD (especially when corrections are made for its reduced volume in depression) (Drevets, 2001). Moreover, the intensity of sadness in MDD has been associated with elevated blood flow into the sgACC and anterior insula (Mayberg et al., 1999). Furthermore, the extent of aberrant sgACC–amygdala connectivity also correlates with depressive illness duration (Menon, 2011). Finally, convergent lines of evidence make a connection between normalization of anomalous ACC activity and treatment response in MDD (Mayberg, 2003). Moreover, a greater pretreatment rACC activity may predict positive treatment response to antidepressants, sleep deprivation, and rTMS. Structural studies have predominantly found reductions in sgACC volume of up to 48%, especially in patients suffering from familial depression, compared to controls (Drevets, 2001).

The DMN is involved in processing social information, self-reflection, reminiscing, and planning future activities (Bressler and Menon, 2010). In addition to the posterior cingulate cortex (PCC), the DMN incorporates other midline cortical structures such as the ventromedial PFC (vmPFC), dorsomedial PFC (DMPFC), Inferior Parietal lobule, Lateral temporal cortex (LTC), medial temporal lobe (MTL) (including the hippocampal formation), and angular gyrus (Menon, 2011).

Patients suffering from MDD tend to exhibit elevated DMPFC activity, relative to controls (Sheline et al., 2010). Increased DMPFC activity in MDD has been linked to excessive self-focus, and rumination about negative past events, at the expense of adaptive problem solving (Johnson et al., 2009, Lemogne et al, 2011). Furthermore, MDD patients have a greater grey matter volume decline in the DMPFC compared to healthy controls (Frodl et al., 2008).

Under physiological circumstances VMPFC plays a role in suppressing maladaptive amygdala activity. Paradoxically, in MDD, increased VMPFC metabolism is associated with greater amygdala firing (Urry et al., 2006). Similar to other DMN regions, the VMPFC has elevated activity in individuals with MDD relative to normal controls (Fitzgerald et al., 2008). Increased VMPFC activity in MDD patients has been linked with melancholy ruminations, hopelessness, magnitude of negative affect, and overall severity of depression (Grimm et al., 2009). Moreover, poorly modulated VMPFC activity in MDD has also been associated with diminished capacity for positive or hopeful thinking (Johnson et al., 2009). In addition to abnormal function, imaging studies have discovered significant reductions in VMPFC volume (up to 32%) in MDD patients compared to healthy controls (Bremner et al., 2002).

The hippocampus is another important DMN component, and has a key role in regulating the stress response, including hypothalamic and HPA axis modulation. Furthermore, the hippocampus participates in mood regulation and declarative, spatial, and episodic memory processes (Sheline, 2000). Reduction of hippocampal volume is among the most common imaging findings in MDD patients (Vythilingam et al., 2004). Not surprisingly, decline of hippocampal volume has been linked to impaired executive function in MDD patients (Frodl et al., 2006). A three-year longitudinal study has documented a significant reduction in hippocampal grey matter volume in MDD patients relative to healthy controls. This reduction in grey matter has been associated with duration of untreated depression and lack of remission (Frodl et al., 2008). On the other hand, successful MDD treatment resulting in remission may either arrest further hippocampal structural decline, or even increase its volume (Vythilingam et al., 2004).

The dorsolateral prefrontal cortex (DLPFC) and posterior parietal cortex are principal components of the cognitive-executive network (CEN) (Menon, 2011). The dorsal ACC (dACC) and VLPFC are also sometimes included as CEN components (Drevets et al., 1998). The DLPFC and VLPFC are the main participants in 'top-down' regulation of maladaptive limbic activity, presumably associated with negative affect (Ray and Zald, 2012). Moreover, diminished DLPFC activity in MDD has been associated with duration of depression, increased amygdala reactivity following an emotional challenge, intensity of one's sadness, psychomotor slowing, poor planning, and degree of cognitive impairment (Steele et al., 2007, Zhou et al., 2010). Suggesting that

MDD-related disease process may be deleterious to DLPFC volume, a recent three-year prospective study reported significantly greater DLPFC grey matter decline in un-remitted MDD patients compared to the control subjects and to MDD subjects who attained remission (Frodl et al., 2008). Additionally, reduction of DLPFC grey matter volume correlates with greater depression severity (Vasic et al., 2008).

Elevated VLPFC activity is one of the most consistent imaging findings in MDD. Although it is subject to interpretation, increased VLPFC activity in depression is most likely a compensatory attempt of top-down regulation of excessive limbic activity, reflected by feelings of sadness and despair. Furthermore, functional imaging studies correlate the degree of VLPFC activity with symptom severity in MDD patients (Zhou et al., 2010). Moreover, meta-analyses have reported a significant reduction in VLPFC grey matter volume of MDD patients relative to healthy subjects (Lorenzetti et al., 2009,). Reduction in VLPFC grey matter volume was also associated with greater severity of depression and impaired executive function (Vasic et al., 2008).

In addition to changes in grey matter volume, MDD is also characterized by compromised structure and function of white matter tracts connecting prefrontal and limbic brain areas. While white matter reduction in MDD does not appear to be age related, this reduction is present during the earliest stages of the illness and may even precede it, advancing further with the progression of the disease (Sheline et al., 2008).

Recent publications highlight the fact that white matter pathology in MDD patients involves the principal cortical and limbic areas including the DLPFC, VMPFC, amygdala, insula, and hippocampus; these are the same as those implicated in the pathophysiology of depression. Furthermore, imaging findings of white matter abnormalities in depressed patients coincide with reported genetic vulnerabilities, which are reflected in deficient myelination, axonal growth, and synaptic function (Tham et al., 2011).

In physiological circumstances, perceived loss or impending threat would elevate SN activity, followed by increased connectivity with the CEN. Greater CEN engagement would then refocus attention on the issue at hand, and initiate problem-solving behaviour. However, in MDD, a negative effect is associated with a 'short-circuiting' between the SN and the DMN, leading to inward focus, non-productive rumination, and elaboration of the negative event (Berman et al., 2011). Furthermore, components of SN, such as the subgenual anterior cingulate cortex (sgACC) and insula, manifest hyper-connectivity with DMN formations, such as the PCC, precuneus, and DMPFC, leading to amplification of the negative affect, and ensuing interference with cognitive tasks (Leibenluft and Pine, 2013, Bartova et al, 2015). Moreover, duration of a depressive episode may intensify co-activation between the sgACC and the DMN, possibly reflecting the biological underpinning of disease progression (Greicius et al., 2007).

Imaging studies have established a consensus on the crucial role of the amygdala, ACC, and insula in the pathophysiology of anxiety disorders (Damsa et al., 2009). Other studies have also implicated the hippocampus, ventral striatum, DLPFC and mPFC in etiopathogenesis of anxiety disorders (Oathes et al., 2015). With some exceptions, panic disorder tends to be characterized by amygdala hyper-responsivity to subtle environmental cues triggering a major threat response; this is due to insufficient top-down governance from higher cortical areas (Kent and Rauch, 2003). In addition to amygdala hyperactivity, functional imaging studies have demonstrated elevated metabolic activity in the hippocampus, thalamus, cerebellum, midbrain, and brainstem of panic disorder patients, compared to controls. Moreover, increased metabolic activity in these brain regions normalized after successful behavioural or pharmacologic therapy, suggesting a state-dependent increase in their activation (Martin et al., 2009). Additionally, patients suffering from social anxiety disorder also exhibited exaggerated activity in the amygdala and associated medial temporal lobe areas (Veit et al., 2002). Furthermore, even adolescent patients afflicted by generalized anxiety disorder (GAD) exhibited an elevated right amygdala response which correlated positively with symptom severity (Martin et al., 2009). Extending these findings, other authors have reported aberrant functional connectivity between ventral PFC, ACC, and the amygdala in GAD patients compared to controls (Etkin et al., 2010). Additionally, more recent research has established excessive sgACC-ventral striatum activity as a hallmark indicator of 'anxious arousal', while greater limbic/paralimbic activity represents a substrate for 'general distress' in anxiety disorders and MDD (Oathes et al., 2015).

Altered neurotransmission in MDD and anxiety disorders

In spite of decades of research and elaboration, the 'monoamine hypothesis' of MDD remains beset with controversies. Principal support for this hypothesis stems from the therapeutic efficacy of antidepressant agents that modulate 5HT, dopamine (DA), and norepinephrine (NE) (Schildkraut, 1965). Yet, if inadequate monoamines are the primary abnormality in MDD, it is difficult to understand why in large studies, using standardized antidepressant treatments, the majority of patients fail to reach remission (Trivedi et al., 2008). Furthermore, a study using pharmacologic 'probes' to assess the integrity of monoamine systems in MDD concluded that approximately 40% of depressed patients had no demonstrable NE or 5HT abnormality (Duval et al., 2000).

In support of the monoamine hypothesis, studies have reported differences in NE and 5HT receptor density in cortical and limbic formations as well as elevated levels of MAO-A in the brains of depressed patients when compared to controls (Delgado, 2000). Additionally, changes in platelet 5HT and NE receptor density and reduction in the number of NE and 5HT neurons have also been noted in depressed and suicidal patients, relative to controls (Baumann and Bogerts, 2001). Studies evaluating CSF levels of NE and 5HT metabolites have yielded equivocal results. The majority of evidence suggests that levels of 5-hydroxyindoleacetic acid (5-HIAA) are decreased in depressed patients, especially in patients who have made violent suicide attempts (Delgado, 2000). Likewise, 3-methoxy-4-hydroxyphenylglycol (MHPG), a principal NE metabolite, was found to be increased in the plasma of agitated and anxious depressed patients, while depressed individuals with psychomotor retardation had reduced MHPG and homovanillic acid (HVA) (a primary dopamine metabolite) levels, relative to controls. Furthermore, studies of salivary MHPG and 5-HIAA noted their reduction only in melancholy MDD patients, but not in other subtypes (Cubala et al., 2014b) (Cubala et al., 2014a). Levels of MHPG and 5-HIAA were unrelated to duration or severity of symptoms. Additionally, a study reported increased plasma

HVA levels in patients suffering from psychotic depression (Okamoto et al., 2008). Furthermore, studies sampling blood from the internal jugular vein found reduced NE and DA levels, and increased 5HT turnover in depressed patients, relative to controls (Lambert et al., 2000).

Monoamine uptake may be disrupted by MDD. Patients suffering from depression have reduced dopamine transporter (DAT) and elevated 5HT transporter (5-HTT) binding potential when compared to controls (Meyer et al., 2002, Meyer, 2007). In addition to these findings, acute monoamine depletion studies indicate that therapeutic benefits of antidepressants may be rapidly and selectively reversed by depletion of the monoamine affected by a particular antidepressant (Delgado, 2004). It is quite possible that depressed patients have an elevated turnover of monoamine metabolites, which may be an indicator of insufficient neurotransmission that could be normalized with successful antidepressant treatment. Remarkably consistent evidence points to reductions in NE and 5HT turnover in depressed patients taking antidepressants, compared to their pretreatment levels (Desireddi et al., 2008). Furthermore, not only do monoamines influence each other via complex interactions, but GABA and Glu tend to have a bidirectional regulatory influence on monoamines (Tao and Auerbach, 2000, Lee et al, 2008). In summary, cumulative evidence supports the view of a complex dysregulation of interrelated neurotransmitter systems and significant biological heterogeneity within the MDD diagnosis, rather than a simple deficit of monoamine signalling (Stone et al., 2008).

Studies evaluating peripheral glutamate levels in MDD patients had inconclusive outcomes (Kugaya and Sanacora, 2005). Contemporary magnetic resonance spectroscopy (MRS) studies mostly report reduced Glx signals (a combined measure of glutamate, GABA, and glutamine spectroscopic signatures) in the ACC and amygdala in depressed patients of all ages. However, new imaging evidence suggests that glutamatergic transmission may become progressively reduced with duration of illness (Portella et al., 2011). Furthermore, these abnormalities may normalize with successful electro-convulsive therapy (ECT) treatment (Kugaya and Sanacora, 2005). These findings are extended by reports of changes in the NMDA receptor glycine binding site and NMDA subunits in depressed patients. Moreover, the function of glutamatergic projections from the vmPFC to monoaminergic brainstem nuclei may be compromised in MDD patients (Hansel and von Kanel, 2008). A positive controlled, randomized trial of ketamine, a glutamatergic agent, in treatment resistant depression supports the utility of glutamatergic treatment interventions in MDD (Zarate et al., 2006).

There is convergent evidence of GABA dysfunction in MDD. In addition to a reduction of plasma GABA levels, post-mortem studies described a decrease in GABA neurons in the lateral orbital PFC (LOPFC) and DLPFC of MDD patients (Kalueff and Nutt, 2007). Furthermore, there is corroborating evidence from an MRS study which described reductions in GABA levels in DLPFC, dmPFC, and ACC of MDD patients relative to controls (Hasler et al., 2007). These reports are of particular interest, given the role of the DLPFC and LOPFC in cognition and volitional regulation of emotion, and the role of the dmPFC and ACC in automatic regulation of affect. Preliminary studies have indicated that altered cortical GABA and Glu concentrations may not only set apart MDD patients from controls, but may also differentiate between depressive subtypes (Sanacora et al., 2004). Finally, several preclinical and clinical studies have linked the improvement in depressive symptomatology in response to antidepressants and ECT treatment with normalization of GABA deficits (Krystal et al., 2002).

We will refrain from discussion of the role of acetylcholine and neuropeptide transmitters in the pathophysiology of MDD due to limited clinical data and space constraints.

Anxiety disorders are associated with complex disturbances of multiple neurotransmitters and their matching receptors in cortical and limbic areas. Altered noradrenergic activity has emerged as a key element in many aspects of pathological anxiety. Panic disorder patients experienced a surge of panic-like anxiety in response to administration of yohimbine (an alpha-2 noradrenergic receptor antagonist), while administration of clonidine (an alpha-2 noradrenergic receptor agonist) produced a blunted growth hormone response, both indicative of aberrant adrenergic transmission in panic disorder (Charney et al., 1982, Gurguis and Uhde, 1990).

Elevated norepinephrine (NE) activity is believed to be responsible for many symptoms of pathologic anxiety, including hyperarousal, startle response, insomnia, and panic attacks (Charney et al., 1987). Much like in panic disorder patients, yohimbine elicits panic-like symptoms in PTSD patients, relative to controls (Kent et al., 2002). Additionally, some PTSD symptoms may be mediated by an aberrant interaction between glucocorticoids and NE (Hurlemann, 2008).

Serotonin (5-HT) release may have both anxiolytic and anxiogenic effects depending on receptor subtype and the brain region involved (Graeff, 2004). Proper functioning of primarily inhibitory 5-HT1A receptors is required for normal development of the neural circuits regulating anxiety. Patients suffering from panic disorder have a lower density of 5-HT1A receptors in their limbic structures (Neumeister et al., 2004). Although the majority of studies found no difference in 5HT concentration or the number of serotonin transporter (5HTT) sites in GAD patients relative to controls, one group reported a negative correlation between 5HTT binding and anxiety symptoms in GAD (Hilbert et al., 2014). Patients suffering from social anxiety disorder may have an overactive presynaptic serotonin system, which is characterized by increased serotonin synthesis and transporter density (Frick et al., 2015).

Although dopamine has an important role in regulation of neural circuitry involved in anxiety and reward processing, there is a dearth of clinical research linking insufficient dopamine signalling with symptoms of anxiety disorders.

In addition to monoamines, several polypeptides, such as cholecystokinin, vasopressin, oxytocin, galanin, neuropeptide Y, and corticotropin-releasing hormone (CRH) have been implicated in the pathophysiology of anxiety disorders (Martin et al., 2009).

The regulation of fear and anxiety is significantly impacted by the balance between the excitatory neurotransmitter glutamate and GABA in key limbic and cortical areas. Increased activity in emotion-processing brain regions in individuals suffering from anxiety disorders could be a result of either decreased inhibitory GABA signalling or increased glutamatergic excitatory neurotransmission (Jardim et al., 2005). In general, agents that inhibit GABA receptors tend to be anxiogenic while those that increase GABA receptor activity are anxiolytic (Kalueff and Nutt, 2007). Panic disorder patients manifest a GABA receptor deficit, with the greatest decrease in receptor numbers evident in cortical areas. Moreover, severity of anxiety symptoms correlates with the deficit in GABA receptors in the orbitofrontal cortex (Hasler et al., 2008).

Autonomic and endocrine alterations in MDD and anxiety disorders

Convergent evidence supports autonomic abnormalities in MDD that are manifested by increased sympathetic nervous system (SNS) and reduced parasympathetic nervous system (PNS) tone. This evidence includes elevated resting heart rate in response to stress, higher blood pressure and systemic vascular resistance, increased whole-body sympathetic activity as reflected by norepinephrine (NE) release and clearance, decreased heart rate variability (HRV) and high frequency HRV (a measure of parasympathetic tone), impaired baro-reflex, and longer ventricular repolarization time (Bassett, 2015, Agelink et al., 2001, Barton et al., 2007). Although there is some variability, study outcomes show that different treatments, including antidepressants, psychotherapy, repetitive transcranial magnetic stimulation (TMS), and ECT, may 'normalize' the sympathetic/parasympathetic imbalance by reducing SNS activity and/ or elevating vagal tone (Chambers and Allen, 2002). Moreover, there appears to be an association between peripheral sympathetic hyperactivity and elevated central arousal. A recent study reported a relationship between SSRI-related remission/response and decline in CNS arousal at rest (Olbrich et al., 2016). Furthermore, it has been suggested that use of biofeedback to correct ANS disturbances may also improve depressive symptoms, indicating that ANS perturbations may play a causal role in depressive symptomatology (Hassett et al., 2007).

Multiple studies suggest that HPA hyperactivity in MDD may be a consequence of elevated hypothalamic corticotropin-releasing factor (CRF) secretion, possibly in response to higher brain areas emitting distress signals (Owens and Nemeroff, 1991). In addition to elevated cerebrospinal fluid (CSF) CRF concentrations and increased CRF mRNA and protein in the hypothalamus of depressed individuals, studies have also registered blunted ACTH response to CRF, likely reflecting down-regulation of cognate receptors (Nemeroff et al., 1988, Gold et al,1995). Furthermore, MDD is also frequently associated with hypercortisolemia, as evidenced by increased number of cortisol and adrenocorticotropin (ACTH) secretory pulses over the course of circadian cycle, an amplified cortisol response to ACTH, and the hypertrophy of pituitary and adrenal glands (Rubin et al., 1987, Gold et al., 1988, Nemeroff, 1996).

Convergent data demonstrate that glucocorticoid receptors (GR) have reduced activity in MDD, which leads to insufficient cortisol signalling, even in the presence of elevated cortisol levels (Pariante and Miller, 2001,). A strong correlation between peripheral cortisol levels and reduced GR sensitivity in MDD is indicative of relative GR resistance and therefore inadequate glucocorticoid signalling (Thase, 2000). Moreover, insufficient glucocorticoid anti-inflammatory influence may be responsible for excessive inflammatory signalling in MDD (Raison and Miller, 2003).

Rates of impaired glucocorticoid signalling in MDD vary from approximately 25% to 50% (Holsboer, 2000). The highest rates of elevated cortisol accompanied by a dexamethasone non-suppression test (DST) are found in melancholic subtypes of MDD, while atypical depression may be associated with normal or mildly elevated cortisol signalling (O'Keane et al., 2012). While melancholy depression can be interpreted as an exaggeration of response to stress, atypical depression may be understood as manifestation of excessive inhibition of stress response (Gold, 2015). Although melancholy and atypical depression are treated as separate subtypes, the majority of depressed patients will experience both types of episodes at some point (O'Keane et al., 2012). Furthermore, atypical episodes tend to be associated with more frequent recurrence, positive family history, and chronicity of MDD. Both the DST and its more sensitive variant DEX-CRF test have been demonstrated to robustly predict treatment response and depressive relapse (Greden et al., 1983, Ising et al, 2007).

In addition to well-documented HPA disturbance, there may also be a reciprocal relationship between thyroid dysfunction and MDD (Duntas and Maillis, 2013). Neuroendocrine and autonomic dysregulation associated with MDD may also contribute to circadian disruption, which frequently accompanies this condition (Gold, 2015).

Common somatic symptoms of anxiety disorders, such as hot flashes, rapid heart rate, difficulty breathing, and increased respiratory rate, may be a reflection of altered autonomic control. Moreover, many of the panic disorder symptoms are remindful of the fight or flight response to threat. Studies have reported elevated plasma norepinephrine in response to stress in GAD patients, compared to healthy controls (Hilbert et al., 2014).

CRH is a principal mediator of the stress response, and CRH-containing neurons are located in the brainstem monoaminergic nuclei, the amygdala, the prefrontal and cingulate cortices, the stria terminalis, the nucleus accumbens, and the periaqueductal grey (Steckler and Holsboer, 1999). Panic disorder patients manifest increased serum CRH concentrations associated with elevated basal cortisol levels (Martin et al., 2009). Additionally, CRH is hypothesized to serve as a mediator of cognitive and physical symptoms of anxiety by enhancing transmission through major structures involved in the stress response and emotional regulation (Sullivan et al., 1999). Furthermore, elevated baseline plasma cortisol concentrations were correlated with the risk for a panic attack after lactate 'challenge' administration. This finding suggests that increased baseline plasma cortisol may be a correlate of anticipatory anxiety, rather than panic attacks themselves (Kent et al., 2002). Changes in cortisol levels in GAD patients have been an inconsistent finding. While some studies reported higher evening cortisol levels in GAD patients relative to the control group, other studies have found no difference in cortisol levels (Hilbert et al., 2014).

Immune disturbance in MDD and anxiety disorders

Patients suffering from MDD manifest multiple features of inflammation, including increase of inflammatory cytokines, their soluble receptors, acute phase proteins, chemokines, adhesion molecules, and prostaglandins in the periphery, as well as CSF (Alesci et al., 2005, Miller et al, 2009). Moreover, recent reports have established an association between peripheral levels of inflammatory mediators and depressive symptom severity, cognitive performance, and metabolic derangements in individuals suffering from MDD (Kop et al., 2002, Miller and Raison, 2015). Furthermore, CSF concentration of inflammatory cytokines in MDD is robustly correlated with aberrant monoamine turnover and suicide risk in depressed individuals (Lindqvist et al., 2009). A recent study found that abnormal IL-6 production across the circadian cycle may be a contributing factor to circadian disturbance in depressed patients (Alesci et al., 2005). In addition to a well-documented alteration in the innate immune response (mediated by inflammatory cytokines, chemokines and macrophages), emerging evidence points to an additional disturbance of acquired immunity (mediated by T and B lymphocytes) in MDD patients. Research has also uncovered increased markers of T cell activation (e.g. soluble IL-2 receptor) in depressed patients, compared to controls (Mossner et al., 2007).

Inflammatory molecules may serve as biomarkers, potentially guiding antidepressant selection and indicating successful treatment of a depressive episode (Miller and Raison, 2015). Peripheral cytokine levels may 'normalize' following successful treatment and remission of an MDD episode (O'Brien et al., 2007). Furthermore, treatment-resistant depressed patients manifesting elevated peripheral inflammation (hsCRP>5mg/L) may have a greater antidepressant response when an infliximab infusion (a TNF-alpha antagonist) is combined with their standard antidepressant medication, relative to depressed individuals with lower inflammation and the control group (Raison et al., 2013). Astonishingly, infliximab is a large molecule which never enters the brain, yet effectively ameliorates depression by suppressing peripheral inflammation! Finally, a preliminary study found that depressed patients with elevated peripheral inflammation, as indicated by hsCRP>3mg/L, may have a more favourable response to a noradrenergic antidepressant vs. an SSRI (Uher et al., 2014).

It has been hypothesized that chronic stress during the course of anxiety disorders may precipitate an increase in pro-inflammatory signalling (O'Donovan et al., 2010). Furthermore, studies have found an association between elevated levels of C-reactive protein (CRP) in men and somatic and cognitive symptoms of anxiety disorders. In contradistinction to increased CRP levels, higher IL-6 and TNF alpha levels were only associated with somatic symptoms of anxiety disorders (Duivis et al., 2013). Although lifestyle factors, especially BMI may be partially responsible for the association between anxiety symptoms and inflammation levels, studies have reported greater elevation of CRP levels in anxious men and women, compared to controls even after adjustment for BMI (Liukkonen et al., 2011).

Cellular oxidative and neuroplastic changes in MDD and anxiety disorders

The most prominent pathohistological finding in MDD is the reduction of glial density and numbers in several brain areas involved in mood regulation and stress response. A greater decrease in astroglia and oligodendroglia numbers and density has been found in the sgACC, DLPFC, orbitofrontal cortex and amygdala of unmedicated MDD patients, relative to controls (Rajkowska et al, 2007). A recent transcriptional study of MDD patients discovered aberrant expression of 17 genes related to oligodendroglia function, suggesting that reduced oligodendroglia numbers may be a consequence of genetic vulnerability (Aston et al., 2005). Given the role of oligodendroglia in myelination of long white matter tracts, these cytological findings may echo imaging reports of disrupted connectivity between key prefrontal and limbic areas involved in emotional regulation. Furthermore, a significant decrease in glial density in the dentate gyrus of the hippocampus in MDD subjects (Stockmeier et al., 2004) may partially explain its diminished competency in HPA regulation.

A post-mortem study using immunohistochemistry evaluated the microglial density in the DLPFC, the ACC, the mediodorsal thalamus, and the hippocampus of mood disordered patients. The authors hypothesized that significant microgliosis (i.e. increased number of microglia) in depressed patients who committed suicide, relative to depressed individuals who died due to other causes, may be a marker of pre-suicidal stress (Steiner et al., 2008).

Unlike widespread glial abnormalities, neuronal alterations in MDD appear to more discrete and subtle. A number of post-mortem studies noted a greater reduction in pyramidal cell size in the hippocampus, ACC, DLPFC (BA 9), and OPFC (BA 47) of MDD patients, compared to controls (Chana et al., 2003, Stockmeier et al., 2004). The distribution of neuronal pathology remarkably mirrors glial reductions and findings from structural imaging studies.

In response to dysregulated peripheral inflammatory signalling in MDD, microglia may become activated and start releasing copious amounts of IL-1, IL-6, TNF-alpha, PGs, NO, and H_2O_2, which in turn prompts astrocytes to release more of the similar inflammatory molecules (Miller et al., 2009). Due to aberrant astroglia-microglia communication, oligodendroglia are likely to suffer oxidative damage related to overexposure to reactive oxygen and nitrogen species (ROS and RNS). Furthermore, TNF-alpha released by microglia and astrocytes, combined with reduced BDNF support, has a toxic effect on oligodendroglia, most likely contributing to demyelination and compromised communication within and between mood-modulatory networks (Miller et al., 2009) (see Fig. 5.1).

Moreover, aberrant microglia function in MDD may be central to inflammatory, neurotrophic, and neurotransmitter disturbance. Proinflammatory cytokines and prostaglandins jointly induce indoleamine 2,3- dioxygenase (IDO), an enzyme which subsequently converts tryptophan to kynurenine and quinolinic acid (QUIN), thereby reducing its availability for 5-HT and melatonin synthesis (Felger and Lotrich, 2013). Proinflammatory cytokines may additionally disrupt serotonergic and dopaminergic neurotransmission by accelerating their reuptake from the synaptic cleft (Miller and Raison, 2015).

QUIN is a robust NMDA agonist and stimulator of Glu release, which disrupts glutamategic transmission and increases the risk of excitotoxicity (Felger and Lotrich, 2013). Additionally, activation of IDO in astrocytes may propagate conversion of tryptophan into kynurenic acid (KA), a known antagonist of dopamine and NMDA receptor activity.

Astrocyte dysfunction may alter GABA/glutamate balance in another important way. Recent research has identified astrocytes as an important source of GABA in the CNS (Lee et al., 2011). In addition to its role in transmission, GABA may act as an anti-inflammatory molecule by attenuating microglial release of inflammatory cytokines (Lee et al., 2011). Accumulation of inflammatory and oxidative compounds

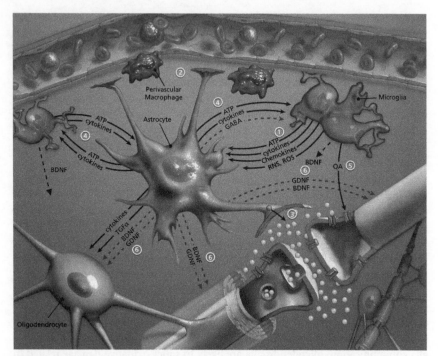

Fig. 5.1 Full lines indicate increased release of mediators, while interrupted lines designate reduced signalling. Abbreviations: RNS, reactive nitrogen species; ROS, reactive oxygen species; ATP, adenosine triphosphate; BDNF, brain-derived neurotrophic factor; GDNF, glial cell-derived neurotrophic factor; GABA, gamma aminobutyric acid; TGFα, transforming growth factor alpha

Reproduced from *Frontiers in Psychiatry*, 5, 2014, Maletic and Raison, 'Integrated neurobiology of bipolar disorder'. This is an open-access article distributed under the terms of the Creative Commons Attribution License (http://creativecommons.org/licenses/by/3.0/)

in MDD may cause astrocytic apoptosis (van Kralingen et al., 2013) and precipitate a shift in the microglia/astroglia balance, favouring microglial activity, thus producing excessive glutametergic transmission relative to GABA output and perpetuating a pro-inflammatory milieu (Maletic and Raison, 2009). Furthermore, since microglia and astrocytes are principal sources of BDNF, their compromised function and numbers may contribute to alterations in neurotrophic signalling in MDD (Maletic and Raison, 2014).

Several convergent factors present in MDD (e.g., loss of diurnal rhythm of cortisol secretion, elevation of inflammatory signals, and impaired astroglia function) jointly impede BDNF synthesis and signalling (Miller and Raison, 2015). Astrocytes activated by inflammatory signals release Glu almost exclusively into the extrasynaptic space, where it binds to extrasynaptic NMDA receptors (Haydon and Carmignoto, 2006). In contradistinction with activation of synaptic NMDA receptors, which lead to enhancement of BDNF synthesis and release, glutamate binding to extrasynaptic NMDA receptors robustly suppresses BDNF synthesis (Hardingham et al., 2002).

Although the majority of studies reported lower peripheral BDNF levels in MDD patients when compared to healthy controls, correlation with the severity of depression and disease recurrence has been inconsistent (Karege et al., 2002; Molendijk et al., 2011). A recent study discovered an association between CSF BDNF levels and suicidal ideation in depressed patients (Martinez et al., 2012). Different antidepressant treatments, including tricyclic and heterocyclic antidepressants, monoamine oxydase inhibitors (MAOIs), SSRIs, SNRIs and selective norepinephrine reuptake inhibitors (NRIs), ketamine (an NMDA-R antagonist), as well as ECT, repetitive transcranial magnetic stimulation (rTMS), exercise, and even psychotherapy have demonstrated evidence of BDNF modulation (Russo-Neustadt and Chen, 2005; Hunsberger et al., 2009; Hanson et al., 2011). Peripheral BDNF levels may even predict antidepressant response. A contemporary study reported that increase in serum BDNF levels to 126% of baseline, after a week of antidepressant treatment, combined with 50% reduction in their $HAMD_{17}$, over the same time period, predicted the ultimate treatment response with 100% specificity (Dreimuller et al., 2012)! However, despite successful antidepressant treatment, peripheral BDNF levels in remitted depressed patients most often lag behind BDNF concentrations in healthy controls (Sen et al., 2008).

Glia-derived neurotrophic factor (GDNF) plays an important role in the maintenance of neuronal health and cognitive function. A recent study reported reduced serum levels of GDNF in depressed patients compared to healthy controls. Furthermore, eight weeks of antidepressant treatment was associated with significant increase in serum GDNF in depressed patients, relative to controls (Zhang et al., 2008).

Reports of changes in the peripheral vascular endothelial growth factor (VEGF) levels in MDD have been very inconsistent. Several studies found elevated plasma and serum VEGF levels in the peripheral blood cells of depressed patients, relative to healthy controls, while others found no such difference (Clark-Raymond and Halaris, 2013).

In summary, disturbed neuron-glia relationships in MDD may result in diminished neurotrophic support, altered bioenergetics and oxidative regulation, excessive glutamate releases, and accumulation of ROS and RNS, all of which may jointly contribute to neurotoxicity and aggravated depressive symptoms (Miller et al., 2009).

There is a paucity of studies evaluating neurotrophic levels, oxidative stress, and cytopathology in anxiety disorders. Although not fully consistent, reports have found correlation between met66met homozygous BDNF genotype in early-onset panic disorder patients and anxiety scores (Konishi et al., 2014), a lack of correlation between val66met BDNF genotype and peripheral BDNF levels (Carlino et al., 2015), lower plasma BDNF in OCD and GAD patients (Wang et al, 2015), decreased BDNF in females with GAD and males with social anxiety and specific phobias, lower serum BDNF in OCD patients but not ones treated with medication (Wang et al., 2011), and a positive correlation between serum GDNF and antidepressant dosage (Tunca et al., 2015).

Moreover, emerging evidence has noted elevated indicators of oxidative damage in GAD (Emhan et al., 2015) and white matter microstructural changes in OCD patients, pointing to likely oligodendroglial dysfunction (Fan et al., 2012).

Conclusion: Integration of neurobiological findings

MDD and anxiety disorders are biologically heterogeneous neuropsychiatric conditions with clear endocrine, autonomic, and immune manifestations. Somatic manifestations of MDD and anxiety disorders are not just epiphenomena, but rather bodily immune and endocrine perturbations provide a feedback signal to the brain, and thus actively shape depressive and anxious symptomatology. While there are substantial similarities in the peripheral manifestations of anxiety disorders and MDD, there are also significant differences in the pattern of altered communication between key brain networks. These significant differences in brain function and microstructural alterations are most likely reflected in differing clinical manifestations of MDD and anxiety disorders. Better understanding of neurobiological underpinning of MDD and anxiety disorders may produce advancements in treatment approaches, and more timely identification and treatment of medical comorbidities.

References

Agelink MW, Majewski T, Wurthmann C, Postert T, Linka T, Rotterdam S, and Klieser E. (2001). Autonomic neurocardiac function in patients with major depression and effects of antidepressive treatment with nefazodone. *J Affect Disord*, 62/3: 187–98.

Alesci S, Martinez PE, Kelkar S, Ilias I, Ronsaville DS, Listwak SJ, Ayala AR, Licinio J, Gold HK, Kling MA, Chrousos GP, and Gold PW. (2005). Major depression is associated with significant diurnal elevations in plasma interleukin-6 levels, a shift of its circadian rhythm, and loss of physiological complexity in its secretion: clinical implications. *J Clin Endocrinol Metab*, 90/5: 2522–30.

Aston C, Jiang L, and Sokolov BP. (2005). Transcriptional profiling reveals evidence for signaling and oligodendroglial abnormalities in the temporal cortex from patients with major depressive disorder. *Mol Psychiatry*, 10/3: 309–22.

Barton DA, Dawood T, Lambert EA, Esler MD, Haikerwal D, Brenchley C, Socratous F, Kaye DM, Schlaich MP, Hickie I, and Lambert GW. (2007). Sympathetic activity in major depressive disorder: identifying those at increased cardiac risk? *J Hypertens*, 25/10: 2117–24.

Bartova L, Meyer BM, Diers K, Rabl U, Scharinger C, Popovic A, Pail G, Kalcher K, Boubela RN, Huemer J, Mandorfer D, Windischberger C, Sitte HH, Kasper S, Praschak-Rieder N, Moser E, Brocke B, and Pezawas L. (2015). Reduced default mode network suppression during a working memory task in remitted major depression. *J Psychiatr Res*, 64: 9–18.

Bassett D. (2015). A literature review of heart rate variability in depressive and bipolar disorders. *Aust N Z J Psychiatry*, 50/6: 511–9.

Baumann B and Bogerts B. (2001). Neuroanatomical studies on bipolar disorder. *Br J Psychiatry Suppl*, 41: s142–7.

Berman MG, Peltier S, Nee DE, Kross E, Deldin PJ, and Jonides J. (2011). Depression, rumination and the default network. *Soc Cogn Affect Neurosci*, 6/5: 548–55.

Bradley RG, Binder EB, Epstein MP, Tang Y, Nair HP, Liu W, Gillespie CF, Berg T, Evces M, Newport DJ, Stowe ZN, Heim CM, Nemeroff CB, Schwartz A, Cubells JF, and Ressler KJ. (2008). Influence of child abuse on adult depression: moderation by the corticotropin-releasing hormone receptor gene. *Arch Gen Psychiatry*, 65/2: 190–200.

Bremner JD, Vythilingam M, Vermetten E, Nazeer A, Adil J, Khan S, Staib LH, and Charney DS. (2002). Reduced volume of orbitofrontal cortex in major depression. *Biol Psychiatry,* 51/4: 273–9.

Bressler SL and Menon V. 2010. Large-scale brain networks in cognition: emerging methods and principles. *Trends Cogn Sci,* 14: 277–90.

Carlino D, Francavilla R, Baj G, Kulak K, D'Adamo P, Ulivi S, Cappellani S., Gasparini P, and Tongiorgi E. (2015). Brain-derived neurotrophic factor serum levels in genetically isolated populations: gender-specific association with anxiety disorder subtypes but not with anxiety levels or Val66Met polymorphism. *PeerJ,* 3: e1252.

Caspi A, Sugden K, Moffitt TE, Taylor A, Craig IW, Harrington H, McClay J, Mill J, Martin J, Braithwaite A, and Poulton R. (2003). Influence of life stress on depression: moderation by a polymorphism in the 5-HTT gene. *Science,* 301/5631: 386–9.

Chambers AS and Allen JJ. (2002).Vagal tone as an indicator of treatment response in major depression. *Psychophysiology,* 39/6: 861–4.

Chan SW, Norbury R, Goodwin GM, and Harmer CH. (2009). Risk for depression and neural responses to fearful facial expressions of emotion. *Br J Psychiatry,* 194/2: 139–45.

Chana G, Landau S, Beasley C, Everall IP, and Cotter D. (2003).Two-dimensional assessment of cytoarchitecture in the anterior cingulate cortex in major depressive disorder, bipolar disorder, and schizophrenia: evidence for decreased neuronal somal size and increased neuronal density. *Biol Psychiatry,* 53/12: 1086–98.

Charney DS, Heninger GR, Sternberg DE, Hafstad KM, Giddings S, and Landis DH. (1982).Adrenergic receptor sensitivity in depression. Effects of clonidine in depressed patients and healthy subjects. *Arch Gen Psychiatry,* 39/3: 290–4.

Charney DS, Woods SW, Goodman WK, and Heninger GR. (1987). Neurobiological mechanisms of panic anxiety: biochemical and behavioral correlates of yohimbine-induced panic attacks. *Am J Psychiatry,* 144/8: 1030–6.

Clark-Raymond A and Halaris A. (2013).VEGF and depression: a comprehensive assessment of clinical data. *J Psychiatr Res,* 47/8: 1080–7.

Cubala WJ, Landowski J, and Chrzanowska A. (2014a). Salivary 5-hydroxyindole acetic acid (5-HIAA) in drug-naive patients with short-illness-duration first episode major depressive disorder. *Neuro Endocrinol Lett,* 35/8: 746–9.

Cubala WJ, Landowski J, Wielgomas B, and Czarnowski W. (2014b). Low baseline salivary 3-methoxy-4-hydroxyphenylglycol (MHPG) in drug-naive patients with short-illness-duration first episode major depressive disorder. *J Affect Disord,* 161: 4–7.

Damsa C, Kosel M, and Moussally J. (2009). Current status of brain imaging in anxiety disorders. *Curr Opin Psychiatry,* 22/1: 96–110.

Dannlowski U, Ohrmann P, Bauer J, Kugel H, Arolt V, Heindel W, and Suslow T. (2007). Amygdala reactivity predicts automatic negative evaluations for facial emotions. *Psychiatry Res,* 154/1: 13–20.

Delgado PL. (2000). Depression: the case for a monoamine deficiency. *J Clin Psychiatry,* 61 Suppl 6: 7–11.

Delgado PL. (2004). How antidepressants help depression: mechanisms of action and clinical response. *J Clin Psychiatry,* 65 Suppl 4: 25–30.

Demirkan A, Lahti J, Direk N, Viktorin A, Lunetta KL, Terracciano A, Nalls MA, Tanaka T, Hek K, Fornage M, Wellman J, Cornelis MC, Ollila HM, Yu L, Smith JA, Pilling LC, Isaacs A, Palotie A, Zhuang WV, Zonderman A, Faul JD, Sutin A, Meirelles O, Mulas A, Hofman A, Uitterlinden A, Rivadeneira F, Perola M, Zhao W, Salomaa V, Yaffe K, Luik

AI, NABEC, Liu Y, Ding J, Lichtenstein P, Landen M, Widen E, Weir DR, Llewellyn DJ, Murray A, Kardia SL, Eriksson JG, Koenen K, Magnusson PK, Ferrucci L, Mosley TH, Cucca F, Oostra BA, Bennett DA, Paunio T, Berger K, Harris TB, Pedersen NL, Murabito JM, Tiemeier H, Van Duijn CM, and Raikkonen K. (2016). Somatic, positive and negative domains of the Center for Epidemiological Studies Depression (CES-D) scale: a meta-analysis of genome-wide association studies. *Psychol Med*, 46/8: 1613–23.

Desireddi NV, Campbell PL, Stern JA, Sobkoviak R, Chuai S, Shahrara S, Thumbikat P, Pope RM, Landis JR, Koch AE, and Schaeffer AJ. (2008). Monocyte chemoattractant protein-1 and macrophage inflammatory protein-1alpha as possible biomarkers for the chronic pelvic pain syndrome. *J Urol*, 179/5: 1857–61; discussion 1861–2.

Dreher JC, Kohn P, Kolachana B, Weinberger DR, and Berman KF. (2008). Variation in dopamine genes influences responsivity of the human reward system. *Proc Natl Acad Sci USA*: doi: 10.1073/pnas.0805517106.

Dreimuller N, Schlicht KF, Wagner S, Peetz D, Borysenko L, Hiemke C, Lieb K, and Tadic A. (2012). Early reactions of brain-derived neurotrophic factor in plasma (pBDNF) and outcome to acute antidepressant treatment in patients with major depression. *Neuropharmacology*, 62/1: 264–9.

Drevets WC, Ongur D, and Price JL. (1998). Neuroimaging abnormalities in the subgenual prefrontal cortex: implications for the pathophysiology of familial mood disorders. *Mol Psychiatry*, 3/3: 220–6, 190–1.

Drevets WC. (2001). Neuroimaging and neuropathological studies of depression: implications for the cognitive-emotional features of mood disorders. *Curr Opin Neurobiol*, 11/2: 240–9.

Drevets WC, Price JL, Bardgett ME, Reich T, Todd RD, and Raichle ME. (2002). Glucose metabolism in the amygdala in depression: relationship to diagnostic subtype and plasma cortisol levels. *Pharmacol Biochem Behav*, 71: 431–47.

Duivis HE, Vogelzangs N, Kupper N, DeJonge P, and Penninx BW. (2013). Differential association of somatic and cognitive symptoms of depression and anxiety with inflammation: findings from the Netherlands Study of Depression and Anxiety (NESDA). *Psychoneuroendocrinology*, 38/9: 1573–85.

Duntas LH and Maillis A. (2013). Hypothyroidism and depression: salient aspects of pathogenesis and management. *Minerva Endocrinol*, 38/4: 365–77.

Duval F, Mokrani MC, Bailey P, Correa H, Crocq MA, Son Diep T, and Macher JP. (2000). Serotonergic and noradrenergic function in depression: clinical correlates. *Dialogues Clin Neurosci*, 2/3: 299–308.

Emhan A, Selek S, Bayazit H, Fatih Karababa I, Kati M, and Aksoy N. (2015). Evaluation of oxidative and antioxidative parameters in generalized anxiety disorder. *Psychiatry Res*, 230/3: 806–10.

Epstein J, Pan H, Kocsis HJ, Yang Y, Butler T, Chusid J, Hochberg H, Murrough J, Strohmayer E, Stern E, and Silberswieg DA. (2006). Lack of ventral striatal response to positive stimuli in depressed versus normal subjects', *Am J Psychiatry*, 163/10: 1784–90.

Etkin A, Prater KE, Hoeft F, Menon V, and Schatzberg AF. (2010). Failure of anterior cingulate activation and connectivity with the amygdala during implicit regulation of emotional processing in generalized anxiety disorder. *Am J Psychiatry*, 167/5: 545–54.

Fan Q, Yan X, Wang J, Chen Y, Wang X, Li C, Tan L, You C, Zhang T, Zuo S, Xu D, Chen K, Finlayson Burden JM, and Xiao Z. (2012). Abnormalities of white matter microstructure in unmedicated obsessive-compulsive disorder and changes after medication. *PLoS One*, 7/4: doi: 10.1371/journal.pone.0035889

Felger JC and Lotrich FE. (2013). Inflammatory cytokines in depression: neurobiological mechanisms and therapeutic implications. *Neuroscience,* **246**: 199–229.

Fitzgerald PB, Laird AR, Maller J, and Daskalakis ZJ.(2008). A meta-analytic study of changes in brain activation in depression. *Hum Brain Mapp,* **29**: 683–95.

Franic S, Middeldorp CM, Dolan CV, Ligthart L, and Boomsma DI. (2010). Childhood and adolescent anxiety and depression: beyond heritability. *J Am Acad Child Adolesc Psychiatry,* **49/8**: 820–9.

Frick A, Ahs F, Engman J, Jonasson M, Alaie I, Bjorkstrand J, Frans O, Faria V, Linnman C, Appel L, Wahlstedt K, Lubberink M, Fredrikson M, and Frumark T. (2015). Serotonin synthesis and reuptake in social anxiety disorder: a positron emission tomography study. *JAMA Psychiatry,* **72/8**: 794–802.

Frodl T, Schaub A, Banac S, Charypar M, Jager M, Kummler P, Bottlender R, Zetzsche T, Born C, Leinsinger G, Reiser M, Moller HJ, and Meisenzahl EM. (2006). Reduced hippocampal volume correlates with executive dysfunctioning in major depression. *J Psychiatry Neurosci,* **31**: 316–23.

Frodl TS, Koutsouleris N, Bottlender R, Born C, Jager M, Scupin I, Reiser M, Moller HJ, and Meisenzahl EM. (2008). Depression-related variation in brain morphology over 3 years: effects of stress? *Arch Gen Psychiatry,* **65/10**: 1156–65.

Frokjaer VG, Mortensen EL, Nielsen FA, Haugbol S, Pinborg H, Adams KH, Svarer C, Hasselbalch SG, Holm S, Paulson OB, and Knudsen GM. (2008). Frontolimbic serotonin 2A receptor binding in healthy subjects is associated with personality risk factors for affective disorder. *Biol Psychiatry,* **63/6**: 569–76.

Gold PW, Goodwin FK, and Chrousos GP. (1988). Clinical and biochemical manifestations of depression. Relation to the neurobiology of stress (1). *New England Journal of Medicine,* **319/6**: 348–53.

Gold PW, Licinio J, Wong ML, and Chrousos GP. (1995). Corticotropin releasing hormone in the pathophysiology of melancholic and atypical depression and in the mechanism of action of antidepressant drugs. *Annals of the New York Academy of Sciences,* **771/1**: 716–29.

Gold PW. (2015). The organization of the stress system and its dysregulation in depressive illness. *Mol Psychiatry,* **20/1**: 32–47.

Goodkind M, Eickhoff SB, Oathes DJ, Jiang Y, Chang A, Jones Hagata LB, Ortega BN, Zaiko YV, Roach EL, Korgaonkar MS, Grieve SM, Galatzer Levy I, Fox PT, and Ekin A. (2015). Identification of a common neurobiological substrate for mental illness', *JAMA Psychiatry,* **72/4**: 305–15.

Graeff FG. (2004). Serotonin, the periaqueductal gray and panic. *Neurosci Biobehav Rev,* **28/3**: 239–59.

Greden JF, Gardner R, King D, Grushaus L, Carroll BJ, and Kronfol Z. (1983). Dexamethasone suppression tests in antidepressant treatment of melancholia. The process of normalization and test-retest reproducibility. *Archives of General Psychiatry,* **40/5**: 493–500.

Greicius MD, Flores BH, Menon V, Glover GH, Solvason HB, Kenna H, Reiss AL, and Schatzberg AF. (2007). Resting-state functional connectivity in major depression: abnormally increased contributions from subgenual cingulate cortex and thalamus. *Biol Psychiatry,* **62/5**: 429–37.

Grimm S, Boesiger P, Beck J, Schuepbach D, Bermpohl F, Walter M, Ernst J, Hell D, Boeker H, and Northoff G. (2009). Altered negative BOLD responses in the default-mode network during emotion processing in depressed subjects. *Neuropsychopharmacology: official publication of the American College of Neuropsychopharmacology,* **34/4**: 932–43.

Gurguis GN and Uhde TW. (1990). Plasma 3-methoxy-4-hydroxyphenylethylene glycol (MHPG) and growth hormone responses to yohimbine in panic disorder patients and normal controls. *Psychoneuroendocrinology,* 15/3: 217–24.

Haavik J, Blau N, and Thony B. (2008). Mutations in human monoamine-related neurotransmitter pathway genes. *Hum Mutat,* 29/7: 891–902.

Hajek T, Kopecek M, Kozeny J, Gunde E, Alda M, and Hoschl C. (2009). Amygdala volumes in mood disorders--meta-analysis of magnetic resonance volumetry studies. *J Affect Disord,* 115/3: 395–410.

Hänsel A and von Känel R. (2008). The ventro-medial prefrontal cortex: a major link between the autonomic nervous system, regulation of emotion, and stress reactivity? *Biopsychosoc Med,* 2/1: 21.

Hanson ND, Owens MJ, and Nemeroff CB. (2011). Depression, antidepressants, and neurogenesis: a critical reappraisal. *Neuropsychopharmacology,* 36/13: 2589–602.

Hardingham GE, Fukunaga Y, and Bading H. (2002). Extrasynaptic NMDARs oppose synaptic NMDARs by triggering CREB shut-off and cell death pathways. *Nat Neurosci,* 5/5: 405–14.

Hasler G, Nugent AC, Carlson PJ, Carson RE, Geraci M, and Drevets WC. (2008). Altered cerebral gamma-aminobutyric acid type A-benzodiazepine receptor binding in panic disorder determined by [11C]flumazenil positron emission tomography. *Arch Gen Psychiatry,* 65/10: 1166–75.

Hasler G, Van der Veen JW, Tumonis T, Meyers N, Shen J, and Drevets WC. (2007). Reduced prefrontal glutamate/glutamine and gamma-aminobutyric acid levels in major depression determined using proton magnetic resonance spectroscopy. *Arch Gen Psychiatry,* 64/2: 193–200.

Hassett AL, Radvanski DC, Vaschillo EG, Vaschillo B, Sigal LH, Karavida MK, Buyske S, and Lehrer PM. (2007). A pilot study of the efficacy of heart rate variability (HRV) biofeedback in patients with fibromyalgia. *Appl Psychophysiol Biofeedback,* 32/1: 1–10.

Haydon PG and Carmignoto G. (2006). Astrocyte control of synaptic transmission and neurovascular coupling. *Physiol Rev,* 86/3: 1009–31.

Hilbert K, Lueken U, and Beesdo Baum K. (2014). Neural structures, functioning and connectivity in Generalized Anxiety Disorder and interaction with neuroendocrine systems: a systematic review. *J Affect Disord,* 158: 114–26.

Hohoff C, Mullings EL, Heatherley SV, Freitag CM, Neumann LC, Domschke K, Krakowitzky P, Rothermundt M, Keck ME, Erhardt A, Unschuld PG, Jacob C, Fritze J, Bandelow B, Maier W, Holsboer F, Rogers PJ, and Deckert J. (2010). Adenosine A(2A) receptor gene: evidence for association of risk variants with panic disorder and anxious personality. *J Psychiatr Res,* 44/14: 930–7.

Holsboer F. (2000). The corticosteroid hypothesis of depression. *Neuropsychopharmacology,* 23/5: 477–501.

Hunsberger J, Austin DR, Henter ID, and Chen G. (2009). The neurotrophic and neuroprotective effects of psychotropic agents. *Dialogues Clin Neurosci,* 11/3: 333–48.

Hurlemann R. (2008). Noradrenergic-glucocorticoid mechanisms in emotion-induced amnesia: from adaptation to disease. *Psychopharmacology (Berl),* 197/1: 13–23.

Ionescu DF, Niciu MJ, Mathews DC, Richards EM, and Zarate CA. (2013). Neurobiology of anxious depression: a review. *Depress Anxiety,* 30/4: 374–85.

Ising M, Horstmann S, Kloiber S, Lucae S, Binder EB, Kern N, Kunzel HE, Pfennig A, Uhr M, and Holsboer F. (2007). Combined dexamethasone/corticotropin releasing hormone test predicts treatment response in major depression—a potential biomarker? *Biol Psychiatry*, 62/1: 47–54.

Jardim MC, Aguiar DC, Moreira FA, and Guimaraes FS. (2005). Role of glutamate ionotropic and benzodiazepine receptors in the ventromedial hypothalamic nucleus on anxiety. *Pharmacol Biochem Behav*, 82/1: 182–9.

Johnson MK, Nolen Hoeksema S, Mitchell KJ, and Levin Y. (2009). Medial cortex activity, self-reflection and depression. *Social cognitive and affective neuroscience*, 4: 313–27.

Kalueff AV and Nutt DJ. (2007). Role of GABA in anxiety and depression. *Depress Anxiety*, 24/7: 495–517.

Karege F, Perret G, Bondolfi G, Schwald M, Bertschy G, and Aubry J. (2002). Decreased serum brain-derived neurotrophic factor levels in major depressed patients. *Psychiatry Res*, 109/2: 143–8.

Kendler KS, Gardner CO, and Lichtenstein P. (2008). A developmental twin study of symptoms of anxiety and depression: evidence for genetic innovation and attenuation. *Psychol Med*, 38/11: 1567–75.

Kendler KS, Kuhn JW, Vittum J, Prescott CA, and Riley B. (2005). The interaction of stressful life events and a serotonin transporter polymorphism in the prediction of episodes of major depression: a replication. *Arch Gen Psychiatry*, 62/5: 529–535.

Kent JM, Mathew SJ, and Gorman JM. (2002). Molecular targets in the treatment of anxiety. *Biol Psychiatry*, 52/10: 1008–30.

Kent JM and Rauch SL. (2003). Neurocircuitry of anxiety disorders. *Curr Psychiatry Rep*, 5/4: 266–73.

Klerman GL, Weissman MM, Ouellette R, Johnson J, and Greenwald S. (1991). Panic attacks in the community. Social morbidity and health care utilization. *JAMA*, 265/6: 742–6.

Konishi Y, Tanii H, Otowa T, Sasaki T, Kaiya H, Okada M, and Okazaki Y. (2014). The association of BDNF Val66Met polymorphism with trait anxiety in panic disorder. *J Neuropsychiatry Clin Neurosci*, 26/4: 344–51.

Kop WJ, Gottdiener JS, Tangen CM, Fried LP, McBurnie MA, Walston J, Newman A, Hirsch C, and Tracy RP. (2002). Inflammation and coagulation factors in persons > 65 years of age with symptoms of depression but without evidence of myocardial ischemia. *American Journal of Cardiology*, 89/4: 419–24.

Korte SM, Prins J, Krajnc AM, Hendriksen H, Oosting RS, Westphal KG, Korte Bouws GA, and Olivier B. (2015). The many different faces of major depression: it is time for personalized medicine. *Eur J Pharmacol*, 753: 88–104.

Krystal JH, Sanacora G, Blumberg H, Anand A, Charney DS, Marek G, Epperson CN, Goddard A, and Mason GF. (2002). Glutamate and GABA systems as targets for novel antidepressant and mood-stabilizing treatments. *Mol Psychiatry*, 7 Suppl 1: S71–80.

Kugaya A and Sanacora G. (2005). Beyond monoamines: glutamatergic function in mood disorders. *CNS Spectr*, 10/10: 808–19.

Lambert G, Johansson M, Agren H, and Friberg P. (2000). Reduced brain norepinephrine and dopamine release in treatment-refractory depressive illness: evidence in support of the catecholamine hypothesis of mood disorders. *Arch Gen Psychiatry*, 57/8: 787–93.

Lavretsky H, Siddarth P, Kumar A, and Reynolds CF, III. (2008). The effects of the dopamine and serotonin transporter polymorphisms on clinical features and treatment response in geriatric depression: a pilot study. *Int J Geriatr Psychiatry*, 23/1: 55–9.

Lee BT, Seong Whi C, Hyung Soo K, Lee BC, Choi IG, Lyoo IK, and Ham BJ. (2007). The neural substrates of affective processing toward positive and negative affective pictures in patients with major depressive disorder. *Prog Neuropsychopharmacol Biol Psychiatry,* 31/7: 1487–92.

Lee JJ, Hahm ET, Lee CH, and Cho YW. (2008). Serotonergic modulation of GABAergic and glutamatergic synaptic transmission in mechanically isolated rat medial preoptic area neurons. *Neuropsychopharmacology,* 33/2: 340–52.

Lee M, Schwab C, and McGeer PL. (2011). Astrocytes are GABAergic cells that modulate microglial activity. *Glia,* 59/1: 152–65.

Leibenluft E and Pine DS. (2013). Resting state functional connectivity and depression: in search of a bottom line. *Biol Psychiatry,* 74/12: 868–9.

Lemogne C, Gorwood P, Bergouignan L, Pelissolo A, Lehericy S, and Fossati P. (2011). Negative affectivity, self-referential processing and the cortical midline structures. *Social cognitive and affective neuroscience,* 6/4: 426–33.

Lindqvist D, Janelidze S, Hagell P, Erhardt S, Samuelsson M, Minthon L, Hansson O, Bjorkqvist M, Traskman Bendz L, and Brundin L. (2009). Interleukin-6 is elevated in the cerebrospinal fluid of suicide attempters and related to symptom severity. *Biol Psychiatry,* 66/3: 287–92.

Liukkonen T, Rasanen P, Jokelainen J, Leinonen M, Jarvelin MR, Meyer Rochow VB, and Timonen M. (2011). The association between anxiety and C-reactive protein (CRP) levels: results from the Northern Finland 1966 birth cohort study. *Eur Psychiatry,* 26/6: 363–9.

Lorenzetti V, Allen NB, Fornito A, and Yucel M. (2009). Structural brain abnormalities in major depressive disorder: a selective review of recent MRI studies. *J Affect Disord,* 117/1–2: 1–17.

Major Depressive Disorder Working Group of the Psychiatric GWAS Consortium. (2012). A mega-analysis of genome-wide association studies for major depressive disorder. *Mol Psychiatry* 18/4: 497–511.

Maletic V and Raison C. (2014). Integrated neurobiology of bipolar disorder. *Front Psychiatry,* 5/98: doi: 10.3389/fpsyt.2014.00098

Maletic V and Raison CL. (2009). Neurobiology of depression, fibromyalgia and neuropathic pain. *Front Biosci,* 14: 5291–338.

Manji HK and Duman RS. (2001). Impairments of neuroplasticity and cellular resilience in severe mood disorders: implications for the development of novel therapeutics. *Psychopharmacol Bull,* 35/2: 5–49.

Manji HK, Drevets WC, and Charney DS. (2001). The cellular neurobiology of depression. *Nat Med,* 7: 541–7.

Martin EI, Ressler KJ, Binder E, and Nemeroff CB. (2009). The neurobiology of anxiety disorders: brain imaging, genetics, and psychoneuroendocrinology. *Psychiatr Clin North Am,* 32/3: 549–75.

Martinez JM, Garakani A, Yehuda R, and Gorman JM. (2012). Proinflammatory and 'resiliency' proteins in the CSF of patients with major depression. *Depress Anxiety,* 29/1: 32–8.

Mayberg HS. (2003). Modulating dysfunctional limbic-cortical circuits in depression: towards development of brain-based algorithms for diagnosis and optimised treatment. *Br Med Bull,* 65: 193–207.

Mayberg HS, Liotti M, Brannan SK, McGinnis S, Mahurin RK, Jerabek PA, Silva JA, Tekell JL, Martin CC, Lancaster JL, and Fox PT. (1999). Reciprocal limbic-cortical function and negative mood: converging PET findings in depression and normal sadness. *Am J Psychiatry,* 156/5: 675–82.

Menon V. (2011). Large-scale brain networks and psychopathology: a unifying triple network model. *Trends Cogn Sci,* **15**/10: 483–506.

Meyer JH, Goulding VA, Wilson AA, Hussey D, Christensen BK, and Houle S. (2002). Bupropion occupancy of the dopamine transporter is low during clinical treatment. *Psychopharmacology (Berl),* **163**/1: 102–5.

Meyer JH. (2007). Imaging the serotonin transporter during major depressive disorder and antidepressant treatment. *J Psychiatry Neurosci,* **32**/2: 86–102.

Miller AH, Maletic V, and Raison CL. (2009). Inflammation and its discontents: the role of cytokines in the pathophysiology of major depression. *Biol Psychiatry,* **65**/9: 732–41.

Miller AH and Raison CL. (2015). The role of inflammation in depression: from evolutionary imperative to modern treatment target. *Nat Rev Immunol,* **16**/1: 22–34.

Molendijk ML, Bus BA, Spinhoven P, Penninx BW, Kenis G, Prickaerts J, Voshaar RC, and Elzinga BM. (2011). Serum levels of brain-derived neurotrophic factor in major depressive disorder: state-trait issues, clinical features and pharmacological treatment. *Mol Psychiatry,* **16**/11: 1088–95.

Mossner R, Mikova O, Koutsilieri E, Saoud M, Ehlis AC, Muller N, Fallgatter AJ, and Rieederer P. (2007). Consensus paper of the WFSBP Task Force on Biological Markers: biological markers in depression. *World Journal of Biological Psychiatry,* **8**/3: 141–74.

Nemeroff CB. (1996). The corticotropin-releasing factor (CRF) hypothesis of depression: new findings and new directions. *Molecular Psychiatry,* **1**/4: 336–42.

Nemeroff CB, Owens MJ, Bissette G, Andorn AC, and Stanley M. (1988). Reduced corticotropin releasing factor binding sites in the frontal cortex of suicide victims. *Archives of General Psychiatry,* **45**/6: 577–9.

Neumeister A, Bain E, Nugent AC, Carson RE, Bonne O, Luckenbaugh DA, Eckelman W, Herscovitch P, Charney DS, and Drevets WC. (2004). Reduced serotonin type 1A receptor binding in panic disorder. *J Neurosci,* **24**/3: 589–91.

Oathes DJ, Patenaude B, Schatzberg AF, and Etkin A. (2015). Neurobiological signatures of anxiety and depression in resting-state functional magnetic resonance imaging. *Biol Psychiatry,* **77**: 385–93.

O'Brien SM, Scully P, Fitzgerald P, Scott LV, and Dinan TG. (2007). Plasma cytokine profiles in depressed patients who fail to respond to selective serotonin reuptake inhibitor therapy. *J Psychiatr Res,* **41**/3–4: 326–31.

O'Donovan A, Hughes BM, Slavich GM, Lynch L, Cronin MT, O'Farrelly C, and Malone KM. (2010). Clinical anxiety, cortisol and interleukin-6: evidence for specificity in emotion-biology relationships. *Brain Behav Immun,* **24**/7: 1074–7.

O'Keane V, Frodl T, and Dinan TG. (2012). A review of atypical depression in relation to the course of depression and changes in HPA axis organization. *Psychoneuroendocrinology,* **37**/10: 1589–99.

Okamoto T, Yoshimura R, Ikenouchi Sugita A, Hori H, Umene Nakano W, Inoue Y, Ueda N, and Nakamura J. (2008). Efficacy of electroconvulsive therapy is associated with changing blood levels of homovanillic acid and brain-derived neurotrophic factor (BDNF) in refractory depressed patients: a pilot study. *Prog Neuropsychopharmacol Biol Psychiatry,* **32**/5: 1185–90.

Olbrich S, Trankner A, Surova G, Gevirtz R, Gordon E, Hegerl U, and Arna M. (2016). CNS- and ANS-arousal predict response to antidepressant medication: Findings from the randomized iSPOT-D study. *J Psychiatr Res,* **73**: 108–15.

Owens MJ and Nemeroff CB. (1991). Physiology and pharmacology of corticotropin-releasing factor. *Pharmacological Reviews*, 43/4: 425–73.

Pariante CM and Miller AH. (2001). Glucocorticoid receptors in major depression: relevance to pathophysiology and treatment. *Biological Psychiatry*, 49/5: 391–404.

Pezawas L, Meyer Lindenberg A, Drabant EM, Verchinski BA, Munoz EK, Kolachana BS, Egan MF, Mattay VS, Hariri AR, and Weinberger DR. (2005). 5-HTTLPR polymorphism impacts human cingulate-amygdala interactions: a genetic susceptibility mechanism for depression. *Nat Neurosci*, 8/6: 828–34.

Pezawas L, Verchinski BA, Mattay VS, Callicott JH, Kolachana BS, Straub RE, Egan MF, Meyer Lindenberg A, and Weinberger DR. (2004). The brain-derived neurotrophic factor val66met polymorphism and variation in human cortical morphology. *J Neurosci*, 24/45: 10099–102.

Pizzagalli DA. (2011). Frontocingulate dysfunction in depression: toward biomarkers of treatment response. *Neuropsychopharmacology*, 36/1: 183–206.

Portella MJ, de Deigo-Adeliño J, Gomez-Ansón B, Morgan-Ferrando R, Vives Y, Puigdemont D, Pérez-Egea R, Ruscalleda J, Enric Á, and Pérez V. (2011). Ventromedial prefrontal spectroscopic abnormalities over the course of depression: a comparison among first episode, remitted recurrent and chronic patients. *J Psychiatr Res*, 45/4: 427–34.

Raison CL and Miller AH. (2003). When not enough is too much: the role of insufficient glucocorticoid signaling in the pathophysiology of stress-related disorders. *Am J Psychiatry*, 160/9: 1554–65.

Raison CL, Rutherford RE, Woolwine BJ, Shuo C, Schettler P, Drake DF, Haroon E, and Miller AH. (2013). A randomized controlled trial of the tumor necrosis factor antagonist infliximab for treatment-resistant depression: the role of baseline inflammatory biomarkers. *JAMA Psychiatry*, 70/1: 31–41.

Rajkowska G, O'Dwyer G, Teleki Z, Stockmeier CA, and Miguel Hildago, JJ. (2007). GABAergic neurons immunoreactive for calcium binding proteins are reduced in the prefrontal cortex in major depression. *Neuropsychopharmacology*, 32/2: 471–82.

Ray RD and Zald, DH. (2012). Anatomical insights into the interaction of emotion and cognition in the prefrontal cortex. *Neurosci Biobehav Rev*, 36/1: 479–501.

Rubin RT, Poland RE, Lesser IM, Winston RA, and Blodgett AL. (1987). Neuroendocrine aspects of primary endogenous depression. I. Cortisol secretory dynamics in patients and matched controls. *Archives of General Psychiatry*, 44/4: 328–36.

Rush AJ, Trivedi MH, Wisniewski SR, Nierenberg AA, Stewart JW, Warden D, Niederehe G, Thase ME, Lavori PW, Lebowitz BD, McGrath PJ, Rosenbaum JF, Sackeim HA, Kupfer DJ, Luther J, and Fava M. (2006). Acute and longer-term outcomes in depressed outpatients requiring one or several treatment steps: a STAR*D report. *Am J Psychiatry*, 163/11: 1905–17.

Russo-Neustadt AA and Chen MJ. (2005). Brain-derived neurotrophic factor and antidepressant activity. *Curr Pharm Des*, 11/12: 1495–510.

Sanacora G, Gueorguieva R, Epperson CN, Wu YT, Appel M, Rothman DL, Krystal JH, and Mason GF. (2004). Subtype-specific alterations of gamma-aminobutyric acid and glutamate in patients with major depression. *Arch Gen Psychiatry*, 61/7: 705–13.

Schildkraut JJ. (1965). The catecholamine hypothesis of affective disorders: a review of supporting evidence. *Am J Psychiatry*, 122/5: 509–22.

Schosser A, Butler AW, Uher R, Ng MY, Cohen-Woods S, Craddock N, Owen MJ, Korszun A, Gill M, Rice J, Hauser J, Henigsberg N, maier W, Mors O, Placentino A, Rietschel M,

Souery D, Preisig M, Craig IW, Farmer AE, Lewis CM, and McGuffin P. (2013). Genome-wide association study of co-occurring anxiety in major depression. *World J Biol Psychiatry*, 14/8: 611–21.

Sen S, Duman R, and Sanacora G. (2008). Serum brain-derived neurotrophic factor, depression, and antidepressant medications: meta-analyses and implications. *Biol Psychiatry*, 64/6: 527–32.

Sequeira A, Mamdani F, Ernst C, Vawter MP, Bunney WE, Lebel V, Rehal S, Klempan T, Gratton A, Benkelfat C, Rouleau GA, Mechawar N, and Turecki G. (2009). Global brain gene expression analysis links glutamatergic and GABAergic alterations to suicide and major depression. *PLoS ONE*, 4: doi:10.1371/journal.pone.0006585

Sheline Y. (2000). 3D MRI studies of neuroanatomic changes in unipolar major depression: The role of stress amd medical comorbidity. *Biol Psychiatry*, 48/8: 791–800.

Sheline, YI, Barch DM, Donnelly JM, Ollinger JM, Snyder AZ, and Mintun MA. (2001). Increased amygdala response to masked emotional faces in depressed subjects resolves with antidepressant treatment: an fMRI study. *Biol Psychiatry*, 50/9: 651–8.

Sheline YI, Price JL, Vaishnavi SN, Mintun MA, Barch DM, Epstein AA, Wilkins CH, Snyder AZ, Couture L, Schechtman K, and McKinstry RC. (2008). Regional white matter hyperintensity burden in automated segmentation distinguishes late-life depressed subjects from comparison subjects matched for vascular risk factors. *Am J Psychiatry*, 165/5: 524–32.

Sheline YI, Price JL, Yan Z, and Mintun MA. (2010). Resting-state functional MRI in depression unmasks increased connectivity between networks via the dorsal nexus. *Proceedings of the National Academy of Sciences of the United States of America*, 107/24: 11020–5.

Shimada-Sugimoto M, Otowa T, and Hettema JM. (2015). Genetics of anxiety disorders: Genetic epidemiological and molecular studies in humans. *Psychiatry Clin Neurosci*, 69/7: 388–401.

Sprengelmeyer R, Steele JD, Mwangi B, Kumar P, Christmas D, Milders M, and Matthews K. (2011). The insular cortex and the neuroanatomy of major depression. *J Affect Disord*, 133/1–2: 120–7.

Steckler T and Holsboer F. (1999). Corticotropin-releasing hormone receptor subtypes and emotion. *Biol Psychiatry*, 46/11: 1480–508.

Steele JD, Currie J, Lawrie SM, and Reid I. (2007). Prefrontal cortical functional abnormality in major depressive disorder: a stereotactic meta-analysis. *J Affect Disord*, 101/1–3: 1–11.

Steiner J, Bielau H, Brisch R, Danos P, Ullrich O, Mawrin C, Bernstein HG, and Bogerts B. (2008). Immunological aspects in the neurobiology of suicide: elevated microglial density in schizophrenia and depression is associated with suicide. *J Psychiatr Res*, 42/2: 151–7.

Stockmeier CA, Mahajan GJ, Konick LC, Overholser JC, Jurjus GJ, Meltzer HY, Uylings HB, Friedman L, and Rajkowska G. (2004). Cellular changes in the postmortem hippocampus in major depression. *Biol Psychiatry*, 56/9: 640–50.

Stone EA, Lin Y, and Quartermain D. (2008). A final common pathway for depression? Progress toward a general conceptual framework. *Neurosci Biobehav Rev*, 32/3: 508–24.

Sullivan GM, Coplan JD, Kent JM, and Gorman JM. (1999). The noradrenergic system in pathological anxiety: a focus on panic with relevance to generalized anxiety and phobias. *Biol Psychiatry*, 46/9: 1205–18.

Sullivan PF, Neale MC, and Kendler KS. (2000). Genetic epidemiology of major depression: review and meta-analysis. *Am J Psychiatry*, 157/10: 1552–62.

Sumner JA, Powers A, Jovanovic T, and Koenen KC. (2016). Genetic influences on the neural and physiological bases of acute threat: A research domain criteria (RDoC) perspective. *Am J Med Genet B Neuropsychiatr Genet*, 171B/1: 44–64.

Takahashi T, Yucel M, Lorenzetti V, Tanino R, Whittle S, Suzuki M, Walterfang M, Pantelis C, and Allen NB. (2010). Volumetric MRI study of the insular cortex in individuals with current and past major depression. *J Affect Disord*, 121/3: 231–8.

Tao R and Auerbach SB. (2000). Regulation of serotonin release by GABA and excitatory amino acids. *J Psychopharmacol*, 14/2: 100–13.

Tham MW, Woon PS, Sum MY, Lee TS, and Sim K. (2011). White matter abnormalities in major depression: evidence from post-mortem, neuroimaging and genetic studies. *J Affect Disord*, 132/1–2: 26–36.

Thase ME. (2000). Mood Disorders: Neurobiology. *In:* BJ Sadock and VA Sadock, eds, *Kaplan & Sadock's Comprehensive Textbook of Psychiatry*. Philadelphia: Lippincott Williams & Wilkins.

Trivedi MH, Hollander E, Nutt D, and Blier P. (2008). Clinical evidence and potential neurobiological underpinnings of unresolved symptoms of depression. *J Clin Psychiatry*, 69/2: 246–58.

Tunca Z, Kivircik Akdede B, Özerdem A, Alkin T, Polat S, Ceylan D, Bayin M, Cengizçetin Kocuk N, Şimşek S, Resmi H, and Akan P. (2015). Diverse glial cell line-derived neurotrophic factor (GDNF) support between mania and schizophrenia: a comparative study in four major psychiatric disorders. *Eur Psychiatry*, 30/2: 198–204.

Uher T, Ransey KE, Dew T, Maier W, Mors O, Hauser J, Dernovsek MZ, Henigsberg N, Souery D, Farmer A, and McGuffin P. (2014). An inflammatory biomarker as a differential predictor of outcome of depression treatment with escitalopram and nortriptyline. *Am J Psychiatry*, 171/12: 1278–86.

Urry HL, Van Reekum CM, Johnstone T, Kalin NH, Thurow ME, Schcaefer JS, Jackson CA, Frye CJ, Greischar LL, Alexander AL, and Davidson RJ. (2006). Amygdala and ventromedial prefrontal cortex are inversely coupled during regulation of negative affect and predict the diurnal pattern of cortisol secretion among older adults. *J Neurosci*, 26/16: 4415–25.

Van Kralingen C, Kho DT, Costa J, Angel CE, and Graham ES. (2013). Exposure to inflammatory cytokines IL-1beta and TNFalpha induces compromise and death of astrocytes; implications for chronic neuroinflammation. *PLoS One*, 8/12: doi:10.1371/journal.pone.0084269

Vasic N, Walter H, Hose A, and Wolf RC. (2008). Gray matter reduction associated with psychopathology and cognitive dysfunction in unipolar depression: a voxel-based morphometry study. *J Affect Disord*, 109/1–2: 107–16.

Veit R, Flor H, Erb M, Hermann C, Lotze, M, Grodd W, and Birbaumer N,. (2002). Brain circuits involved in emotional learning in antisocial behavior and social phobia in humans. *Neurosci Lett*, 328/3: 233–6.

Vythilingam M, Vermetten E, Anderson GM, Luckenbaugh D, Anderson ER, Snow J, Staib LH, Charney DS, and Bremner JD. (2004). Hippocampal volume, memory, and cortisol status in major depressive disorder: effects of treatment. *Biol Psychiatry*, 56/2: 101–12.

Wacker J, Dillon DG, and Pizzagalli DA. (2009). The role of the nucleus accumbens and rostral anterior cingulate cortex in anhedonia: integration of resting EEG, fMRI, and volumetric techniques. *Neuroimage*, 46/1: 327–37.

Wang Y, Mathews CA, Li Y, Lin Z, and Xiao Z. (2011). Brain-derived neurotrophic factor (BDNF) plasma levels in drug-naive OCD patients are lower than those in healthy people, but are not lower than those in drug-treated OCD patients. *J Affect Disord*, 133/1–2: 305–10.

Wang Y, Zhang H, Li Y, Wang Z, Fan Q, Yu S, Lin Z, and Xiao Z. (2015). BDNF Val66Met polymorphism and plasma levels in Chinese Han population with obsessive-compulsive disorder and generalized anxiety disorder. *J Affect Disord*, 186: 7–12.

Wong ML, Dong C, Maestre-Mesa J, and Licinio J. (2008). Polymorphisms in inflammation-related genes are associated with susceptibility to major depression and antidepressant response. *Mol Psychiatry*, 13/8: 800–12.

Xu Y, Li F, Huang X, Sun N, Zhang F, Liu P, Yang H, Luo J, Sun Y, and Zhang K. (2009). The norepinephrine transporter gene modulates the relationship between urban/rural residency and major depressive disorder in a Chinese population. *Psychiatry Res*, 168/3: 213–7.

Zarate CA, Jr, Singh JB, Carlson PH, Brutsche NE, Ameli R, Luckenbaugh DA, Charney DS, and Manji HK. (2006). A randomized trial of an N-methyl-D-aspartate antagonist in treatment-resistant major depression. *Arch Gen Psychiatry*, 63/8: 856–64.

Zhang X, Zhang Z, Xie C, Xi G, Zhou H, Zhang Y, and Sha W. (2008). Effect of treatment on serum glial cell line-derived neurotrophic factor in depressed patients. *Prog Neuropsychopharmacol Biol Psychiatry*, 32/3: 886–90.

Zhou Y, Yu C, Zheng H, Liu Y, Song M, Qin W, Li K, and Jiang T. (2010). Increased neural resources recruitment in the intrinsic organization in major depression. *Journal of affective disorders*, 121: 220–30.

Chapter 6

The DSM-5: What should general practitioners know?

Joel Paris

Introduction to the DSM-5

Medicine has always required diagnostic procedures to classify the diseases that physicians treat. The World Health Organization (1993) publishes an International Classification of Diseases (ICD), standard throughout the world, with a new edition (ICD-11) planned for 2017. In psychiatry, the Diagnostic and Statistical Manual of Mental Disorders (DSM), published by the American Psychiatric Association (APA), whose diagnoses can be translated into ICD coding, has had great influence on research and practice.

The DSM manuals, originally developed for statistical purposes, have been popular as guides to diagnosis ever since the third edition (American Psychiatric Association, 1980). DSM has also changed the way physicians think about mental disorders. This is because diagnoses can be made by relatively simple algorithms of observable symptoms, as opposed to the complex prototypes used in the past (which are still used in the ICD system). An algorithmic structure was intended to make DSM-based diagnoses more reliable, at least in principle (Decker, 2013). However, field trials have found troublingly low reliability for even the most common diagnoses, such as major depression (Regier et al, 2013). These problems may reflect the heterogeneity of diagnostic categories, as well as an unclear boundary with normal psychological variations.

The fifth edition (DSM-5; American Psychiatric Association, 2013) retains much the same format as previous versions. Initially, DSM-5 was intended be a major revision based less on clinical signs and symptoms, and instead could be based on dimensions of psychopathology and scored on standard scales that are thought to be more readily linked to neuroscience (Kupfer and Regier, 2011).

However, many of the proposed changes in DSM-5 proved controversial, and were, in the end, not adopted. One reason was that some proposed categories might lead to over-diagnosis in patients who do not need to be treated. Another issue was that proposed changes from categorical to dimensional diagnosis had never been systematically tested for reliability and validity. Therefore, it would have been unwise to introduce such measures in the absence of solid research.

In the end, the feeling among most experts was that any radical revisions would require very strong evidence. Thus, the final DSM-5 was less different from previous editions than most clinicians expected. This chapter reviews the changes that were eventually made, as well as their rationale.

The system of algorithmic diagnosis introduced on DSM-III assumed that if categories could be made more reliable, they would become more valid. Proof of validity would then allow diagnoses to become guides to a etiology and treatment, as is the case in other medical specialties. However, research exploring whether DSM categories have specific causes, or whether they predict treatment responses, has been disappointing. We are a long way from developing a system of categorization that is based on an understanding of the mechanisms behind disease. This is inevitable, given the enormous complexity of the human brain. Thus, in spite of progress in basic neuroscience research, little more is known about the causes of major mental disorder than was the case 30 years ago (Hyman, 2007; 2010).

Moreover, DSM categories have a worrying tendency to be heterogeneous and to overlap with each other (Paris, 2015a). This is probably because definitions are based almost entirely on patient self-report and clinical observation. The history of medicine suggests that progress in diagnosis has often been the result of a deeper understanding of mechanisms driven by endophenotypes (Gottesman, 2003). Yet until now, research in psychiatry has not been able to identify the underlying mechanisms behind phenotypes clinicians can recognize.

It is unlikely that this situation will change in the foreseeable future. We are only at the beginning of neuroscience research. The Human Genome Project was a scientific success, but has been of little help to psychiatry, in which the most important disorders have no coherent pattern of genetic association. Similarly, while neuroimaging is a promising method for the future, it has thus far revealed little about the causes of major mental disorders (Hyman, 2010).

Furthermore, research at the level of neuronal activity and neurochemistry is unlikely to fully explain complex psychological mechanisms that are best studied at a mental level (Gold, 2009). For example, claims that genetics will be the basis for 'precision medicine', an approach currently being explored for diseases like cancer, is not feasible in mental disorders, which are associated with a large number of small changes in the genome, each of which only has a small effect (Jablensky, 2015).

Finally, the idea that mental disorders are associated with 'chemical imbalances', and that can be effectively treated through pharmacological interventions has only been partially successful (Paris, 2010). We do not know whether such imbalances exist, and we are also not quite sure how those drugs that are effective actually work in the brain. It may take many decades before there is sufficient progress in basic research for neuroscience to become clinically relevant. Similarly, the idea that psychopathology is better described by dimensional scores of symptom intensity than by illness categories is of uncertain validity.

Although plans to radically change diagnosis in DSM-5 proved abortive, the National Institute of Mental Health developed its own system of classification, the Research Domain Criteria (RDoC), intended to guide future research (Insel et al, 2014). Yet, at this point the RDoC system is almost entirely theoretical, has not been developed in any detail, and has little clinical relevance (Lilienfeld, 2014).

Another problem for the DSM system lies in how mental disorders can be separated from normality (Frances, 2013). There are hundreds of diagnoses in the manual, some of which could be variants of normal behaviour. In fact, the use of the term 'disorder' (rather than 'disease' or 'illness') implicitly acknowledges that categories listed in the manual do not have the same status as medical conditions like hepatitis or multiple sclerosis.

In spite of all these difficulties, the DSM system has real advantages. It is familiar to most providers, and is reasonably user-friendly. As an accepted standard, it allows clinicians to communicate more easily about cases. Moreover, we are not likely to find out the causes of the disorders we treat for decades to come. That is why DSM will probably continue to be the common language of psychiatry for some time to come.

A quick look at changes in DSM-5

Details of all these changes can be found either in the manual itself, or in a companion volume (Black, 2014).

Psychoses

Schizophrenia is placed in a chapter of the manual that also includes brief psychoses and delusional disorder. There are no major changes in the overall algorithm for diagnosis of schizophrenia, which requires abnormalities in one or more of the following domains: delusions, hallucinations, disorganized thinking (and/or speech), disorganized or abnormal motor behaviour, and negative symptoms. However, the classical subtypes (e.g. paranoid schizophrenia) have been dropped due to lack of evidential support.

A proposal to include 'risk psychosis', i.e. a sub-clinical form that appears early in development, was not accepted, mainly because most of these patients never develop schizophrenia. It would be unwise to treat this group with antipsychotic drugs that have such a wide range of side effects.

Bipolar disorder

Bipolar disorders require the presence of a manic episode (in Bipolar-I) or a hypomanic episode (in bipolar-II). They are now placed in a separate chapter from depression, with no major changes in their diagnostic algorithms.

Family practitioners should be aware that there is a controversy as to whether these disorders, particularly bipolar-II, are being over-diagnosed (Paris, 2015b). The reason is that unstable mood is found in many other conditions, particularly borderline personality disorder. Enthusiasm for bipolar diagnoses may be based on the effectiveness of mood stabilizers in classical cases, but these drugs are not very useful in patients who fall within a broader spectrum (what DSM-5 calls 'bipolar disorder, unspecified').

DSM-5 discourages the diagnosis of bipolar disorder in pre-pubertal children. The concept of bipolarity in childhood (as opposed to its well-known presentation in adolescence) was a new diagnostic practice based on a symptomatic resemblance. These cases, characterized by mood instability and impulsivity, are considered by DSM-5 to fit better into a new category of disruptive mood dysregulation disorder (DMDD). This diagnosis describes children with behaviour disorders that are unusually difficult to manage, and was introduced to discourage clinicians from treating them with antipsychotic drugs.

Depressive disorders

The only changes in the definition of major depressive disorder in DSM-5 is the removal of an exclusion for depression following bereavement, on the grounds that extended and severe periods of low mood after a loss should not automatically be considered normal. This decision has been controversial (Kleinman, 2012), and practitioners are advised to be cautious in separating grief from depression.

However, it is not clear why grief was ever regarded as an exception to the diagnostic rules. Most depressed patients have good reasons to feel low, but the use of a 'major' diagnosis implies that their response to life stressors is excessive.

Persistent depressive disorder is a new label, replacing 'dysthymia', i.e. chronic, low-grade depression. Pre-menstrual dysphoric disorder (PMDD), formerly in a section of disorders requiring further study, has now been accepted for full status as a diagnosis in DSM-5.

Anxiety disorders

There are no changes in the definitions of panic disorder, generalized anxiety disorder, or social phobia. Separation anxiety disorder is listed separately, and is usually applied to children who refuse to go to school. Some diagnoses (obsessive-compulsive disorder, post-traumatic stress disorder) that were formally grouped with these classical presentations now have their own chapters.

Obsessive-compulsive disorder

The diagnosis of obsessive-compulsive disorder (OCD) has the same criteria as in past editions, but, in view of its severe psychopathology, is no longer viewed as an anxiety disorder. This new chapter also includes a 'spectrum' of related conditions, including body dysmorphic disorder, hoarding disorder, and trichotillomania.

Trauma and stressor-related disorders

This group of symptomatic reactions to stressful events includes post-traumatic stress disorder (PTSD), acute stress disorder, and adjustment disorder. The criteria for PTSD have often been questioned on the grounds of being too broad, but in DSM-5, the diagnosis has been further expanded to include witnessing or learning about traumatic events. Nonetheless, clinicians should be aware that PTSD should not be diagnosed just because symptoms occur after traumatic events. The criteria continue to require certain characteristic clinical features such as intrusive memories and avoidance.

Substance use

The main change in this chapter of DSM-5 is the elimination of the traditional distinction between drug abuse and addiction. The rationale is that these phenomena are not separate, but lie on a continuum of severity. However, some have expressed concern that the term 'addiction' now has a much wider definition (Frances, 2013), losing distinctions between physical and psychological dependence.

Eating disorders

The only change in the definition of anorexia nervosa is the elimination of amenorrhea as a requirement. Bulimia nervosa retains the same criteria as in previous editions. However, a new category of binge eating disorder (which must occur at least once a week) has been added. This decision has been criticized for describing phenomena that are common and close to normal (Frances, 2013).

Sexual disorders

As in previous editions, various types of sexual dysfunctions are described. More controversial categories such as gender dysphoria are in a separate chapter, but with the same criteria. Paraphilic disorders also have their own chapter, with no changes to the diagnostic criteria.

Somatic symptom disorders

This term replaces a number of older terms ('psychosomatic', 'conversion', 'somatization', 'hypochondriasis') that have been used to describe patients who present with somatic symptoms of various kinds. Diagnosis requires a prominence of these symptoms, associated with significant distress and impairment.

Neurocognitive disorders

This term replaces older concepts ('dementia' and 'delirium'). Disorders can be subclassified by severity and by aetiology (if known). Notably, DSM-5 eliminates almost all diagnoses attached to the physicians who first identified them; for this reason, the well-known term 'Alzheimer' is not to be found in the manual.

Neurodevelopmental disorders

This grouping includes intellectual deficiency (formerly 'mental retardation'), as well as a range of other learning disabilities. Psychological testing is recommended to add a quantitative aspect to their assessment.

This chapter also includes attention-deficit hyperactivity disorder (ADHD), a category whose diagnosis has increased markedly. The popularity of ADHD is largely due to the effectiveness of stimulants. However, there are many causes for decreased attention, so ADHD may be overdiagnosed, particularly in adults (Paris, 2015b). While all adult cases must be shown to begin in childhood, DSM-5 expands the criteria somewhat by allowing its age of onset to be prior to puberty (as opposed to age 7 in previous editions). This somewhat expands the range of the diagnosis in adults.

This group also includes autism spectrum disorders. The term 'Asperger's syndrome' has been removed, as DSM-5 prefers both to avoid names, and to define spectra that vary in severity.

Disruptive, impulsive, and conduct disorders

This group includes the common diagnoses of conduct disorder and oppositional defiant disorder. While these diagnoses are first made in children, DSM-5 avoids having a separate section on childhood disorders, largely because these conditions tend to be continuous with adult diagnoses, including anxiety, mood, and personality disorders.

Personality disorders

This chapter attracted attention because it was slated to be radically revised. In addition to an overall definition of personality disorder, there have been a traditional group of ten categories (plus a common form of disorder that fits none but can be called 'unspecified'). The idea was to replace these categories with scores based on ratings of personality traits, and to retain only six of the ten, in which case diagnosis would also be based on trait dimensions. This would have allowed for some classical categories (antisocial, borderline) to find a place in the manual. The broader intention of the DSM-5 editors was to use personality disorder as a 'poster child' for dimensional diagnosis, in which all psychopathology would be based on dimensional scores.

However, many personality disorder researchers opposed this change, partly because it was complex for clinicians to use, and partly because only a limited amount of research existed to support it (Paris, 2015c). But late in the process of developing the manual, an external review concluded that the new system was too radical a change. As a result, all ten DSM-IV categories were retained, and the proposal for a new system has been placed in Section III of the manual (reserved for diagnoses that require further study). It remains to be seen whether some form of this 'alternative model' will be used to diagnose personality disorders in future editions.

It is worth noting that, contrary to what many clinicians believe, personality disorders usually begin in adolescence, and DSM allows them to be diagnosed them at that stage if they have been present for a year or more. (This is not allowed for antisocial personality, which must still be called conduct disorder until age 18.)

Another misconception is that personality disorders are permanent and incurable. Rather, these conditions gradually remit over the course of adult life (Paris, 2003), and there are now several efficacious treatments for borderline personality disorder (Paris, 2015b).

Other disorders

Any system of classification has to end up with folders that do not fit, and that can only be described as 'other', and a few are listed in a separated chapter in DSM-5. Also, several chapters in the manual describe categories that are rarely seen by psychiatrists, for example, sleep-wake disorders (which must not be the symptoms of another mental disorder). There is also a separate chapter on the contentious diagnosis of dissociative disorders, although many psychiatrists consider dissociation to be an artefact of specific kinds of psychotherapy (Paris, 2015a).

The five-axis system

The five-axis system, introduced several decades ago in DSM-III, has been eliminated in DSM-5. Thus personality disorders are no longer separated on 'Axis II', but are listed in the same way as other diagnoses. Also, 'Axis V', a scoring of patient functioning used in past editions, has been eliminated on the grounds of poor reliability. Instead, since clinicians are sometimes asked to make functional ratings for insurance, the manual recommends using another system, the World Health Organization Disability Assessment Schedule (Narrow and Kuhl, 2011).

How to use DSM-5

Since a diagnostic manual is the standard way of communicating about mental disorders in practice, it would be a good idea to have a copy of the pocket edition of DSM-5 on your bookshelf or your computer. But DSM-5 is not designed to be a guide to daily practice. Physicians are always pressed for time, and are unlikely to carefully count criteria in the way that researchers do. Such procedures should be reserved for cases in which diagnosis is not obvious, and in which differential diagnosis is tricky. In that scenario, it is valuable to look up criteria listed in the manual, and to follow a structured procedure that clarifies a diagnostic conclusion. If there is sufficient time to spend an hour with a patient, that time could be better used obtaining a detailed life history.

DSM-5 was originally planned as a paradigm shift that would classify mental disorder on the basis of neuroscience instead of based on signs and symptoms. Current evidence has proven insufficient for such a change. Development of a system based on the a etiology of mental disorders will have to be put on hold. It may take many decades for research to unravel these complex problems. The RDoC developed by the National Institute of Mental Health, while it could be of some value to neuroscientists, is only beginning to be researched in clinical settings (Lilienfeld, 2014).

As it stands, since DSM-5 offers continuity with past editions, general practitioners who are familiar with previous versions should find it easy to apply the new edition. And given the elimination of the five-axis system, it may actually be easier to use DSM-5 than DSM-IV. However, it should not be considered, as it sometimes has been called, 'Psychiatry's Bible'. It is a rough-and-ready guide to a complex area of medicine in which research is still at an early stage. An overly literal view of the system has also created a serious problem with overdiagnosis of categories such as major depression, bipolar disorder, ADHD, and PTSD (Paris, 2015c).

On the other hand, we need a classification system that allows physicians to communicate with each other, and DSM-5 fills that bill. But we do not know the causes of most mental disorders. Reducing mental disorders to brain disorder may or may not be possible, and current attempts to do so have undermined the humanistic traditions of psychiatry (Kirmayer and Gold, 2012). In this light, DSM-5 can only be considered as a provisional and convenient guide to the exploration of a vast territory.

References

American Psychiatric Association. (1980). *Diagnostic and Statistical Manual of Mental Disorders* (3rd edn). Washington, DC: American Psychiatric Publishing.

American Psychiatric Association. (2013). *Diagnostic and Statistical Manual of Mental Disorders*, (5th edn). Washington, DC: American Psychiatric Publishing.

Black, D. (2014). *DSM-5 Guidebook: The Essential Companion to the Diagnostic and Statistical Manual of Mental Disorders, Fifth Edition*. Washington DC: American Psychiatric Publishing.

Decker, HS. (2013). *The Making of the DSM-III: A Diagnostic Manual's Conquest of American Psychiatry*. New York: Oxford University Press.

Frances, A. (2013). *Saving Normal: An Insider's Revolt Against Out-of-Control Psychiatric Diagnosis, DSM-5, Big Pharma, and the Medicalization of Ordinary Life*. New York, William Morrow.

Gold, I. (2009). Reduction in psychiatry. *Canadian Journal of Psychiatry*, **54**: 506–12

Gottesman II and Gould TD. (2003). The endophenotype concept in psychiatry: etymology and strategic intentions. *American Journal of Psychiatry*, **160**: 636–645.

Hyman S. (2007). Can neuroscience be integrated into the DSM-V? *Nature Reviews Neuroscience*, **8**: 725–32.

Hyman, S. (2010). The diagnosis of mental disorders: the problem of reification. *Annual Review of Clinical Psychology*, **6**: 155–79.

Insel TR, Cuthbert B, Garvey M, Heinssen R. Pine DS, Quinn K, Sanislow C, and Wang, P. (2010). Research Domain Criteria (RDoC): toward a new classification framework for research on mental disorders. *American Journal of Psychiatry*, **167**: 748–51

Jablensky, A. (2015). Schizophrenia or schizophrenias? The challenge of genetic parsing of a complex disorder. *American Journal of Psychiatry*, **172**: 105–7

Kirmayer LJ and Gold I. (2012). Critical neuroscience and the limits of reductionism. In: S Choudury, J Slaby, eds. *Critical Neuroscience: A Handbook of the Social and Cultural Contexts of Neuroscience*. New York, Wiley-Blackwell, 307–30.

Kleinman A. (2012). Bereavement, culture and psychiatry. *Lancet*, **379**: 608–9.

Kupfer DJ and Regier DA. (2011). Neuroscience, clinical evidence, and the future of psychiatric classification in DSM-5. *American Journal of Psychiatry*, **168**: 172–4.

Lilienfeld SO. (2014). The Research Domain Criteria (RDoC): An analysis of methodological and conceptual challenges. *Behaviour Research and Therapy*, **62**: 129–39.

Narrow WE and Kuhl EA. (2011). Clinical significance and disorder thresholds in DSM-V: the role of disability and distress. In: D Regier, WE Narrow, E. Kuhl, and DJ Kupfer, eds. *The Conceptual Evolution of DSM-5*. Washington, DC: American Psychiatric Publishing, 147–62.

Paris J. (2003). *Personality Disorders Over Time*. Washington, DC: American Psychiatric Press.

Paris J. (2010). *The Use and Misuse of Psychiatric Drugs: An Evidence-Based Critique*. Oxford: John Wiley & Sons, Ltd.

Paris J. (2015a). *The Intelligent Clinician's Guide to DSM-5, revised and expanded edition*. New York: Oxford University Press.

Paris J. (2015b). *Overdiagnosis in Psychiatry*. New York: Oxford University Press.

Paris J. (2015c). *A Concise Guide to Personality Disorders*. Washington, DC: American Psychological Association.

Regier DA, Narrow WE, Clarke D, Kraemer HC, Kuramoto SJ, Kuhl EA, and Kupfer DJ. (2013). DSM-5 field trials in the United States and Canada, Part II: test-retest reliability of selected categorical diagnoses. *American Journal of Psychiatry*, **170**: 159–70.

Chapter 7

Anxiety disorders in primary care

Markus Dold and Siegfried Kasper

Introduction

With a lifetime prevalence of about 29% (Kessler et al., 2005), anxiety disorders are one of the most common psychiatric disorders and the one-year prevalence rates are estimated at 14–18% (Baldwin et al., 2014; Bandelow et al., 2008, 2012). In Europe, approximately 61.5 million people suffer from anxiety disorders (Wittchen et al, 2011). According to a review of prevalence studies, the median 12-month prevalence rate for the different anxiety disorders varies between 1.2% for panic disorder and agoraphobia, 2.0% for social phobia and generalized anxiety disorder, and 4.9% for specific phobias (Wittchen et al., 2011). Costs associated with the various anxiety disorders represent approximately one-third of the total expenditures for mental illness.

Usually, people with anxiety disorders are frequent users of emergency medical services and consult their general practitioners often. Nevertheless, according to a large number of epidemiological surveys, anxiety disorders are underdiagnosed in primary care (Ormel et al., 1991; Wittchen et al., 2002; Calleo et al., 2009). This is mainly caused by the fact that the patients often present predominant symptoms other than anxiety (e.g. patients with panic attacks report chest pain) when consulting their doctor.

Anxiety patients in general are at a high risk for suicide attempts (Weissman et al., 1989). Both unipolar and bipolar depressive disorders represent a frequent comorbidity of the various anxiety disorders (Wittchen and Jacobi, 2005), and the simultaneous presence of anxiety and depressive disorder is associated with lower successful response to antidepressant treatment (Bennabi et al., 2015; Souery et al., 2007). Another common comorbidity is substance abuse (Brady and Lydiard, 1993).

With respect to the aetiology of anxiety disorders it should be taken into account that some somatic diseases can cause anxiety symptoms. Cardiovascular (e.g. angina pectoris, arrhythmia, heart failure, hypertonia, or myocardial infarct), respiratory (e.g. asthma, COPD, or pneumonia), neurological (e.g. encephalopathies, essential tremor, or dizziness), and metabolic (e.g. hyperthyroidism) diseases may possibly provoke anxiety symptoms.

Generalized anxiety disorder

The lifetime prevalence of generalized anxiety disorder (GAD) according to the *DSM-5* ranges from 4.3–5.9% and the one-year prevalence ranged in epidemiological studies between 1.2–3.1% (Baldwin et al., 2014; Bandelow et al., 2008, 2012; Wittchen et al., 2011). GAD occurs in females twice as much as in males and the most common age range for GAD is 45–59 years. Without adequate treatment, GAD can become a chronic disorder.

GAD is characterized by excessive, inappropriate, uncontrollable worries and unrealistic concerns with regard to everyday life, e.g. health, work, family, and financial issues. The anxiety is present although there is no trigger, and/or the worries are out of proportion to the likelihood of the anticipated events. This excessive anxiety is characteristically chronic (more than a few months) and not limited to a specific environment or to particular circumstances. The anxiety and the worries can be regarded as 'free-floating' and usually cause clinically meaningful distress or impairment in social, occupational, or other important areas of functioning (Fig. 7.1). Key symptoms include restlessness, fatigue, concentration difficulties, irritability, muscle tension, and sleep difficulties. To consider a diagnosis of GAD, these symptoms must not be caused by any other mental or somatic disorder.

Many of the GAD symptoms overlap with depression, which complicates diagnosing this disorder. Therefore, it can be assumed that in a primary care setting, many GPs do not adequately recognize their GAD, and thus GAD patients are often misdiagnosed due to the focus being on the somatic complaints. This is mainly caused by the fact that the main complaint is often not the anxiety itself, but instead pain or disturbed sleep. Frequent comorbidities of GAD are major depressive disorder, bipolar disorder, other anxiety disorders, obsessive-compulsive disorder (OCD), or substance abuse.

According to the guidelines of the World Federation of Societies of Biological Psychiatry (WFSBP), the recommended pharmacological first-line treatments for

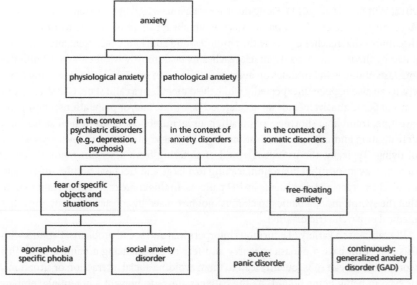

Fig. 7.1 Algorithm for exploring the various anxiety disorders

GAD include selective serotonin-reuptake inhibitors (SSRIs) (escitalopram, paroxetine, and sertraline), serotonin-norepinephrine-reuptake inhibitors (SNRIs) (venlafaxine and duloxetine), and the calcium channel modulator pregabalin (see Table 7.1). Trial results with the second-generation antipsychotic drug quetiapine were positive but should be regarded as preliminary. Other treatment options include, for instance, a pharmacotherapy with buspirone and hydroxyzine. Benzodiazepines should only be used for long-term treatment when other drugs or a course of cognitive behaviour therapy (CBT) had failed (Bandelow, 2008; Bandelow et al., 2013). Furthermore, an absence of a history of dependency should be ensured before treatment initiation. However, they can be combined with antidepressant drugs in the first couple of weeks of treatment before the onset of efficacy of the antidepressant compounds.

In therapy-resistant GAD, an augmentation treatment of SSRIs with second-generation antipsychotic drugs (risperidone or olanzapine) is commonly employed. Additionally, as a psychological treatment strategy, CBT and associated techniques are well-established in the treatment of GAD. CBT is based on cognitive models stressing the role of worrying, cognitions, and avoidance behaviour.

Panic disorder and agoraphobia

The most important change in the newly introduced DSM-5 with regard to the classification of anxiety disorders contains the separation of panic disorder (PD) and agoraphobia. These two disorders are no longer grouped together as one diagnostic entity and they are now recognized as two separate disorders. The American Psychiatric Association (APA) justifies this measure due to evidence that a majority of patients with agoraphobia do not experience panic symptoms (APA, 2013).

The lifetime prevalence of PD in epidemiological surveys is about 4.7% and the one-year prevalence amounts to 2.7% (Baldwin et al., 2014; Bandelow et al., 2008, 2012; Wittchen et al., 2011). Panic disorder is characterized by recurrent panic attacks. According to the DSM-5, a panic attack is 'an abrupt surge of intense fear or intense discomfort that reaches a peak within minutes', and attacks are recurrent and unanticipated by the patient. A panic attack reaches its peak mostly within about 10 minutes and lasts about 30–45 minutes on average. While it can occur because of existing anxiety, it can also happen unexpectedly while the patient is in a calm state. Classical symptoms of panic attacks include an accelerated heart rate and/or palpitations, chest pain, sweating, trembling, shortness of breath, nausea, numbness, chills or heat sensations, derealisation and/or depersonalization, fear of losing control, and, in severe cases, fear of dying. Typically, the patient is afraid of suffering from a serious medical condition such as myocardial infarction, leading to a large and frequent number of visits to medical emergency departments by PD patients. In this context, it is important to note that the symptoms of a panic attack must not be caused by substance use or any other medical or psychiatric disorder.

PD can cause a variety of enormous interpersonal and social problems. Patients with this condition have a persistent worry and fear of experiencing a panic attack. This worry and fear can subsequently lead to them avoiding social interaction or situations, or even to being home bound. As the patient's aim is to prevent a potentially embarrassing attack, PD is often accompanied with social withdrawal.

Table 7.1 Recommended doses for psychiatric drugs in the pharmacological treatment of the various anxiety disorders according to the recommendations of the WFSBP

Drug	GAD	Panic disorder	Social anxiety disorder
Benzodiazepines			
Alprazolam		1.5–8	
Clonazepam		1–4	1.5–8
Diazepam	5–15	5–20	
Lorazepam	2–8	2–8	
Calcium channel modulators			
Pregabalin	150–600		
Monoamine oxidase inhibitors (MAOIs)			
Moclobemide			300–600
Tranylcypromine			
Norepinephrine-dopamine-reuptake inhibitors (NDRIs)			
Bupropion			
Norepinephrine-reuptake inhibitors (NARIs)			
Reboxetine			
Noradrenergic and specific serotonergic antidepressants (NaSSAs)			
Mianserine			
Mirtazapine			
Other antidepressants			
Tianeptine			
Vortioxetine			
Selective serotonin reuptake inhibitors (SSRIs)			
Citalopram		20–60	20–40
Escitalopram	10–20	10–20	10–20
Fluoxetine		20–40	20–40
Fluvoxamine	50	100–300	100–300
Paroxetine	20–50	20–60	20–50
Sertraline	50–150	50–150	50–150
Serotonin antagonist and reuptake inhibitors (SARIs)			
Trazodone			

(continued)

Table 7.1 Continued

Drug	GAD	Panic disorder	Social anxiety disorder
Serotonin-norepinephrine reuptake inhibitors (SNRIs)			
Duloxetine	60–120		
Milnacipran			
Venlafaxine	75–225	75–225	75–225
Tricyclic antidepressants (TCAs)			
Amitriptyline			
Clomipramine		75–250	
Desipramine			
Imipramine			
Nortriptyline			
Trimipramine			

Adapted from *World Journal of Biological Psychiatry*, 9, Bandelow B. et al., 'World Federation of Societies of Biological Psychiatry (WFSBP) Guidelines for the Pharmacological Treatment of Anxiety, Obsessive-Compulsive and Post-Traumatic Stress Disorders – First Revision', pp. 248–312. Copyright (2008) with permission from Taylor & Francis.

On the other hand, agoraphobia is characterized by significant and persistent fear in the presence (or anticipation) of at least two specific situations. Such situations may include usually being in crowds, public places, public transportation, being outside of the home, open spaces, or standing in line. Following the DSM-5 criteria, a patient must exhibit avoidance behaviours when a specific situation associated with agoraphobia is present. Furthermore, no other psychiatric disorder may be responsible for the anxiety and panic symptoms caused by the specific situation. The DSM-5 retains the features of agoraphobia necessary for diagnosis, but at least two different specific agoraphobia situations are now needed in order to provide a clear distinction from specific phobias. Moreover, the DSM-5 criteria for agoraphobia are extended to be consistent with these for the other anxiety disorders (e.g. clinical judgment that the fear is out of proportion to the actual danger in the situation, and the need for the presence of the symptoms over a minimum duration of 6 months).

Many of the symptoms of agoraphobia mirror those of a panic attack, including nausea, dizziness, sweating, rapid heart rate, stomach upset, chest pains, and diarrhoea. All in all, it can be estimated that about two-thirds of all patients with panic disorder suffer from agoraphobia, which suggests a large overlap between both disorders.

SSRIs and venlafaxine can be regarded as first-line pharmacological treatments for both panic disorder and agoraphobia. Additionally, the efficacy of tricyclic antidepressants (TCAs) like clomipramine and imipramine is verified in a number of clinical trials, even if SSRIs/SNRIs should be preferred because of their favourable risk profile. Moreover, TCAs can potentially lead to overdose. In treatment-resistant conditions, a medication with benzodiazepines (alprazolam, clonazepam, diazepam, lorazepam) can be established if the patient does not have a history of dependency. Also, they can be combined with antidepressants in the first weeks of treatment before the onset of efficacy of the antidepressants. For the antidepressant mirtazapine, preliminary evidence from non-randomized trials is available. According to open studies, combination treatments of TCAs with fluoxetine, olanzapine monotherapy, and the augmentation of SSRIs with olanzapine were effective in the management of therapy resistance.

Within an acute panic attack, the reassurance of the patient might be sufficient in most cases. In severe attacks, the administration of (preferably short-acting) benzodiazepines may be necessary. After remission, the pharmacotherapy should be continued for at least several months in order to prevent relapses. SSRIs, venlafaxine, TCAs, benzodiazepines, and other drugs have shown long-term efficacy in clinical trials. With regard to SSRIs and SNRIs, the same doses administered to adequately treat the acute phase are used in the maintenance treatment.

In terms of non-pharmacological treatment options, there is a large body of evidence for the efficacy of CBT in both PD and agoraphobia. Furthermore, exposure therapy is efficacious in the management of agoraphobia. Altogether, the best results indicate a combination of CBT/exposure therapy and psychopharmacotherapy.

Specific phobia

Specific phobia is characterized by excessive or unreasonable fear of single people, objects, or situations (e.g. flying, heights, various animals, seeing blood, dentists, etc.). Subsequently, the fear usually provokes avoidance behaviour in the patient. The lifetime prevalence rate amounts to 12.5% and the 12-month prevalence rate is 6–9% (Baldwin et al., 2014; Bandelow et al., 2008, 2012; Wittchen et al., 2011). Usually, patients suffering from a specific phobia consult a psychiatrist or other medical professional only if the phobia has greatly reduced their quality of life.

The efficacy of exposure therapy in the management of a specific phobia is well established and is the first choice for therapy. Psychopharmacological drugs are not recognized as standard treatment in simple cases of specific phobia. Only if the phobia is associated with a meaningfully diminished quality of life psychopharmacotherapy should be considered. However, there is a lack of evidence with regard to pharmacological interventions in specific phobia. In a small preliminary randomized controlled trial (RCT), the SSRI paroxetine was superior to placebo, and in another small RCT (n = 12), escitalopram did not differentiate significantly from placebo in.

Social anxiety disorder

The annual prevalence of social anxiety disorder is about 7% and the lifetime prevalence is about 12% (Baldwin et al., 2014; Bandelow et al., 2008, 2012; Wittchen et al., 2011). The median age of onset of social anxiety disorder is about 13 years, and onset can be either abrupt or gradual.

Social phobia is characterized by enormous, persistent, and unreasonable fear of being evaluated negatively by other persons when in social performances or social interactions (for instance speaking in public or speaking to unfamiliar people). Usually, various somatic and cognitive symptoms occur in social anxiety disorder. The concern about being embarrassed or judged negatively results in fear and/or anxiety, which is typically accompanied by autonomic arousal including symptoms like increased sweating, apnoea, tremors, tachycardia, and nausea. The feared situations are avoided or endured with intense anxiety or distress. The discomfort that people with social anxiety disorder experience can expand to routine activities such as eating in front of others or using a public bathroom. Usually, patients desire social contacts and want to participate in social situations, but their anxiety has become unbearable. Therefore, in many cases, social anxiety disorder can lead to social isolation.

According to the WFSBP guidelines, the mainstay of the pharmacological management of social anxiety disorder includes SSRIs (escitalopram, fluvoxamine, paroxetine, and sertraline) and the SNRI venlafaxine. There is a lack of evidence for successful pharmacotherapy using TCAs and benzodiazepines in social anxiety disorder. On the other hand, the irreversible monoamine oxidase inhibitor (MAOI) phenelzine can be an option in case of treatment resistance. As social anxiety disorder is generally a chronic disorder, long-term treatment is recommended in order to prevent relapses. Among psychological therapies, evidence-based research indicates that exposure therapy and CBT are both successful in treating social anxiety disorder.

Benzodiazepines can be used in therapy-refractory cases in absence of a history of dependency. Like in other anxiety disorders, they can be combined with antidepressants in the first weeks of treatment before the onset of efficacy of the antidepressant agents. For citalopram and gabapentin, preliminary positive evidence is available based on RCTs, and based on case series for olanzapine, tranylcypromine, tiagabine, topiramate, and levetiracetam.

Conclusion

- The lifetime prevalence of all anxiety disorders is up to 29%.

- Anxiety disorders are underdiagnosed in primary care as the anxiety symptoms are often not the presenting symptoms when the patients consult their GP.

- Selective serotonin-reuptake inhibitors (SSRIs) and serotonin-norepinephrine-reuptake inhibitors (SNRIs) are the mainstay in the pharmacological management of generalized anxiety disorder (GAD), panic disorder, agoraphobia, and social anxiety disorder.

- Pregabalin is recommended for the pharmacotherapy of GAD.

- Benzodiazepines should be used only in absence of a history of dependency. They are often combined with antidepressant drugs in the first weeks of treatment before the onset of efficacy of the antidepressants.

- Specific phobias should be preferentially treated with psychotherapy.

- With regard to psychotherapeutic interventions, cognitive behavioural therapy (CBT) and/or exposure therapy can be considered as evidence-based treatment options and should therefore be preferred.

References

American Psychiatric Association. (2013). Diagnostic and Statistical Manual of Mental Disorders—DSM-5. 5th edn. Washington, DC: American Psychiatry Publishing.

Baldwin DS, Anderson IM, Nutt DJ, Allgulander C, Bandelow B, den Boer JA, Christmas DM, Davies S, Fineberg N, Lidbetter N, Malizia A, McCrone P, Nabarro D, O'Neill C, Scott J, van der Wee N, and Wittchen HU. (2014). Evidence-based pharmacological treatment of anxiety disorders, post-traumatic stress disorder and obsessive-compulsive disorder: a revision of the 2005 guidelines from the British Association for Psychopharmacology. *J Clin Psychopharmacol*, 28: 403–39.

Bandelow B, Boerner RJ, Kasper S, Linden M, Wittchen HU, and Möller HJ. (2013). The diagnosis and treatment of generalized anxiety disorder. *Dtsch Arztebl Int*, 110: 300–10: doi: 10.3238/arztebl.2013.0300.

Bandelow B. (2008). The medical treatment of obsessive-compulsive disorder and anxiety. *CNS Spectr*, 13: 37–46.

Bandelow B, Zohar J, Hollander E, Kasper S, and Moller HJ. (2008). World Federation of Societies of Biological Psychiatry (WFSBP) guidelines for the pharmacological treatment of anxiety, obsessive-compulsive and post-traumatic stress disorders—first revision. *World J Biol Psychiatry*, 9: 248–312.

Bandelow B, Sher L, Bunevicius R, Hollander E, Kasper S, Zohar J, Moller HJ, and WFSBP Task Force on Anxiety Disorders, OCD, and PTSD. (2012). Guidelines for the pharmacological treatment of anxiety disorders, obsessive-compulsive disorder and posttraumatic stress disorder in primary care. *Int J Psychiatry Clin Pract*, 16: 77–84.

Bennabi D, Aouizerate B, El-Hage W, Doumy O, Moliere F, Courtet P, Nieto I, Bellivier F, Bubrovsky M, Vaiva G, Holztmann J, Bougerol T, Richieri R, Lancon C, Camus V, Saba G, Haesbaert F, d'Amato T, Charpeaud T, Llorca PM, Leboyer M, and Haffen E. (2015). Risk factors for treatment resistance in unipolar depression: a systematic review. *J Affect Disord*, 171: 137–41.

Brady KT and Lydiard RB. (1993). The association of alcoholism and anxiety. *Psychiatr Q*, 64: 135–49.

Calleo J, Stanley MA, and Greisinger A. (2009). Generalized anxiety disorder in older medical patients: diagnostic recognition, mental health management and service utilization. *J Clin Psychol Med Settings*, 16: 178–85.

Kessler RC, Berglund P, Demler O, Jin R, Merikangas KR, and Walters EE. (2005). Lifetime prevalence and age-of-onset distributions of DSM-IV disorders in the National Comorbidity Survey Replication. *Arch Gen Psychiatry*, 62: 593–602.

Ormel J, Koeter MWJ, and Vandenbrink W. (1991). Recognition, management, and course of anxiety and depression in general practice. *Arch Gen Psychiatry*, 48: 700–6.

Souery D, Oswald P, Massat I, Bailer U, Bollen J, Demyttenaere K, Kasper S, Lecrubier Y, Montgomery S, Serretti A, Zohar J, Mendlewicz J, and Group for the Study of Resistant Depression. (2007). Clinical factors associated with treatment resistance in major depressive disorder: results from a European multicenter study. *J Clin Psychiatry*, 68: 1062–70.

Weissman MM, Klerman GL, Markowitz JS, and Ouellette R. (1989). Suicidal ideation and suicide attempts in panic disorder and attacks. *New Engl J Med*, 321: 1209–14.

Wittchen HU, Kessler RC, and Beesdo K. (2002). Generalized anxiety and depression in primary care: prevalence, recognition, and management. *J Clin Psychiatry*, 63: 24–34.

Wittchen HU and Jacobi F. (2005). Size and burden of mental disorders in Europe—a critical review and appraisal of 27 studies. *Eur Neuropsychopharmacol*, **15**: 357–76.

Wittchen HU, Jacobi F, Rehm J, Gustavsson A, Svensson M, and Jonsson B. (2011). The size and burden of mental disorders and other disorders of the brain in Europe 2010. *European Neuropsychopharmacology*, **21**: 655–79.

Chapter 8

ADHD across the lifespan

David W. Goodman

Introduction

Attention Deficit Hyperactivity Disorder (ADHD) is an internationally acknowledged neuropsychiatric disorder. Recognized by the World Health Organization, ADHD expert organizations around the world have published consensus guidelines for diagnosis and treatment of ADHD in children and adolescents. With the growing body of adult ADHD research, diagnosis and treatment guidelines for adults with ADHD have been published in the UK, European Consensus, Canada, and Scotland. (Geller et al., 2007; Kooij et al., 2010; CADDRA, 2011; SIGN, 2009; NICE, 2009).

Prevalence Rates for ADHD

A meta-analytic review of 41 child and adolescent studies conducted in 27 countries from every world region found a prevalence estimate of ADHD in the general population of 3.4% (range 0.85–10%) (Polanczyk et al., 2015). In the US, the Centers for Disease Control (CDC) estimates the US child and adolescent prevalence rate at 8.8% (Visser et al., 2014). For adults, the US estimate of ADHD prevalence rate is 4.4% with the international prevalence range between 0.5–4.4% (Fayyad et al., 2007). Due to changes in diagnostic criteria over time and the methods of ADHD assessment across studies, the prevalence rates are estimates for epidemiologic consideration.

Screen patients for ADHD complaining of mental symptoms

A screener is a list of ADHD symptoms that allows for a brief inquiry thus raising consideration for a more thorough assessment. While these screeners can be administered to all patients, the sensitivity and specificity of screeners may lead to mis- and over-diagnosis and, subsequently, inappropriate treatment. Given the high comorbidity rate of ADHD with other psychiatric disorders, screeners are a time-efficient method for sorting psychiatric symptoms in patients who present with any behavioural and mental health complaints. Parents, teachers, or patients prior to the clinical interview can complete these screeners, thus saving the clinician's time. The World Health Organization (WHO) has developed a 6-question adult rated screener for adult ADHD to be completed by the patient. The Adult Self-Report ADHD Scale (ASRS) is an expanded questionnaire for adults listing all 18 symptoms from the Diagnostic and

Statistical Manual 5 (DSM-5) (Kessler et al., 2005) and is rated on a frequency basis as an assessment of symptoms that can be used at baseline and then throughout the course of treatment. The sensitivity for detection of adult ADHD is 68.7% and specificity is 99.5%. However, some adults with ADHD under-report their symptoms. This discrepancy is evident when a close family member reports greater frequency, severity, and impairment than the patient. In these cases, it is helpful to include the observer in periodic reviews of treatment benefit, assuming a priori patient consent. Both adult scales are readily available on the Internet and additional useful tools can be found at www.caddra.ca, www.adhdeurope.eu, and adhdinadults.com.

Evaluating patients over the age of 50 for ADHD

Two studies in Europe have found prevalence rates of ADHD in adults over age 50 to be 2.8–3.5% (Michielsen et al., 2012; de Zwaan et al., 2012). Understanding that ADHD is a chronic and life-long disorder, adult complaints of longstanding inattention, disorganization, and inability to sustain attention should lead to consideration of ADHD, regardless of age (Goodman et al. 2016). The onset of new cognitive changes in adulthood without childhood symptoms requires a medical evaluation for other aetiologies.

Diagnostic criteria for ADHD

Several specific changes have occurred with the development of the new edition of the Diagnostic and Statistical Manual (DSM-5) diagnostic criteria for ADHD (APA, 2013). First, the age of onset criterion before age 7 has been increased to age 12 to better account for predominantly inattentive children. Second, symptom descriptors have been modified to apply to adults. Third, impairments have been defined as 'interfering with, or reducing the quality of social, academic, or occupational functioning'. This definition of impairments allows for a broader interpretation of impairment across different age groups.

The International Classification of Mental and Behavioural Disorders (ICD-10) (WHO, 1993) uses the term 'hyperkinetic disorder' and requires both inattention *and* hyperactivity to be present prior to age seven. These diagnostic criteria are stricter than the DSM-5 both for age of onset and the lack of recognition of the inattentive presentation. This may, in part, explain differences in prevalence rates between European and North American surveys.

Obtaining clinical information from outside informants

When assessing children, it is helpful to obtain information from parents and teachers as they observe the children in different settings. Often, symptom checklists rated by teachers (in the structured school setting) and parents (in the unstructured home setting) aid in the identification of a child's symptoms/impairments. Collateral observer information is important to corroborate the child's description of symptoms. Adults may be better able to identify their cognitive symptoms, mental experience, and resultant impairments during the day. When possible for the adult, an ADHD symptom checklist from a parent or another close relative documenting childhood symptoms provides collateral information, which may aid in diagnostic assessment. The citation of symptoms/impairments by others may enable a more appropriate clinical judgment of the severity of ADHD-related symptoms/impairments.

Medical illnesses that may mimic ADHD

Prior to the establishment of a diagnosis of ADHD, the clinician should consider other medical conditions that may present with similar cognitive and/or behavioural symptoms and complaints. Medical conditions including but not limited to fetal alcohol syndrome, fragile X syndrome, lead poisoning, learning disabilities, mental retardation, metabolic disorders, narcolepsy, pervasive developmental disorders, sleep apnoea/sleep deprivation, concussive injury, thyroid disorder, or vision/hearing impairment may encompass behavioural and/or cognitive symptoms, which should be considered in the differential diagnosis of ADHD. In adults, medical illnesses that might present with cognitive and/or behavioural symptoms similar to ADHD often have the hallmark of symptomatic onset in adulthood. Therefore, the onset of symptoms similar to ADHD in adulthood without child onset of symptoms is often explained by other medical/psychiatric disorders.

Thorough assessment of concurrent mental disorders

Preschoolers

A US study of 302 pre-schoolers (ages 3–6) with ADHD found that only 34.1% of those with ADHD had no psychiatric comorbidity. The rest of this sample had at least one psychiatric comorbid disorder: ADHD plus oppositional defiant disorder 52.3%, ADHD plus communication disorder 21.9%, ADHD plus anxiety 12.3%, ADHD with other comorbidities 4.3% (Posner et al., 2007).

Children

The CDC estimates the rate of lifetime childhood diagnosis of ADHD is 9.5% (Pastor et al., 2015). The Multimodal Treatment Study, a US study of 579 children ages 7–10, found that no comorbidity occurred in 31% of ADHD children (MTA Cooperative, 1999). Prevalence rates of concurrent mental disorders were: ADHD plus oppositional defiant disorder 40%, ADHD plus anxiety disorder 34%, ADHD plus contact disorder 14%, ADHD plus Tic disorder 11%, ADHD plus mood disorder 4% (Jensen et al., 2001).

Adults

The National Comorbidity Survey Replication, a large US epidemiologic study surveying 3199 adults ages 18–44, found a prevalence rate of ADHD in the adult population of 4.4% (Kessler et al., 2006). Prevalence rates of 12-month comorbid DSM-IV mental disorder among adult respondents with ADHD were: mood disorders (38.3%);

bipolar disorder (19.4%), major depression (18.6%), dysthymia (12.8%), anxiety disorders (47%), social anxiety (29.3%), posttraumatic stress disorder (11.9%), panic disorder (8.9%), generalized anxiety disorder (8.0%), agoraphobia (4.0%), and obsessive-compulsive disorder (2.7%). This study also found the prevalence rate of ADHD with active concurrent DSM-IV substance abuse disorder was 15.2%.

These studies indicate that the majority of ADHD patients, regardless of age, will present with comorbid psychiatric disorders which require evaluation and concurrent treatment.

Executive functioning

Executive functioning (EF) is characterized by set shifting (the ability to move smoothly from one task to another), working memory (the ability to hold and manipulate information in your head), organization (the ability to efficiently sequence steps of a task), and response inhibition (the ability to consider and resist an impulse) (Seidman, 2006). While some experts consider executive dysfunction subsumed under ADHD, others consider executive dysfunction a separate entity that frequently co-occurs with ADHD (Biederman et al., 2006). The presence of executive dysfunction with ADHD leads to greater academic impairments beyond the effect of ADHD, per se. Therefore, in addition to diagnosing ADHD, it is helpful to evaluate the degree of executive dysfunction present. The assessment of EF may be more properly performed after the optimal management of ADHD symptoms in order to quantify the residual executive dysfunction. While the core symptoms of ADHD are very responsive to medication, executive dysfunction symptoms are less responsive to medication, but could be managed through behavioural therapy approaches (Swanson et al., 2011). Notwithstanding, the management of executive dysfunction is still needed in the treatment of ADHD (Hosenbocus and Chahal, 2012).

Neuropsychological testing

Often requested, neuropsychological testing in children and adults is not required to make an ADHD diagnosis by DSM-5 or ICD 10 criteria. Nevertheless, neuropsychological testing may be helpful in determining intelligence level, associated learning disorders, and EF. Most often, neuropsychological tests are administered in a quiet environment with a test administrator, which may reduce the detection of deficits and may not accurately reflect deficits that would occur in a setting normal to the patient. While specific cognitive deficits may be present on testing, the extrapolation and correlation to daily functioning remains controversial (Barkley and Fischer, 2011). Though counter-intuitive, the absence of deficits on neuropsychological testing does not rule out ADHD.

Treatment algorithm

Following the completion of a comprehensive psychiatric assessment, which should encompass the evaluation of all comorbid psychiatric and medical, a diagnostic prioritization of these disorders will enable the formulation of a treatment algorithm. In

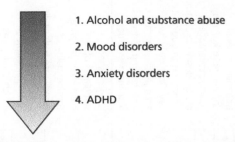

1. Alcohol and substance abuse

2. Mood disorders

3. Anxiety disorders

4. ADHD

Order of treatment considers the severity of the concurrent disorders

Fig. 8.1 Diagnostic prioritization for pharmacotherapy order of treatment
Reproduced from Goodman, D.W, 'Treatment and assessment of ADHD in adults', in: *ADHD Across the Lifespan: an Evidence-Based Understanding From Research to Clinical Practice*, edited by Biederman, J. Copyright (2006) with permission from Veritas Institute for Medical Education.

children, it is recommended to treat the most severely impairing disorder first and then re-evaluate other conditions (Pliszka et al., 2006). For adults, in whom there is a greater likelihood of concurrent psychiatric and medical illnesses, diagnostic prioritization is more nuanced. The order of treatment is severe alcohol/substance use disorders, then severe mood disorders, then severe anxiety disorders, and finally ADHD (see Fig. 8.1) (Goodman, 2006). This diagnostic prioritization is established for two reasons. First, the cognitive symptoms of ADHD may also be present in the other untreated psychiatric disorders. Therefore, acute psychiatric comorbidity should be stabilized prior to the evaluation of cognitive symptoms specific to ADHD. Secondly, ADHD medications may exacerbate the symptoms of other untreated psychiatric disorders. For example, the adult ADHD patient with unrecognized bipolar disorder may experience mood destabilization when prescribed stimulant medication in monotherapy.

Treatment of concurrent medical conditions that might be exacerbated by ADHD medication (e.g. hypertension and migraine) and treatment should occur prior to starting ADHD medications.

Medication Options

While there are several classes of medication, approved and off-label (see Tables 8.1–8.3) stimulant medications are endorsed by five international guidelines as first-line treatment for ADHD across the lifespan. While there are some differences in the recommended stimulant compound (methylphenidate or amphetamine) depending upon the age of the patient, such differences should be considered as a function of available agents in specific countries at the time of the guideline publication. For example, National Institute for Health and Care Excellence (NICE) recommends methylphenidate as first-line medication for adults with ADHD, while the Canadian ADHD Resource Alliance (CADDRA) recommendation for adult ADHD is lisdexamfetamine. Atomoxetine is listed as treatment for children, adolescents, and adults in most of the guidelines.

Stimulant medications, classified by the US Food and Drug Administration (FDA) as controlled drugs, exist as two compounds: methylphenidate and amphetamine.

Table 8.1 Medications approved by the FDA for ADHD

Brand name (manufacturer)	Dose form	Typical starting dose	FDA max/daily (mg)	Off-label max/day	Comments
Amphetamine preparations					
Short-acting					
Adderall*	5, 7.5, 10, 12.5, 15, 20, 30 mg tablets	3–5 years: 2.5 mg qD; ≥6 years: 5 mg qD-bid	40	>50 kg: 60 mg	Short-acting stimulants often used as initial treatment in small children (<16 kg), may have disadvantage of bid-tid dosing to control symptoms throughout day. Once daily, long acting stimulants are now recommended as first line medication.
Dexedrine	5 mg capsules	3–5 years: 2.5 mg qD	40	>50 kg: 60 mg	
DextroStat	5, 10 mg capsules	≥6 years: 5 mg qD-bid	60	>50 kg: 60 mg	
Procentra	5 mg/5 mL liquid	3–5 years: 2.5 mg qD-bid, increase by 2.5 mg/d qwk; >6 years: 5 mg qD in bid, increase by 5 mg/d qwk	3–5 years: 40 mg/d; >6 years: 60 mg/d	n/a	
Long-acting					
Dexedrine spansule	5, 10, 15 mg capsules	≥6 years: 5–10 mg qD-bid	40	>50 kg: 60 mg	Longer acting stimulants offer greater convenience, confidentiality, and compliance with single daily dosing but may have greater problematic effects on daytime appetite and sleep; Except for Adzenys, all three medications may be opened and sprinkled on soft foods.
Adderall XR*	5, 10, 15, 20, 25, 30 mg capsules	≥6 years: 10 mg qD	30	>50 kg: 60 mg	
Adzenys XR-ODT	3.1, 6.3, 9.4, 12.5, 15.7, 18.8 mg dissolving tablet	≥6 years: 6.3 mg qD; adult: 12.5mg qD	6–12 years: 18.8 mg; 13–17 years: 12.5	Not yet determined	
Vyvanse	20, 30, 40, 50, 60, and 70 mg capsules	30 mg qD	70	Not yet determined	

Methylphenidate preparations

Short-acting	Focalin*	2.5, 5, 10 mg capsules	2.5 mg bid	20	50 mg	Short-acting stimulants often used as initial treatment in small children (<16 kg), may have disadvantage of bid-tid dosing to control symptoms throughout day. Once-daily, long acting stimulants are now recommended as first line medication.
	Methylin*	5, 10, 20 mg tablets	5 mg bid	60	>50 kg: 100 mg	
	Ritalin*	5, 10, 20 mg tablets	5 mg bid	60	>50 kg: 100 mg	
Intermediate-acting	Metadate ER	20 mg tablet	10 mg qAM	60	>50 kg: 100 mg	Longer acting stimulants offer greater convenience, confidentiality, and compliance with single daily dosing but may have greater problematic effects on daytime appetite and sleep.
	Methylin ER	10, 20 mg tablets	10 mg qAM	60	>50 kg: 100 mg	
	Ritalin SR*	20 mg tablet	10 mg qAM	60	>50 kg: 100 mg	
Long-acting	Metadate CD IR:ER-30%:70%	10, 20, 30, 40, 50, 60 mg capsules	20 mg qAM	60	>50 kg: 100 mg	Metadate CD, Aptensio XL, Ritalin LA caps may be opened and sprinkled on soft food.
	Ritalin LA IR:ER-50%:50%	10, 20, 30, 40 mg capsules	20 mg qAM	60	>50 kg: 100 mg	
	Aptensio XR IR:ER-40%:60%	10, 20, 30, 40, 50, 60 mg capsules	10 mg qAM	60	n.a.	

(Continued)

Table 8.1 Continued

Brand name (manufacturer)	Dose form	Typical starting dose	FDA max/daily (mg)	Off-label max/day	Comments
Concerta*	18, 27, 36, 54 mg capsules	18 mg qAM	72	108 mg adult trials	Swallow whole with liquids; non-absorbable tablet shell may be seen in stool.
Daytrana patch	10, 15, 20, 30 mg patches	Begin with 10 mg patch qD, then titrate up by patch strength	30	Not yet determined	Recommended wear-time is 9 hours resulting in 12 duration of action. Daily placement by alternating hips. Erythematous rash may limit use.
Focalin XR	5, 10, 15, 20, 25, 30, 35, 40 mg capsules	5 mg qAM	30	50 mg	Can be sprinkled on soft food.
Quillivant	5 mg/ml bottles: 60, 120, 150, 180 ml	>6 years; 20 mg qD, increase by 10–20 mg/d qwk	60 mg/d	n.a.	
SNRI					
Strattera	10, 18, 25, 40, 60, 80, 100 mg capsules	Children and adolescents <70 kg: 0.5 mg/kg day for 4 days; then 1.2 mg/kg day; adult starting dose: 40 mg/day	Lesser of 1.4 mg/kg or 100 mg; adult therapeutic dose: 80–100 mg/day	Lesser of 1.8 mg/kg or 100 mg; adult trials to 120 mg	Not a schedule II medication. Consider if active substance abuse or severe side effects of stimulants (mood lability, tics); give qAM, qhs, or divided doses bid.; do not open capsule; monitor closely for suicidal thinking and behaviour, clinical worsening, or unusual changes in behaviour.

Alpha 2-adrenergic agents

Clonidine preparations

Short-acting	Clonidine*	0.1, 0.2, 0.3 mg tablets	n.a.	27–40.5 kg;0.2 mg/d; 40.5–45kg: 0.3 mg/d; >45 kg: 0.4 mg/d; adults: 0.6 mg/d	May be used alone or as adjuvant to another medication for ADHD. Effective for impulsivity and hyperactivity; modulating mood levels; tics worsening from stimulants; sleep disturbances.
Long-acting	Kapvay	0.1 mg tablets	age>6: 0.1 mg qhs; titrate in 0.1 mg increments every 7 days, qhs or bid dosing.	child: 0.4 mg	n.a.

Guanfacine preparations

Short-acting	Guanfacine	1, 2 mg tablets	<45 kg: 0.5 mg qhs; titrate in 0.5 mg increments q7d bid, tid, qid: >45 kg: 0.1 mg qhs; titrate in 0.1 mg increments q7d bid, tid, qid	27–40.5 kg: 2 mg/d; 40.5–45kg: 3 mg/d; >45 kg: 4 mg/d	n.a.	Review personal and family cardiovascular history. Taper off to avoid rebound hypertension.
Long-acting	Intuniv	1, 2, 3, 4 mg tablets	age 6–17: 1 mg qAM; titrate in increments of 1 mg qd every 7 days.	4 mg QD	n.a.

*Generic formulation available

Adapted from *Journal of the American Academy of Child & Adolescent Psychiatry*, 46, Pliszka S., 'Practice Parameter for the Assessment and Treatment of Children and Adolescents With Attention-Deficit/Hyperactivity Disorder', pp. 894–921. Copyright (2007) with permission from Elsevier.

Table 8.2 Medications used for ADHD, not approved by FDA

Generic class/ brand name	Dose form	Typical starting dose	Max/daily	Comments
Antidepressants				
Bupropion Wellbutrin*	75, 100 mg tablets	Lesser of 3 mg/kg/day or 150 mg/day	Lesser of 6 mg/kg or 300 mg, with no single dose >150 mg	Lowers seizure threshold; contraindicated if current seizure disorder. Usually given in divided doses, bid for children and adolescents for both safety and effectiveness. Obtain baseline ECG before starting imipramine and nortriptyline
Wellbutrin SR*	100, 150, 200 mg tablets	above	450 mg (adults)	
Wellbutrin XL*	150, 300 mg tablets	above	450 mg (adults)	
Imipramine Tofranil*	10, 25, 50, 75 mg tablets	1 mg/kg/day	Lesser of 4 mg/kg or 200 mg	
Nortriptyline Pamelor*	10, 25, 50, 75 mg capsules	0.5 mg/kg/day	Lesser of 2 mg/kg or 100 mg; 150 mg (adults)	

*Generic formulation available.

Table 8.3 FDA-approved medication for adults with ADHD

Medication (daily dose)	Child dosing	Adolescent dosing	Adult dosing	US trials adult max dose	Approval for adult age range (years)
Atomoxetine	0.5 mg/kg (<70kg) max 1.2 mg/kg (max 100 mg)	Same as child dosing	40–100 mg	120 mg	18–65
Dexmethyl-phenidate XR	5–20 mg	Same as child dosing	10–20 mg	40 mg	18–65
Lisdexamfetamine	30–70 mg	Same as child dosing	30–70 mg	70 mg	18–55
Mixed amphetamine salts XR	10–30 mg	Same as child dosing	20+ mg	60 mg	18–65
OROS Methylphenidate HCL	18–54 mg	18–72 mg	18 or 36 mg–72 mg	108 mg	18–65

Data from Food and Drug Administration, U.S. Department of Health and Human Services.

Table 8.4 Stimulant preparations delivery systems

Preparation	Stimulant	Description	Duration of action (hrs) (shortest to longest)
Liquid	Methylphenidate (Methylin), dextroamphetaime (Procentra)	Liquid, immediate delivery	3–4
Immediate release tablet	Methylphenidate (Ritalin, Metadate, Methylin), dexmethylphenidate (Focalin), dextroamphetamine (Dexedrine), mixed amphetamine salts (Adderall)	No delivery system; immediate delivery	3–4
Chewable tablet	Methylphenidate (chewable Methylin)	No delivery system; immediate delivery	3–4
Slow release matrix	Methyphenidate SR (Ritalin SR)	Wax matrix	4–6
Beaded*	Mixed-amphetamine salts XR (Adderall XR); methylphenidate (Metadate CD), (Aptensio XL); dextroamphetamine (Dexedrine spansules)	Double-beaded; immediate release bead followed by 2nd release 4 hours later; ph-dependent polymer	≤12
SODAS	Dexmethylphenidate XR (Focalin XR), methylphenidate LA (Ritalin LA)	SODAS® (Spheroidal Oral Drug Absorption System); immediate release bead then 2nd release bead later	≤12
OROS	Methylphenidate OROS (Concerta)	OROS® (Oral Release Osomotic System); osmotic push devise delivers MPH with an ascending pharmacokinetic profile over 8 hours	≤12
XR-ODT	Amphetamine XR-ODT (Adzenys)	oral dissolving tablet (ODT) mixture of immediate release and polymer-coated, delayed-release resin particles	<12

(continued)

Table 8.4 Continued

Preparation	Stimulant	Description	Duration of action (hrs) (shortest to longest)
Patch	Methylphenidate patch (Daytrana)	DOT® (Delivery Optimized Thermodynamics) Matrix transdermal system; cutaneous gradient diffusion	Variable depending on wear time; 12 with 9 hour wear time
Prodrug'	Lisdexamfetamine (Vyvanse)	No delivery system; duration of action determined by rate-limited enzymatic hydrolysis of lysine from dextroamphetamine	≤13

*Can be sprinkled on soft food

' Can be dissolved in water; duration of action remains the same

The preparation (vehicle of delivery) determines the rate of absorption of the stimulant into the circulation and this determines the duration of action of the medication. The half-life of the compound always remains the same regardless of the vehicle of delivery as it is established once the compound is metabolized in the blood circulation. Adverse events may be related to the compound and/or the preparation. Side effect intolerance to one preparation may not predict sensitivity to another preparation of the same compound. Given the broad range of available preparations, clinicians should be able to find an appropriate choice for their patient

Reproduced from *Primary Psychiatry*, 17, David W. Goodman, 'The Black Book of ADHD'. Copyright (2010) Primary Psychiatry.

Each drug is available as an immediate release with approximate duration of action of 3–5 hours. The immediate release formulations are available as tablet, liquid, chewable, and sprinkle depending on the country. The diverse formulations allow a clinician to find a medication preparation that a child can ingest without objection. Each compound is also available as longer-duration formulation. The technology for extending the duration of action is equally diverse: beaded (immediate and delayed), patch, prodrug, wax matrix, liquid suspension, oral release osmotic system (OROS), spheroidal oral drug absorption system (SODAS). Each formulation introduces the compound into the body for the purpose of extending the duration of action for 8–14 hours, depending on patient variables (see Table 8.4).

In addition to stimulants, there are several alternative classes of medication. Atomoxetine, approved for children and adults, is a non-stimulant whose clinical effects may take 3–4 weeks to be observed. Atomoxetine has been shown to be helpful for ADHD patients with anxiety (Geller et al., 2007) or executive dysfunction (Brown et al., 2011). Alpha 2 agonists (guanfacine and clonidine) are FDA approved in extended formulations for children and adolescents. These agents may be used as monotherapy in stimulant-intolerant patients or in combination with other ADHD medication for residual symptoms (i.e. insomnia, fidgetiness).

Outcomes with medication treatment

A 20-year literature review identified eight long-term controlled trials with durations ranging from one to eight years at follow-up. Their results suggested that combined pharmacological and behavioural interventions, and pharmacological intervention alone are effective in managing core ADHD symptoms and at improving academic performance at 14 months (Parker et al., 2013). Additionally, the Multimodal Treatment Study of ADHD in children funded by the National Institute of Mental Health is often cited as a 14-month comparison of medication treatment, medication, and behavioural therapy (combined treatment), behavioural therapy, and community care (MTA Cooperative, 1999). The study showed that medication alone and combined treatments are significantly more effective than behavioural therapy alone or community care. A secondary analysis reported that combined treatment worked significantly better than pharmacologic treatment or behavioural therapy. It may be that behavioural therapy for ADHD in the presence of coexisting psychiatric disorders provides a benefit beyond medication alone (Conners et al., 2001). Nevertheless, it should be noted that the cost of behavioural therapy was six times greater than the cost of medication alone in this 14-month study (Jensen et al., 2005). Therefore, pursuing behavioural therapy in the absence of medication, while potentially helpful, will require greater time and cost.

Medication side effects

The profiles of side effects for children/adolescents may be different from those seen in adults, as children are more sensitive to some side effects like anorexia and nausea. For children and adolescents, the European ADHD Guidelines Group (EAGG) (Graham et al., 2011) listed the more-frequent side effects and best practice management.

Appetite and growth

Clinicians should plot growth on standard growth charts for children. A quantitative systematic analysis of 18 studies of stimulant medication found a significant effect of stimulants associated with height and weight deficits occurring in treatment up to 3.5 years (Faraone et al., 2008). The study indicated that after discontinuing stimulants, growth rate accelerated and compensated for the initial height and weight deficits within two years. For atomoxetine, a meta-analysis of seven double-blind, placebo-controlled, and six open-label studies found a reduction in mean weight and height at 24 months were, respectively, 2.5 kg and 2.7 cm lower than the expected values (Kratochvil et al., 2006). It is suggested that morning medication be given after the meal so as to not suppress breakfast. High-calorie foods and increased volume of food in evenings may be helpful as the effect of anorexia diminishes. The degree of appetite suppression may vary between compounds and/or preparations (delivery systems) so alternative medication trials may be helpful.

Cardiovascular risks

It is important to screen for patient and familial risk factors, including cardiac structural or electrical abnormalities, sudden death before age 30, history of spontaneous or exercise-induced fainting, or chest pains. At the recommendation of the American Academy of Pediatrics/American Heart Association in 2008, electrocardiograms are not mandatory before starting stimulant medication and should only be obtained when specifically indicated. With the administration of medication, blood pressure and pulse should be monitored regularly. If elevations of blood pressure and pulse occur, assessment of contributing factors like caffeine, decongestants, and over-the-counter supplements need to be assessed before assuming an ADHD medication effect. Management of this elevation may require stimulant dose reduction, use of an alternative stimulant compound, or the prescription of an antihypertensive. In ADHD patients, the use of alpha2 agonists (guanfacine, clonidine) may further reduce ADHD symptoms while controlling blood pressure and pulse.

Insomnia

Although insomnia may be provoked by stimulant medications, many ADHD patients (approximately 40% in the adults (Kooij and Bijlenga, 2013)) have sleep disturbances. Therefore, it is important to establish the patient's sleep pattern prior to starting ADHD medications in order to evaluate pre-existing or medication-induced sleep disturbance. If sleep changes are a result of the stimulant medication, consider stimulant dose reduction, change in timing of dose, melatonin 3–10 mg orally 90 minutes prior to bedtime, alpha-2 agonist, or an antihistamine.

Motor tics

Tics may accompany ADHD as a comorbid condition (e.g. Tourette's) or develop from stimulant medication. A meta-analysis of nine double-blind, randomized, placebo-controlled trials (n = 477 subjects) concluded there was no evidence that methylphenidate worsened tic severity in the short term and that only supra-therapeutic doses of dextroamphetamine worsened tics (Bloch et al., 2009). In a Cochrane review, atomoxetine was found to significantly improve comorbid tics (Pringsheim and Steeves, 2011). The management of stimulant-provoked tics may include stimulant dose reduction, alpha-2 agonist, or a low dose of antipsychotic.

Misuse/abuse/diversion

Medication abuse and misuse is a growing concern in the US due to the increasing number of people who are prescribed stimulant medication for ADHD. Many ADHD treatment guidelines recommend the use of long-acting stimulant medications which can reduce the amount of short-acting stimulant medication available to patients, family members, and the community. The abuse of short-acting medications for the purpose of getting high is best achieved by the rapid introduction into the blood system, which is achieved by snorting, injecting, or inhaling short-acting stimulant medications. Because of this attribute, short-acting stimulant medications may have a higher liability for abuse and contribute to the diversion to non-patients. Misuse of these medications for performance enhancement by non-ADHD people is achieved with both short-acting and long-acting stimulant preparations. Therefore, when prescribing stimulant medications, the clinician ought to assess multiple factors in a household that will contribute to the risk of misuse/abuse/diversion. Psycho-education of patients and families about issues of misuse/abuse/diversion is an important part of diminishing the risks of these behaviours.

Seizures

In children with epilepsy, ADHD is the most frequent psychiatric disorder. Despite warnings in the drug information summaries, in well-controlled epilepsy trials methylphenidate is effective in reducing ADHD symptoms without increasing seizure risk. A review of literature on methylphenidate treatment for ADHD in paediatric patients with epilepsy also supports this conclusion (Baptista-Neto et al., 2008). Data on atomoxetine is sparse and safety has not been established.

Suicidal thoughts and behaviour

Suicidal thoughts and behaviour seem not to be directly associated with ADHD or stimulant medications. While atomoxetine carries a suicide warning, this risk is very low. If suicidal thoughts and/or behaviour occur, assessment for other current psychiatric disorders is necessary and treatment should be instituted accordingly.

Psychotic symptoms

Psychotic symptoms are not associated with ADHD and are rarely associated with ADHD medication treatment in the paediatric population. However, there are isolated case reports of emergent psychosis due to psychostimulants in children (Cherland and Fitzpatrick, 1999) and adults (Kraemer et al., 2010). Therefore, the use of stimulants should be judicious in patients with history of psychotic symptoms or history of family members with psychotic illnesses. Emergence of paranoia needs rapid assessment.

Elevated heart rate and/or blood pressure

Stimulants and atomoxetine may increase heart rate and/or systolic/diastolic blood pressure, although changes are usually mild. If needed, medication reduction, change in compound or preparation, an alpha-2 agonist, or antihypertensive medication may be considered. In adults, baseline vital signs may detect untreated hypertension that requires evaluation and treatment prior to the use of ADHD medication. Treated hypertension need not be an obstacle to ADHD medication use.

Drug interactions

Methylphenidate, amphetamines, and atomoxetine have no inhibitory effects on the cytochrome P450 isoenzymes. The liver does not metabolize methylphenidate.

Amphetamines have multiple metabolic pathways, one of which is 2D6. Atomoxetine is a 2D6 substrate whose metabolism will be altered by 2D6 inhibitors/inducers. Guanfacine and clonidine are 3A4 substrates whose metabolism may change with 3A4 inducers or inhibitors. While pharmacokinetic drug interactions may be limited, pharmacodynamic interactions exist with psychiatric, medical, over-the-counter medications, and herbs/supplements/caffeine. While these drug interactions are too numerous to mention here, clinicians should be mindful of side effects that can arise. It is best to query patients about all prescriptions and over-the-counter drugs (including caffeine) before starting ADHD medication.

Complementary and alternative treatment options

In Australia, 50 families were surveyed regarding their use of complementary and alternative medicine (CAM) and 67.6% of families reported current or past CAM (Sinha and Efron, 2005). Of the 23 different therapies reported, the most common was modified diet (33 families), vitamins and/or minerals (16), dietary supplements (12), aromatherapy (12), and chiropractic manipulation (10). Of the families that participated in the survey, 64% reported that they informed the paediatrician of their CAM use and slightly more than half the families used CAM to avoid medication side effects. Such treatments include neurofeedback, homeopathy, acupuncture, restriction and elimination diets, megavitamins, chiropractic manipulation, omega fatty acids, sugar elimination, pycnogenol, St John's wort, iron supplementation, and others. Clinicians need to assist patients and family in evaluating those treatments shown to be effective by research.

Neurofeedback

In a published meta-analytic review of EEG neurofeedback treatments in children with ADHD, five eligible studies with a total of 263 ADHD patients were identified (Micoulaud-Franchi et al., 2014). While the parent assessment (probably unblinded) showed an overall significant improvement in both inattention and hyperactivity/impulsivity scores, teacher assessment (probably blinded) demonstrated improvement only in inattention scores compared to controls. Holtmann and colleagues (2014) published a stringent meta-analysis of eight randomized controlled trials published in 2013 and found that the effects were stronger for unblinded measures; three recent subsequently published well-controlled trials found no effects for the most blinded ADHD outcome (2014). All the trials were conducted with children and the duration of the trials ranged from 2 weeks to 6 months.

Nutritional supplements

Bloch and Mulqueen (2014) reviewed the literature citing only randomized placebo-controlled trials and found that 15 RCT trials for polyunsaturated fatty acids suggesting a smaller yet real treatment benefit compared to stimulants; zinc (4 studies), iron (1), St John's wort (1), pycnogenol (2), carnitine (3), and melatonin (2) offer little evidence of efficacy.

Restrictive/elimination diets

In a review of diets, 11 review articles and five double-blind randomized trials investigated elimination or challenge diets in children with ADHD (total n = 135) (Nigg and Holton, 2014). The effect size is estimated at 0.3 which, although indicates a mild effect, may have a 10–30% chance in providing a clinically significant benefit.

Acupuncture

A literature review by Li and colleagues (2011) in children and adolescents with ADHD found no published randomized controlled double-blind studies. They concluded there is inadequate evidence to conclude any efficacy in the treatment of ADHD in this age population.

Homeopathy

A Cochrane review of homeopathy treatment for ADHD extracted eligible studies of children (total n = 160) (Coulter and Dean, 2007). The authors concluded that the data did not suggest significant treatment effects from global symptoms, core symptoms, or related outcomes such as anxiety in ADHD.

Meditation

A Cochrane review of meditation treatment for ADHD identified four randomized, placebo-controlled studies (Krisanaprakornkit et al., 2010). Two studies used mantra meditation and two studies used yoga but only two studies were appropriate for meta-analysis. The authors conclude that mantra meditation (mind-based) did not yield significant effects from medications and standard therapy controls. Yoga (physical-based) showed some positive findings, but these were inconsistent.

Psychotherapies

According to the best practice guidelines published in 2011 by the American Academy of Pediatrics, both medication treatment and behavioural therapy are recommended in children ages six and older (Wolraich et al., 2011).

Behaviour therapy

For children, behavioural therapy can be conceptualized in the areas of behavioural parent training, behaviour classroom management, and behavioural peer intervention. Parents and teachers are taught how to shape desirable behaviour with consequences. Consistency of consequences is critical to the success of this therapy. Behavioural peer intervention for the children may help navigate peer relations by reducing intrusion and emotional outbursts, and teaching cooperative reciprocity. For adults, the behaviour therapy paradigm is the same and the consequences leading to behaviour change need to be coordinated with the adult in treatment. Desirable behaviours may be broken down into smaller, achievable steps. Social skills training may also be needed for ADHD adults, who tend to interrupt conversation, intrude on personal space, or react abruptly.

Cognitive therapy

While there are 6 published trials of cognitive behavioural therapy (CBT) in adults with ADHD that show positive results, there is a paucity of cognitive therapy research in children and adolescents (Antshel and Olszewski, 2014). This therapy is a skill-based psychological technique to correct distortions in automatic thoughts that provoke more intense emotional reactions like anxiety and dysthymic moods.

Cognitive training

In contrast to cognitive therapy, cognitive training may be regarded as training the brain. A meta-analysis of clinical and neuropsychological outcomes from 16 randomized controlled trials with children showed no significant improvement in inattention and/hyperactivity/impulsivity symptoms by blinded raters (Cortese et al., 2013). While there were significant effects on laboratory tests for working memory, effects on academic performance were not statistically significant. We want to emphasize the point that unblinded raters found significant improvements across several measures while blinded raters did not note significant changes when compared to a control arm. In a meta-analysis of 12 controlled studies with children and adults evaluating Cogmed cognitive training, the authors noted significant improvement in working memory with a moderate effect size (Spencer-Smith and Klingberg, 2015). Therefore, working memory seems to improve, but behavioural changes and outcomes do not seem to be substantial.

Social skills training

An extensive literature review of randomized trials investigating social skills training for children with ADHD as monotherapy or with medication yields 11 trials with children (total n = 747) aged five–12 (Storebø et al., 2011). The duration of these interventions ranged from eight weeks up to two years, and there was a diverse range of social skills training modalities. Storebø et al conclude that there is not enough evidence to support the use of social skills training for children with ADHD. However, the heterogeneity of the therapies may have reduced the ability to discern benefits.

Psychosocial treatment

A review of the published meta-analysis identified 12 studies on psychosocial treatment (Fabiano et al., 2015). The difficulty in assessing its efficacy across the published studies is that diverse populations (inclusion/exclusion criteria), treatment modalities (e.g. social skills training, cognitive therapy, contingency management, parent management training, biofeedback), and outcome measures were employed. While it may appear to be intuitive to consider psychosocial interventions clinically useful, this review of meta-analysis studies does not offer clear guidance for the support of psychosocial interventions.

Treatment comparisons

In the most extensive review of published studies of pharmacological, non-pharmacological, and combination treatments for ADHD across the lifespan, statistically significant outcomes were reported in 50% (62/111) of pharmacologic trials, 65% (17/26) of non-pharmacologic trials, and 83% (19/23) of combined treatment trials (Arnold et al., 2015). In addition to direct improvement to ADHD core symptoms, all three categories of treatment differentially produced improvements in driving outcomes, self-esteem, social function, academic outcomes, antisocial behaviour, drugged and addictive behaviour, obesity, and occupational outcomes. With 51 studies used to evaluate the treatment effect over two to 13 years, the percentage of outcomes reported to improve was greater for the shorter follow-up time (<3 years) (93%) than with the longer follow-up time (>3 years) (57%). In this study, the highest effect sizes were associated with combined (pharmacological and non-pharmacological) treatments. The outcomes associated with large treatment effect sizes occurred in academic, self-esteem, and social functioning categories.

Patient follow-up

If a patient is prescribed medication, follow-up within two to three weeks is necessary to evaluate medication effects and side-effects, and to discuss any additional clinical information, as well as questions from the patient and/or parents. Medication dose adjustment may occur at this time depending on efficacy and tolerance and should include a subsequent follow-up after a further month. This will give the patient and/or parents adequate time within several environments and across several events to evaluate the medication effect and duration. All follow-up sessions must include checking vital signs and assessing any side effects. Optimal medication dosing is achieved when ADHD symptoms are substantially reduced throughout the entire day and side effects are manageable and tolerable. Using a parent/teacher rating scale for children or the ASRS can help to quickly assess treatment effects over time.

If psychotherapy is started without medication, follow-up may be done after one month to assess progress, gather additional clinical information, and provide support and guidance. If the psychotherapy is not substantially helpful in a defined timeframe (i.e. 3–6 months), reconsideration of medication choice and assessment of parent/patient resistance to medication is warranted.

The parent with ADHD symptoms

Parents may inquire about their own cognitive symptoms in a follow-up session. Given the high heritability (76%) of ADHD, it is not unusual to identify a parent with the disorder. Often, the effective treatment of an ADHD child is facilitated by treating the ADHD parent. With both child and parent treated, a behavioural program in the home is more consistently completed.

Conclusion

ADHD exists at a relatively high prevalence and will be present in patients of all ages seeking treatment in primary care settings. The negative consequences of untreated ADHD persist from childhood to adulthood with increasing cost to the patient, family, and society. Primary care clinicians increasingly will be asked to provide assessment, diagnosis, and treatment as the general public becomes more aware of this disorder. Diagnostic evaluation may be complicated by co-existing medical and psychiatric disorders. Diagnostic prioritization and treatment algorithms need to incorporate co-existing conditions. Prescribed medication needs to be monitored for optimal benefit, tolerability of side effects, long-term safety, and misuse/diversion. International research has established highly effective treatments (both medications and psychotherapeutic intervention) to reduce symptoms, and improve daily function and quality of life.

References

Antshel KM and Olszewski AK. (2014). Cognitive behavioral therapy for adolescents with ADHD. *Child Adolesc Psychiatr Clin N Am*, **23**: 825–42.

American Psychiatric Association (APA). (2013). *Diagnostic and statistical manual of mental disorders*. Arlington, VA: American Psychiatric Association.

Arnold LE, Hodgkins P, Caci H, Kahle J, and Young S. (2015). Effect of treatment modality on long-term outcomes in attention-deficit/hyperactivity disorder: a systematic review. *PLoS One*, **10**: e0116407.

Baptista-Neto L, Dodds A, Rao S, Whitney J, Torres A, and Gonzalez-Heydrich J. (2008). An expert opinion on methylphenidate treatment for attention deficit hyperactivity disorder in pediatric patients with epilepsy. *Expert Opin Investig Drugs*, **17**: 77–84.

Barkley RA and Fischer M. (2011). Predicting impairment in major life activities and occupational functioning in hyperactive children as adults: self-reported executive function (EF) deficits versus EF tests. *Dev Neuropsychol*, **36**: 137–61.

Biederman J, Petty C, Fried R, Fontanella J, Doyle AE, Seidman LJ and Faraone SV. (2006). Impact of psychometrically defined deficits of executive functioning in adults with attention deficit hyperactivity disorder. *Am J Psychiatry*, **163**: 1730–8.

Bloch MH and Mulqueen J. (2014). Nutritional supplements for the treatment of ADHD. *Child Adolesc Psychiatr Clin N Am*, **23**: 883–97.

Bloch MH, Panza KE, Landeros-Weisenberger A, and Leckman JF. (2009). Meta-analysis: treatment of attention-deficit/hyperactivity disorder in children with comorbid tic disorders. *J Am Acad Child Adolesc Psychiatry*, **48**: 884–93.

Brown TE, Holdnack J, Saylor K, Adler L, Spencer T, Williams DW, Padival AK, Schuh K, Trzepacz PT, and Kelsey D. (2011). Effect of atomoxetine on executive function impairments in adults with ADHD. *J Atten Disord*, **15**: 130–8.

Canadian ADHD Resource Alliance (CADDRA). (2011). *Canadian ADHD Practice Guidelines*. Toronto, ON: CADDRA.

Cherland E and Fitzpatrick R. (1999). Psychotic side effects of psychostimulants: a 5-year review. *Can J Psychiatry*, **44**: 811–3.

Conners CK, Epstein JN, March JS, Angold A, Wells KC, Klaric J, Swanson JM, Arnold LE, Abikoff HB, Elliott GR, Greenhill LL, Hechtman L, Hinshaw SP, Hoza B, Jensen PS, Kraemer HC, Newcorn JH, Pelham WE, Severe JB, Vitiello B, and Wigal T. (2001). Multimodal treatment of ADHD in the MTA: an alternative outcome analysis. *J Am Acad Child Adolesc Psychiatry*, **40**: 159–67.

Cortese S, Holtmann M, Banaschewski T, Buitelaar J, Coghill D, Danckaerts M, Dittmann RW, Graham J, Taylor E, and Sergeant J. (2013). Practitioner review: current best practice in the management of adverse events during treatment with ADHD medications in children and adolescents. *J Child Psychol Psychiatry*, **54**: 227–46.

Coulter MK and Dean ME. (2007). Homeopathy for attention deficit/hyperactivity disorder or hyperkinetic disorder. *Cochrane Database Syst Rev*, 17/4: CD005648.

De Zwann M, Gruss B, Muller A, Graap H, Martin A, Glaesmer H, Hilbert A, and Philipsen A. (2012). The estimated prevalence and correlates of adult ADHD in a German community sample. *Eur Arch Psychiatry Clin Neurosci*, 262: 79–86.

Fabiano GA, Schatz NKL, Aloe AM, Chacko A, and Chronis-Tuscano A. (2015). A systematic review of meta-analyses of psychosocial treatment for attention-deficit/hyperactivity disorder. *Clin Child Fam Psychol Rev*, 18: 77–97.

Faraone SV, Biederman J, Morley CP, and Spencer TJ. (2008). Effect of stimulants on height and weight: a review of the literature. *J Am Acad Child Adolesc Psychiatry*, 47: 994–1009.

Fayyad J, De Graff R, Kessler R, Alonso J, Angermeyer M, Demyttenaere K, De Girolamo G, Haro JM, Karam EG, Lara C, Lepine JP, Ormel J, Posada-Villa J, Zaslavsky AM, and Jin R. (2007). Cross-national prevalence and correlates of adult attention-deficit hyperactivity disorder. *Br J Psychiatry*, 190: 402–9.

Geller D, Donnelly C, Lopez F, Rubin R, Newcorn J, Sutton V, Bakken R, Paczkowski M, Kelsey D, and Sumner C. (2007). Atomoxetine treatment for pediatric patients with attention-deficit/hyperactivity disorder with comorbid anxiety disorder. *J Am Acad Child Adolesc Psychiatry*, 46: 1119–27.

Goodman D. (2006). Treatment and assessment of ADHD in adults. In: *ADHD Across the Life Span: From Research to Clinical Practice—An Evidence-Based Understanding*. Joseph Biederman, (ed). Hasbrouck Heights, NJ: Veritas Institute for Medical Education, Inc.

Goodman DW, Mitchell S, Rhodewalt L, and Surman CBH. (2016). Clinical presentation, diagnosis and treatment of attention-deficit hyperactivity disorder (ADHD) in older adults: A review of the evidence and its implications for clinical care. *Drug Aging*, 33(1): 27–36.

Graham J, Banaschewski T, Buitelaar J, Coghill D, Danckaerts M, Dittmann, RW, Dopfner M, Hamilton R, Hollis C, Holtmann M, Hulpke-Wette M, Lecendreux M, Rosenthal E, Rothenberger A, Santosh P, Sergeant J, Simonoff E, Sonuga-Barke E, Wong IC, Zuddas A, Steinhausen HC, and Taylor E. (2011). European guidelines on managing adverse effects of medication for ADHD. *Eur Child Adolesc Psychiatry*, 20: 17–37.

Holtmann M, Sonuga-Barke E, Cortese S, and Brandeis D. (2014). Neurofeedback for ADHD: a review of current evidence. *Child Adolesc Psychiatr Clin N Am*, 23: 789–806.

Hosenbocus S and Chahal R. (2012). A review of executive function deficits and pharmacological management in children and adolescents. *J Can Acad Child Adolesc Psychiatry*, 21: 223–9.

Jensen PS, Garcia JA, Glied S, Crowe M, Foster M, Schlander M, Hinshaw S, Vitiello B, Arnold LE, Elliott G, Hechtman L, Newcorn JH, Pelham WE, Swanson J, and Wells K. (2005). Cost-effectiveness of ADHD treatments: findings from the multimodal treatment study of children with ADHD. *Am J Psychiatry*, 162: 1628–36.

Jensen PS, Hinshaw SP, Kraemer HC, Lenora N, Newcorn JH, Abikoff HB, March JS, Arnold LE, Cantwelll DP, Conners CK, Elliott GR, Greenhill LL, Hechtman L, Hoza B, Pelham WE, Severe JB, Swanson JM, Wells KC, Wigal T, and Vitiello B. (2001). ADHD comorbidity findings from the MTA study: comparing comorbid subgroups. *J Am Acad Child Adolesc Psychiatry*, 40: 147–58.

Kessler RC, Adler L, Ames M, Demler O, Faraone S, Hiripi E, Howes MJ, Jin R, Secnik K, Spencer T, Ustun TB, and Walters EE. (2005). The World Health Organization Adult ADHD Self-Report Scale (ASRS): a short screening scale for use in the general population. *Psychol Med*, 35: 245–56.

Kessler RC, Adler L, Barkley R, Biederman J, Conners CK, Demler O, Faraone SV, Greenhill LL, Howes MJ, Secnik K, Spencer T, Ustun TB, Walters EE, and Zaslavsky A. (2006). The prevalence and correlates of adult ADHD in the United States: results from the National Comorbidity Survey Replication. *Am J Psychiatry*, 163: 716–23.

Kooij JJ and Bijlenga D. (2013). The circadian rhythm in adult attention-deficit/hyperactivity disorder: current state of affairs. *Expert Rev Neurother*, 13: 1107–16.

Kooij SJ, Bejerot S, Blackwell A, Caci H, Casas-Brugue M, Carpentier RP, Edvinsson D, Fayyad J, Foeken K, Fitzgerald M, Gaillac V, Ginsberg Y, Henry C, Krause J, Lensing MB, Manor I, Niederhofer H, Nunes-Filipe C, Ohlmeier MD, Oswald P, Pallanti S, Pehlivanidis A, Ramos-Quiroga JA, Rastam M, Ryffel-Rawak D, Stes S, and Asherson P. (2010). European consensus statement on diagnosis and treatment of adult ADHD: The European Network Adult ADHD. *BMC Psychiatry*, 10: 67.

Kraemer M, Uekermann J, Wiltfang J, and Kis B. (2010). Methylphenidate-induced psychosis in adult attention-deficit/hyperactivity disorder: report of 3 new cases and review of the literature. *Clin Neuropharmacol*, 33: 204–6.

Kratochvil CJ, Wilens TE, Greenhill LL, Gao H, Baker KD, Feldman PD, and Gelowitz DL. (2006). Effects of long-term atomoxetine treatment for young children with attention-deficit/hyperactivity disorder. *J Am Acad Child Adolesc Psychiatry*, 45: 919–27.

Krisanaprakornkit T, Ngamjarus C, Witoonchart C, and Piyavhatkul N. (2010). Meditation therapies for attention-deficit/hyperactivity disorder (ADHD). *Cochrane Database Syst Rev*, 6: CD006507.

Li S, Yu B, Zhou D, He C, Kang L, Wang X, Jiang S, and Chen X. (2011). Acupuncture for Attention Deficit Hyperactivity Disorder (ADHD) in children and adolescents. *Cochrane Database Syst Rev*, 4: CD007839.

Michielsen M, Semeijn E, Comijs HC, van de Ven P, Beekman AT, Deeg DJ, and Kooij JJ. (2012). Prevalence of attention-deficit hyperactivity disorder in older adults in The Netherlands. *Br J Psychiatry*, 201, 201/4: 298–305.

Micoulaud-Franchi JA, Geoffroy PA, Fond G, Lopez R, Bioulac S, and Philip P. (2014). EEG neurofeedback treatments in children with ADHD: an updated meta-analysis of randomized controlled trials. *Front Hum Neurosci*, 8: 906.

The MTA Cooperative Group. (1999). A 14-month randomized clinical trial of treatment strategies for attention-deficit/hyperactivity disorder. Multimodal Treatment Study of Children with ADHD. *Arch Gen Psychiatry*, 56/12: 1073–86.

National Insitute for Health and Care Excellence (NICE). (2009). *Attention Deficit Hyperactivity Disorder: Diagnosis and Management of ADHD in Children, Young People and Adults*. Leicester.

Nigg JT and Holton. (2014). Restriction and elimination diets in ADHD treatment. *Child Adolesc Psychiatr Clin N Am*, 23: 937–53.

Parker J, Wales G, Chalhoub N, and Harpin V. (2013). The long-term outcomes of interventions for the management of attention-deficit hyperactivity disorder in children and adolescents: a systematic review of randomized controlled trials. *Psychol Res Behav Manag*, 6: 87–99.

Pastor P, Reuben C, Duran C, and Hawkins L. 2015. Association between diagnosed ADHD and selected characteristics among children aged 4–17 years: United States, 2011–2013. *NCHS Data Brief*: 1–8.

Pliszka SR, Crismon ML, Hughes CW, Corners CK, Emslie GJ, Jensen PS, McCracken JT, Swanson JM, and Lopez M. (2006). The Texas Children's Medication Algorithm

Project: revision of the algorithm for pharmacotherapy of attention-deficit/hyperactivity disorder. *J Am Acad Child Adolesc Psychiatry,* 45: 642–57.

Polanczyk GV, Salum GA, Sugaya LS, Caye A, and Rohde L. (2015). Annual research review: A meta-analysis of the worldwide prevalence of mental disorders in children and adolescents. *J Child Psychol Psychiatry,* 56: 345–65.

Posner K, Melvin GA, Murray DW, Gugga SS, Fisher P, Skrobala A, Cunningham C, Vitiello B, Abikoff HB, Ghuman JK, Kollins S, Wigal SB, Wigal T, McCracken JT, McGough JJ, Kastelic E, Boorady R, Davies M, Chuang SZ, Swanson JM, Riddle MA, and Greenhill LL. (2007). Clinical presentation of attention-deficit/hyperactivity disorder in preschool children: the Preschoolers with Attention-Deficit/Hyperactivity Disorder Treatment Study (PATS). *J Child Adolesc Psychopharmacol,* 17: 547–62.

Pringsheim T and Steeves T. (2011). Pharmacological treatment for Attention Deficit Hyperactivity Disorder (ADHD) in children with comorbid tic disorders. *Cochrane Database Syst Rev,* 4: CD007990.

Scottish Intercollegiate Guidelines Network (SIGN). (2009). *Management of attention deficit and hyperkinetic disorders in children and young people: A national clinical guide,* Edinburgh: Elliott House.

Seidman L. (2006). Neuropsychological functioning in people with ADHD across the lifespan. *Clin Psychol Rev,* 26: 466–85.

Sinha D and Efron D. 2005. Complementary and alternative medicine use in children with attention deficit hyperactivity disorder. *J Paediatr Child Health,* 41: 23–6.

Spencer-Smith M and Klingberg T. (2015). Benefits of a working memory training program for inattention in daily life: a systematic review and meta-analysis. *PLoS One,* 10: e0119522.

Storebø OJ, Skoog M, Damm D, Thomsen PH, Simonsen E, and Gluud C. (2011). Social skills training for Attention Deficit Hyperactivity Disorder (ADHD) in children aged 5 to 18 years. *Cochrane Database Syst Rev:* CD008223.

Swanson J, Baler RD, and Volkow ND. (2011). Understanding the effects of stimulant medications on cognition in individuals with attention-deficit hyperactivity disorder: a decade of progress. *Neuropsychopharmacology,* 36: 207–26.

Visser SN, Danielson ML, Bitsko RH, Holbrook JR, Kogan MD, Ghandour RM, Perou R, and Blumberg SJ. (2014). Trends in the parent-report of health care provider-diagnosed and medicated attention-deficit/hyperactivity disorder: United States, 2003–2011. *J Am Acad Child Adolesc Psychiatry,* 53: 34–46 e2.

Wolraich M, Brown L, Brown RT, Dupaul G, Earls M, Feldman HM, Ganiats TG, Kaplanek B, Meyer B, Perrin J, Pierce K, Reiff M, Stein MT, and Visser S. (2011). ADHD: clinical practice guideline for the diagnosis, evaluation, and treatment of attention-deficit/hyperactivity disorder in children and adolescents. *Pediatrics,* 128: 1007–22.

World Health Organization (WHO). (1993). *ICD 10 Diagnostic Criteria for Mental and Behavioral Disorders: Clinical descriptions and diagnostic guidelines.* Geneva: World Health Organization.

Chapter 9

Trauma and stressor-related disorders

Andrea Feijo Mello and Mary Sau Ling Yeh

Introduction to trauma and stressor-related disorders

Although the manifestation of psychopathological symptoms after traumatic events has been described since 1860, the term post-traumatic stress disorder (PTSD) first appeared as a nosological entity in the third edition of the Diagnostic and Statistical Manual of Mental Disorders (American Psychiatric Association, 1980). The conceptualization of PTSD evolved from the First World War, when the term 'war neurosis' referred to psychiatric symptoms emerging after a traumatic experience. Soldiers received psychological first aid to help them cope with their traumatic experiences and then return to the front. However, it was only after the Vietnam War, through a political effort by the veterans, that the American Psychiatric Association (APA) coined the term PTSD and included it in the anxiety disorders section (Ringel and Brandel, 2012; Shorter 2005).

Although a period of distress almost always occurs after a traumatic event, the majority of people will not develop a mental disorder. However, some will present with severe distress, and may benefit from a proper diagnosis and early intervention (Wade et al., 2013).

General practitioners (GPs) usually evaluate patients during the acute phase after exposure to car accidents, natural disasters, violence assaults, and a sudden death of a family member, among other events. Therefore, GPs may play a relevant role in the early detection and treatment of trauma and stressor related disorders (Rothbaum et al., 2014). Debriefing immediately after an exposure to major traumatic events has proved to be an ineffective treatment strategy; in some clinical circumstances it may even be deleterious (i.e. it may enhance the consolidation of emotional memories, and also promote a sense of victimization). Thus, providing a sense of safety, calming, and hope is more appropriate in the first weeks following the traumatic event (Rose et al., 2002). In addition, benzodiazepines, which are usually prescribed in the emergency room for individuals with acute stress reactions, may lead to worse clinical outcome, and are not recommended (Gelpin et al., 1996).

The acute extreme response to a traumatic event is referred to as Acute Stress Disorder (ASD) and may occur in approximately 20% of individuals following trauma exposure. The provision of care immediately after exposure to a traumatic event may constitute a 'window of opportunity' for the prevention of PTSD, which is the most severe nosological entity of the chapter in the Trauma and stress-related disorders section of the DSM-5 (American Psychiatric Association, 2013).

ASD is characterized by symptoms of dissociation, avoidance, hyper-arousal, and negative thoughts and/or intrusion after exposure to an extreme traumatic event. The

Table 9.1 Other trauma and stressor-related diagnosis

Disorder	Main symptoms	Prevalence	Differential diagnosis
Reactive attachment (in children before age of five, and at least nine months)	Inhibited, emotionally withdrawn behaviour toward adult caregiver Minimal social and emotional responsiveness, irritability, sadness, fear Experienced neglect, deprivation, lack of stimulation and affection	Less than 10% in foster care or institutionalized children	Autism Depression
Disinhibited social engagement (in children at least nine months)	Child actively approaches and interacts with unfamiliar adults Socially disinhibited behaviour Experienced neglect, deprivation, lack of stimulation and affection	Less than 20% in foster care or institutionalized children	Attention deficit/ hyper activity disorder
Adjustment disorder (within three months of stressor)	Distress out of proportion of the stressor Impairment in social, occupational and other areas of functioning Not normal bereavement Does not last more than six months after the end of stressor Can be with: depressed mood and/or anxiety or conduct/emotion disturbance	Around 5–20% in outpatient mental health services 50% in hospital psychiatric consultations	Major depression PTSD and ASD, personality

Data from *Diagnostic and statistical manual of mental disorder*, 5th ed., 2013, American Psychiatric Association.

symptoms occur within the first month after the trauma. If the symptoms exceed this period of time, the diagnosis of PTSD is considered.

The Trauma and Stress Related Disorders section of the DSM-5 includes seven diagnostic entities: post-traumatic stress disorder, acute stress disorder, adjustment disorders, reactive attachment disorder, disinhibited social engagement disorder, other specific trauma and stressor-related disorder, unspecified trauma and stressor related disorder. This chapter provides a clinical overview of the epidemiology, diagnosis, and treatment of ASD and PTSD, which are the most prevalent DSM-5 trauma and stressor-related disorders. Table 9.1 provides a brief description of the other diagnostic categories.

Risk factors and epidemiology

Several factors may lead to heightened vulnerability to trauma and stressor-related disorders, which may include but are not limited to gender, type of trauma, frequency of exposure, genetic factors, early life trauma and adversities, and a lack of social support (Sayed et al, 2013).

Epidemiological studies have shown that women are nearly twice as susceptible to develop PTSD after exposure to a significant traumatic event. Certain types of trauma, e.g. participating in a war, being taken as a camp prisoner, torture, and rape seem to be more strongly related to the development of PTSD (American Psychiatric Association, 2013). In addition, evidence indicates that exposure to repetitive traumatic events may be associated with a higher risk of PTSD (Moreira et al., 2015). Furthermore, genetic and epigenetic factors confer a more intense and dysfunctional stress response to threat, and PTSD may thus result from complex gene-environment interactions (Rothbaum et al., 2014).

Certain developmental stages (i.e. childhood and adolescence) may be particularly vulnerable to de development of PTSD. Furthermore, exposure to early-life trauma may confer a higher risk to PTSD later in life. Therefore, at least to some extent, neurodevelopmental aspects may contribute to the neurobiology of PTSD. However, early-life trauma (e.g. childhood abuse and neglect) may be considered a non-specific risk factor for several mental disorders, including but not limited to depression, anxiety disorders, borderline personality disorder (BPD), and PTSD (Mello et al., 2009).

Prevalence estimates for PTSD have varied across studies (Santiago et al., 2013). Methodological inconsistencies and differences in the degree of trauma exposure in different countries and populations may contribute to the observed heterogeneity of findings. In the US, the lifetime prevalence of PTSD in the general population is 7.8% (American Psychiatric Association, 2013). For women, rates are around 10% while for men rates range from 5–7%. In Europe, data shows differences between countries, and exposure to traumatic experiences related to war and combat seem to significantly impact the prevalence of PTSD across different populations (Burri and Maercker, 2014). In comparison with the European Study of the Epidemiology of Mental Disorders Croatia showed a prevalence about ten times higher than in other included countries (e.g. Spain, Belgium, France and England) (Wittchen et al., 2011). In the Netherlands, the prevalence was reported to be 7.4% (de Vries and Olff, 2009). In Denmark, Elklit (2002) reported 9% of lifetime prevalence. In Northern Ireland a lifetime prevalence of 8.8% was observed, but prevalence rates increased to 14.6% when only the victims of conflicts (the 'troubles') were considered (Bamford Centre for Mental Health and Wellbeing, 2012). In Algeria studies reported prevalence rates as high as 37% and in Gaza rates of 17.8% have been reported (de Jong et al., 2001) In Brazil, an epidemiological study reported rates of 4.6% for males and 13.6% for females and PTSD was strongly related to urban violence (violent assault) (Ribeiro et al., 2013), while the same correlation between PTSD and interpersonal violence was reported in other Latin and Central America countries.

A recent systematic review showed that the mean prevalence of PTSD 12 months following a traumatic event is 17%, although if the traumatic event was intentional (e.g. terrorist attack, rape, physical assaultive violence) the rates increased to 23.3% (Santiago et al., 2013).

PTSD is also related to certain types of unhealthy behaviours such as alcohol misuse, drug abuse and high mortality rates (Weiss et al., 2015). Studies have indicated that PTSD is associated with hypertension, hyperlipidemia and cardiovascular disease (Cohen et al., 2009). Traumatic stress leads to dysregulation of the hypothalamic pituitary adrenal axis (HPA), increased activity of the autonomic nervous system, and elevation of inflammatory markers (McFarlane et al., 2010). Symptoms related to these comorbidities can be the reason for patients to seek primary care physicians; research findings indicate that subjects exposed to traumatic situations do not access medical care even when it is needed. In addition, low educational levels and low income, besides the stigma attached to mental disorders may contribute to the lack of service use (Ghafoori et al., 2014).

Individuals with PTSD often present with unhealthy behaviours. Therefore, patients should be encouraged to exercise and to seek treatment for smoking as well as alcohol-related disorders (Weiss et al., 2015). After receiving a diagnosis of PTSD, approximately 50% of patients will not achieve full remission even with adequate treatment (Perkonigg et al., 2005). GPs may aid in the early identification and treatment of PTSD and its comorbidities, leading to more favourable long-term outcomes.

Diagnosis

The DSM-IV criteria have been employed for two decades considering PTSD as an anxiety disorder, but with the publication of the DSM-5 a whole section dedicated to trauma and stressor-related disorders was introduced (American Psychiatric Association, 2013).

For both ASD and PTSD, the criterion requisite for diagnosis is very specific: exposure to an extreme traumatic event involving direct personal experience of actual or threatened death or serious injury, or other threat to physical integrity, or witnessing such kind of event or receiving the information of violent death or serious injury of a family member or close associate. The DSM-5 extended this requirement to include events that occurred to someone closely related to the individual as well as to first responders of traumatic events (e.g. police officers, fire-fighters or volunteers) who could be exposed to terrorist attacks, natural disasters, serious traffic accidents, etc. (American Psychiatric Association, 2013).

Additionally, in the DSM-5, for a diagnosis of ASD, symptoms of dissociation are no longer required to fulfil criteria (as in DSM-IV). However, nine out of 14 listed symptoms are now required for a diagnosis of ASD.

For PTSD, the DSM-5 clarifies that the reaction to a traumatic event can occur any time after the experience of trauma, and not necessarily during the event itself. It also now separates numbing from avoidance, while an additional criterion was significantly changed to encompass negative alterations in cognition and mood. Evidence indicates that during the development of PTSD patients frequently report feelings of affective detachment, negative perspectives about the future, irritability with routine activities, and difficulties in concentrating and learning new things. Therefore, this change in the DSM-5 aids in the differentiation of these negative symptoms from depressive symptoms, which may occur with PTSD as a comorbid disorder. In addition, negative

Table 9.2 Symptoms of PTSD

Re-experiencing symptoms (at least one symptom)	• Recurrent intrusive thoughts or memories • Flashbacks, feeling like experiencing the traumatic event again • Nightmares about the traumatic event
Avoidance symptoms (at least one symptom)	• Avoidance of thoughts, memories, or feelings that remind the event • Avoidance of situations, places or people associated with the event
Negative cognitions and mood symptoms (at least two symptoms)	• Marked loss of interest in activities that used to enjoy • Persistent negative beliefs about oneself or the world • Persistent negative emotions such as fear, guilt or shame • Inability to experience positive emotions • Distorted cognitions about the cause or consequences of the event • Inability to remember important parts of the event • Feeling detached or disconnected from other people
Hyperarousal symptoms (at least two symptoms)	• Hypervigilance, constantly alert for signs of danger or threat • Exaggerated startle response • Sleep disturbances such as insomnia • Impaired concentration • Feeling of irritability or angry outbursts • Reckless or self-destructive behaviour

Data from *Diagnostic and Statistical Manual of Mental Disorder*, 5th ed., 2013, American Psychiatric Association.

symptoms also include amnesia, negative beliefs (e.g. foreshortened future), distorted cognition and blame, negative emotions (e.g. fear, anger, horror, guilt, shame), diminished interest, detachment, and inability to experience positive emotions (American Psychiatric Association, 2013).

A fifth criterion is now referred to as arousal and reactivity, and includes an additional item (i.e. reckless and self-destructive behaviour).

In addition to these changes in criteria, the DSM-5 now incorporates two PTSD subtypes: a preschool subtype for children under six years old and a dissociative subtype for people who experience significant depersonalization and derealisation symptoms. The DSM-5 criteria for the diagnosis of children under six years old proved to be more developmentally sensitive than the DSM-IV criteria (Gigengack et al., 2013). The dissociative subtype with depersonalization and derealisation symptoms, which were only considered for ASD in DSM-IV, are extended to PTSD in DSM-5 because of the observed persistence of these type of symptoms in clinical settings with patients during follow-up treatment (Tsai et al., 2015) For a more complete listing of symptoms of PTSD see Table 9.2.

Screening

The utilization of screening tools may aid in the recognition of PTSD in primary care settings (Spoont et al., 2015). General practitioners should be watchful to the possibility of PTSD when patients seek health care complaining of multiple somatic symptoms such as chronic pain, musculoskeletal, gastrointestinal, dermatologic, or sleep disorders (NCCMH, 2005; American Psychiatric Association, 2004). Patients may not spontaneously report a history of trauma exposure, making it essential for primary care clinicians to directly ask about and screen for previous traumatic exposure. When assessing for PTSD, clinicians must be aware that patients may avoid talking about the trauma due to a fear or discomfort of re-experiencing traumatic memories. Fig. 9.1 provides an algorithm for the assessment of PTSD.

Many PTSD screening tools have been evaluated in primary care. Primary care PTSD Screen (PC-PTSD; van Dam et al., 2010) and PTSD Checklist (PCL) (Dickstein et al., 2015) are two of the most studied instruments for screening for PTSD in primary care. Both instruments are self-administered. The PC-PTSD (Fig. 9.2) is currently used to screen for PTSD in the US Veterans Affairs health care system, and a new version is being developed to incorporate diagnostic changes in DSM-5 criteria. There is already an updated DSM-5 version of PTSD Checklist (PCL-5), but this tool's psychometric properties have yet to be established. A two-step procedure has also been suggested, in which clinicians evaluate, in greater detail, the exposure to a traumatic event as well as PTSD symptoms when a patient screening is positive (Dickstein et al., 2015).

It is worth noting that these screening tools are not a substitute of a full clinical diagnostic evaluation. In addition, there is limited evidence to support that the routine screening of PTSD in primary care would lead to better outcomes.

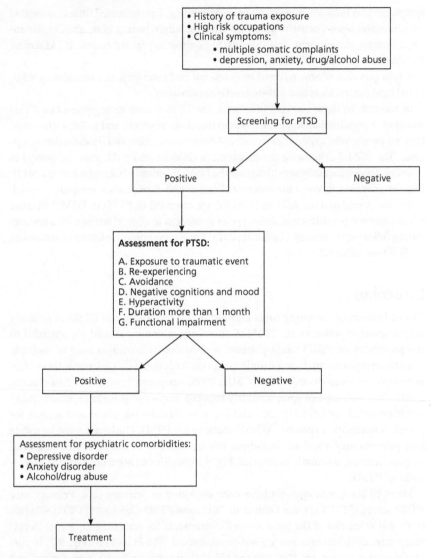

Fig. 9.1 Algorithm for assessment of posttraumatic stress disorder

Treatment

The treatment of PTSD is challenging due to the diversity of symptoms, individual experiences, and vulnerability. Evidence-based treatment of PTSD comprises psychological and pharmacological interventions. The selection of the most appropriate treatment strategy for an individual depends on the severity of symptoms, the presence of any comorbid conditions, and level of functioning.

The UK's National Institute for Health and Care Excellence (NICE) guidelines recommend trauma-focused psychological treatment, such as trauma-focused cognitive

---

Primary Care PTSD Screen (PC-PTSD)

Instructions:
In your life, have you ever had any experience that was so frightening, horrible, or upsetting that, in the past month, you:

	Yes	No
1. Have had nightmares about it or thought about it when your did not want to?		
2. Tried hard not to think about it or went out of your way to avoid situations that reminded you of it?		
3. Were constantly on guard, watchful, or easily startled?		
4. Felt numb or detached from others, activities, or your surroundings?		

PC-PTSD should beconsidered "positive" if a patient anseers "yes" to any three items.

Fig. 9.2 Primary care PTSD screen (PC-PTSD)
Reproduced from Primary Care PTSD Screen (PC-PTSD), Prins, et al, 2003, The National Center for PTSD, US Department of Veterans Affairs. Instrument available online: VA National Center for PTSD. Primary Care PTSD Screen (PC-PTSD). http://www.ptsd.va.gov/professional/assessment/screens/pc-ptsd.asp. Accessed January 9, 2015.

behavioural therapy or eye movement desensitization and reprocessing (EMDR) as first-line PTSD treatment for adults. When drug treatment is required, four drugs are recommended for first-line treatment: paroxetine, mirtazapine, amitriptyline and phenelzine (NCCMH, 2005).

The APA practice guidelines recommend both psychotherapy and pharmacotherapy as the initial treatment and selective serotonin reuptake inhibitors (SSRIs) as first-line pharmacotherapy (American Pyschiatric Association, 2004).

In primary care settings PTSD is usually under-recognized and treatment is not usually available, but some recent studies showed initiatives in the field of collaborative care (mental health professionals working together with primary care physicians helping to recognize acute stress mental symptoms) with promising results, but more large-scale and well-designed studies are still required (Fortney et al., 2015).

Psychological interventions

Fear is a normal reaction when an individual is exposed to danger or threat, and neurophysiological systems are activated in response to stress. Cortisol and noradrenaline released during stress act on the hippocampus, amygdala and prefrontal cortex, which are areas that influence memory function. Studies relate PTSD to maladaptive memory processing: consolidation of a traumatic event, retrieval of a traumatic event and impairment of memory extinction, suggesting memory dysfunction as a core element of PTSD (Trezza and Campolongo, 2013). Therefore, the development of PTSD occurs when trauma-related memories are not properly integrated into memory.

Several psychological interventions have been tried for PTSD treatment. Psychological debriefing intervention focuses on emotional processing by encouraging the recollection of the traumatic incident, which was thought to reduce acute emotional distress and prevent the development of PTSD. However, it has been shown that single-session individual debriefing for patients with ASD may increase the risk of PTSD (Rose et al., 2002).

Several reviews of psychotherapy interventions have been published demonstrating that trauma-focused cognitive-behavioural therapy (TFCBT) and similar exposure psychotherapies are effective in the treatment of ASD and PTSD. TFCBT targets the distorted thoughts and emotions related to traumatic event to desensitize the patient to trauma-related triggers, and it is a first-line treatment for ASD.

Another form of psychotherapy recognized as a treatment for both disorders is EMDR, which combines elements of exposure-based therapy, cognitive behaviour therapy, and concurrent induction of repeated eye movements.

In a Cochrane systematic review, the efficacy of the following categories of psychotherapeutic interventions was evaluated: TFCBT/exposure therapy, stress management, other therapies (supportive therapy, nondirective counselling, psychodynamic therapy, and hypnotherapy), group cognitive behavioural therapy and EMDR. The study concluded that individual and group TFCBT, stress management, and EMDR were more effective than wait list and other therapies (Wessely et al., 2000).

Some research on other lines of psychotherapy that do not emphasize exposure, e.g. interpersonal psychotherapy (Markowitz et al., 2015) and mindfulness (Kearney et al., 2012) has been recently published with positive results. These non-exposure therapies may help PTSD patients to cope with stress management, but there is no consensus in guidelines about them.

Pharmacological treatment

Antidepressants

The SSRIs are considered the first-line pharmacological treatment for PTSD. Large randomized, double-blind trials have shown their efficacy. Paroxetine is the only drug with a current UK product licence recommendation, while sertraline and paroxetine received approval from the US Food and Drug Administration for the treatment of PTSD. Although SSRIs are usually well tolerated and safe, there are side effects such as sexual dysfunction, gastrointestinal disturbances and discontinuation syndrome. SSRIs should be initiated with a low dose and adjusted gradually to avoid a possible ansiogenic side effect in the beginning of the treatment, especially in those patients with accentuated anxiety symptoms. Effective daily dosage has been in the same range as those used for treatment of depression. Response to SSRIs usually occurs after six to twelve weeks (Asnis et al., 2004). Nonetheless, approximately 60% of patients will respond to treatment and only 20–30% of patients will achieve remission (Stein et al., 2002).

Besides the SSRIs, venlafaxine, a serotonin norepinephrine reuptake inhibitor (SNRI), has the most evidence of efficacy in the treatment of PTSD.

A recent systematic review and meta-analysis of 51 randomized controlled trials to determine the efficacy of pharmacological treatment for PTSD found statistically significant evidence for the use of paroxetine, venlafaxine, and fluoxetine (Hoskins et al., 2015).

Early clinical trials with tricyclic antidepressants and monoamine oxidase inhibitors (MAOIs) suggested that these agents might be useful in PTSD treatment. Tricyclic antidepressants (TCAs), such as amitriptyline and imipramine, and monoamine oxidase inhibitors (MAOIs) such as phenelzine, have demonstrated beneficial effects in reducing PTSD symptoms (Davidson et al., 1990; Frank et al., 1988). However, TCAs also block histaminergic, cholinergic, and α_2 noradrenergic receptors, which causes unwanted side effects such as weight gain, dry mouth, constipation, drowsiness, and dizziness. Furthermore, MAOIs can interact with tyramine to cause a potential hypertensive crisis. Therefore, their use in clinical practice is limited by their side effects.

Adrenergic inhibitors

Studies of central nervous system norepinephrine suggest a pathophysiologic role of excessive norepinephrine in PTSD. Noradrenergic hyperactivity is thought to enhance consolidation of traumatic memories and increase risk of developing PTSD. Therefore, adrenergic inhibitors, which modulate noradrenergic activity, have been proposed as PTSD treatment. There are agents that decrease norepinephrine release such as clonidine, and agents that block post-synaptic norepinephrine receptors such as prazosin and propranolol.

Recent studies with prazosin, a central nervous system alpha-1 adrenergic antagonist, demonstrated improvements in PTSD symptoms and clinical efficacy for nightmares and sleep disturbances (Raskind et al., 2007; Raskind et al., 2003). The most common side effects of prazosin were dizziness and postural hypotension.

Case reports and open label trials with clonidine, an alpha-2 adrenergic agonist, have suggested that clonidine is effective in reducing hyperarousal and nightmares in patients with PTSD (Kinzie and Leung, 1989).

Anticonvulsants

The implication of the limbic kindling-like phenomenon in the pathophysiology of PTSD has stimulated clinical research of antiepileptic drugs for the treatment of this disorder. A hypothesis on the aetiology of PTSD has suggested that after exposure to traumatic events, the limbic nuclei may become kindled or sensitized, resulting in increased susceptibility to physiologic arousal (Post et al., 1997). There have been studies with carbamazepine, topiramate, lamotrigine, valproic acid, gabapentine and tiagabine. Topiramate is the anticonvulsant with more controlled studies in the treatment of PTSD and it seems to be effective for PTSD.

Atypical antipsychotics

Atypical antipsychotics may be helpful, particularly as adjunctive therapy, in the treatment of PTSD in cases with marked dissociative symptoms, treatment-resistant PTSD, and comorbid psychosis or bipolar disorder. Only a limited number of controlled clinical trials have investigated the use of olanzapine, risperidone, quetiapine and aripiprazol (Stein et al., 2002).

Although studies suggest promising results, larger controlled studies are necessary to confirm the efficacy of atypical antipsychotic agents for the treatment of PTSD.

Benzodiazepines (not recommended for ASD)

Benzodiazepines act on $GABA_A$ receptors, increasing the inhibitory activity of γ-aminobutyric acid system (GABA) resulting in sedation and also an anxiolytic effect. Although benzodiazepines may reduce anxiety symptoms and improve sleep in individuals with PTSD, clinical reports did not demonstrate long-term efficacy in the treatment of the core symptoms of PTSD nor prevented the development of the disorder (Gelpin et al., 1996; Mellman et al., 2002). Furthermore, benzodiazepine drugs may lead to substance use disorder as well as withdrawal syndrome upon discontinuation, which may exacerbate PTSD symptoms.

Table 9.3 Doses of pharmacological agents in the treatment of PTSD

Antidepressants	Doses (mg/day)
Paroxetine	20–50
Sertraline	50–200
Fluoxetine	20–80
Venlafaxine	75–300
Mirtazapine	15–45
Amitriptyline	50–300
Imipramine	50–300
Phenelzine	15–75
Anticonvulsants	**Doses (mg/day)**
Topiramate	25–500
Lamotrigine	50–500
Carbamazepine	300–1000
Antiadrenergic	**Doses (mg/day)**
Prazosin	2–15
Clonidine	0.2–0.4
Antipsychotics	**Doses (mg/day)**
Risperidone	0.5–6
Olanzapine	5–20
Quetiapine	25–300

Moreover, patients treated with benzodiazepines immediately after stress exposure may even increase the incidence of PTSD. The World Health Organization (WHO) recommends that benzodiazepines should not be used to reduce acute traumatic stress symptoms in the first month after a traumatic event (World Health Organization, 2013). (Table 9.3)

Pharmacological preventive interventions

Propranolol

Preclinical studies have suggested that the administration of β-adrenergic antagonist propranolol immediately after exposure to trauma may reduce the consolidation of traumatic memories. Open-label trials have suggested that propranolol may improve PTSD symptoms. Nevertheless, a subsequent study by Stein and colleague showed contradictory results. They conducted a randomized controlled trial of 14 days of propranolol (n = 17), gabapentin (n = 14) or placebo (n = 17) administered to patients within 48 hours of a traumatic injury. None of the drugs showed a significant benefit over placebo in PTSD prevention (Stein et al., 2007).

Docosahexaenoic acid

Experimental research demonstrated that docosahexaenoic acid (DHA) promoted hippocampal neurogenesis in the brain. It was hypothesized that neurogenesis promoted by omega-3 PUFA supplementation in the peritraumatic period might facilitate the extinction of fear memory and prevent PTSD. Clinical studies have found that DHA reduced PTSD symptoms in trauma exposed individuals. However, a randomized, double-blind, placebo-controlled trial found DHA ineffective when given to immediately after accident-injured patients (Matsuoka et al., 2015).

Conclusion

Individuals with an established diagnosis of PTSD face significant psychological distress, impairment in social and occupational functioning, and lower quality of life. Many people who have experienced a traumatic event may seek help from a primary care practitioner because of symptoms of somatization and the diagnosis of PTSD frequently may be missed. Increasing the ability of GPs to recognize and treat patients with ASD and PTSD can contribute to enhanced patient physical and emotional health.

Unfortunately, after receiving a diagnosis of PTSD, about 50% of patients do not achieve full remission. Even with adequate treatment, efforts to recognize acute symptoms and early intervention are needed to avoid the development of a chronic illness and serious functional impairment.

The first line of treatment includes psychological and pharmacological interventions, and in the primary care setting, although it is still in its development, collaborative care is a promising area of treatment for PTSD.

References

American Psychiatric Association. (1980). *Diagnostic and Statistical Manual of Mental Disorders-DSMIII.* 3rd ed. Washington, DC: American Psychiatric Association.

American Psychiatric Association. (2004). Practice guideline for the treatment of patients with acute stress disorder and post-traumatic stress disorder. Washington, DC: American Psychiatric Association.

American Psychiatric Association. (2013). *Diagnostic and Statistical Manual of mental Disorders-DSM-5.* Arlington: American Psychiatric Association.

Asnis GM, Kohn SR, Henderson M, and **Brown NL.** (2004). SSRIs versus non-SSRIs in post-traumatic stress disorder: an update with recommendations. *Drugs,* **64**/4:383–404.

Bamford Centre for Mental Health and Wellbeing. (2012). *Troubled consequences: a report on mental health impact of the civil conflict in Northern Ireland.* Belfast: Commission for Victims and Survivors. Available from: http://icrt.org.uk/wp-content/uploads/2012/11/2012-Dec-Troubled-Consequences.pdf.

Burri A and **Maercker A.** (2014). Differences in prevalence rates of PTSD in various European countries explained by war exposure, other trauma and cultural value orientation. *BMC Res Notes,* **7**: 407.

Cohen BE, Marmar C, Ren L, Bertenthal D, and **Seal KH.** (2009). Association of cardiovascular risk factors with mental health diagnoses in Iraq and Afghanistan war veterans using VA health care. *JAMA,* **302**/5: 489–92.

van Dam D, Ehring T, Vedel E, and **Emmelkamp PM.** (2010). Validation of the Primary Care Posttraumatic Stress Disorder screening questionnaire (PC-PTSD) in civilian substance use disorder patients. *J Subst Abuse Treat,* **39**/2: 105–13.

Davidson J, Kudler H, Smith R, Mahorney SL, Lipper S, Hammett E, Saunders WB, and **Cavenar JO Jr.** (1990). Treatment of posttraumatic stress disorder with amitriptyline and placebo. Arch Gen Psychiatry, **47**/3: 259–66.

Davidson J, Baldwin D, Stein DJ, Kuper E, Benattia I, Ahmed S, Pedersen R, and **Musgnung J.** (2006). Treatment of posttraumatic stress disorder with venlafaxine extended release: a 6-month randomized controlled trial. *Arch Gen Psychiatry,* **63**/10: 1158–65.

Dickstein BD, Weathers FW, Angkaw AC, Nievergelt CM, Yurgil K, Nash WP, Baker DG, Litz BT, and **Marine Resiliency Study Team.** (2015). Diagnostic Utility of the Posttraumatic Stress Disorder (PTSD) Checklist for Identifying Full and Partial PTSD in Active-Duty Military. *Assessment,* **22**/3: 289–97.

Gelpin E, Bonne O, Peri T, Brandes D, and **Shalev AY.** (1996). Treatment of recent trauma survivors with benzodiazepines: a prospective study. *J Clin Psychiatry,* **57**/9: 390–4.

Elklit A. (2002). Victimization and PTSD in a Danish national youth probability sample. *J Am Acad Child Adolesc Psychiatry,* **41**/2: 174–81.

Fortney JC, Pyne JM, Kimbrell TA, Hudson TJ, Robinson DE, Schneider R, Moore WM, Custer PJ, Grubbs KM, and **Schnurr PP.** (2015). Telemedicine-based collaborative care for posttraumatic stress disorder: a randomized clinical trial. *JAMA Psychiatry,* **72**/1: 58–67.

Frank JB, Kosten TR, Giller EL Jr, and **Dan E.** (1988). A randomized clinical trial of phenelzine and imipramine for posttraumatic stress disorder. *Am J Psychiatry,* **145**/10: 1289–91.

Gigengack MR, van Meijel EP, Alisic E, and **Lindauer RJ.** (2015). Comparing three diagnostic algorithms of posttraumatic stress in young children exposed to accidental trauma: an exploratory study. *Child Adolesc Psychiatry Ment Health,* **9**: 14.

Ghafoori B, Barragan B, and Palinkas L. (2014). Mental health service use among trauma-exposed adults: a mixed-methods study. *J Nerv Ment Dis*, 202/3: 239–46.

Hoskins M, Pearce J, Bethell A, Dankova L, Barbui C, Tol WA, van Ommeren M, de Jong J, Seedat S, Chen H, and Bisson JI. (2015). Pharmacotherapy for post-traumatic stress disorder: systematic review and meta-analysis. *Br J Psychiatry*, 206/2: 93–100.

de Jong JT, Komproe IH, Van Ommeren M, El Masri M, Araya M, Khaled N, van De Put W, and Somasundaram D. (2001). Lifetime events and posttraumatic stress disorder in 4 postconflict settings. *JAMA*, 286/5: 555–62.

Kearney DJ, McDermott K, Malte C, Martinez M, and Simpson TL. (2012). Association of participation in a mindfulness program with measures of PTSD, depression and quality of life in a veteran sample. *J Clin Psychol*, 68/1: 101–16.

Kinzie JD and Leung P. (1989). Clonidine in Cambodian patients with posttraumatic stress disorder. *J Nerv Ment Dis*, 177/9: 546–50.

Markowitz JC, Petkova E, Neria Y, Van Meter PE, Zhao Y, Hembree E, Lovell K, Biyanova T, and Marshall RD. (2015). Is Exposure Necessary? A Randomized Clinical Trial of Interpersonal Psychotherapy for PTSD. *Am J Psychiatry*, 172/5: 430–40.

Matsuoka Y, Nishi D, Hamazaki K, Yonemoto N, Matsumura K, Noguchi H, Hashimoto K, and Hamazaki T. (2015). Docosahexaenoic acid for selective prevention of posttraumatic stress disorder among severely injured patients: a randomized, placebo-controlled trial. *J Clin Psychiatry*, 76/8: e1015–22.

McFarlane AC. (2010). The long-term costs of traumatic stress: intertwined physical and psychological consequences. *World Psychiatry*, 9/1: 3–10.

McLean SA, Clauw DJ, Abelson JL, and Liberzon I. (2005). The development of persistent pain and psychological morbidity after motor vehicle collision: integrating the potential role of stress response systems into a biopsychosocial model. *Psychosom Med*, 67/5: 783–90.

Mellman TA, Bustamante V, David D, and Fins AI. (2002). Hypnotic medication in the aftermath of trauma. *J Clin Psychiatry*, 63/12:1183–4.

Mello MF, Faria AA, Mello AF, Carpenter LL, Tyrka AR, and Price LH. (2009). [Childhood maltreatment and adult psychopathology: pathways to hypothalamic-pituitary-adrenal axis dysfunction]. *Revista brasileira de psiquiatria*, 31/Suppl 2: S41–8.

Moreira FG, Quintana MI, Ribeiro W, Bressan RA, Mello MF, Mari JJ, and Andreoli SB. (2015). Revictimization of violence suffered by those diagnosed with alcohol dependence in the general population. *Biomed Res Int*, 2015: 805424.

NCCMH. (2005). *Post-traumatic Stress Disorder: the Management of PTSD in Adults and Children in Primary and Secondary Care*. Leicester and London: The British Psychological Society and the Royal College of Psychiatrists.

Perkonigg A, Pfister H, Stein MB, Hofler M, Lieb R, Maercker A, and Wittchen HU. (2005). Longitudinal course of posttraumatic stress disorder and posttraumatic stress disorder symptoms in a community sample of adolescents and young adults. Am J *Psychiatry*, 162/7: 1320–7.

Post RM, Weiss SR, Smith M, Li H, and McCann U. (1997). Kindling versus quenching. Implications for the evolution and treatment of posttraumatic stress disorder. *Ann NY Acad Sci*, 821: 285–95.

Raskind MA, Peskind ER, Kanter ED, Petrie EC, Radant A, Thompson CE, et al. (2003). Reduction of nightmares and other PTSD symptoms in combat veterans by prazosin: a placebo-controlled study. *Am J Psych*, 160/2: 371–3.

Raskind MA, Peskind ER, Hoff DJ, Hart KL, Holmes HA, Warren D, Shofer J, O'Connell J, Taylor F, Gross C, Rohde K, and McFall ME. (2007). A parallel group placebo controlled study of prazosin for trauma nightmares and sleep disturbance in combat veterans with post-traumatic stress disorder. *Biol Psychiatry*, 61/8: 928–34.

Ribeiro WS, Mari Jde J, Quintana MI, Dewey ME, Evans-Lacko S, Vilete LM, Figueira I, Bressan RA, de Mello MF, Prince M, Ferri CP, Coutinho ES, and Andreoli SB (2013). The impact of epidemic violence on the prevalence of psychiatric disorders in Sao Paulo and Rio de Janeiro, Brazil. *PLoS One*, 8/5: e63545.

Ringel S and Brandel JR. (2012). *Trauma. Contemporary directions in theory, practice and research*. Thousand Oaks: SAGE Publications.

Rose S, Bisson J, Churchill R, and Wessely S. (2002). Psychological debriefing for preventing posttraumatic stress disorder (PTSD). *Cochrane Database Syst Rev*, 2: (CD000560).

Rothbaum BO, Kearns MC, Reiser E, Davis JS, Kerley KA, Rothbaum AO, Mercer KB, Price M, Houry D, and Ressler KJ. (2014). Early intervention following trauma may mitigate genetic risk for PTSD in civilians: a pilot prospective emergency department study. *J Clin Psychiatry*, 75/12: 1380–7.

Santiago PN, Ursano RJ, Gray CL, Pynoos RS, Spiegel D, Lewis-Fernandez R, Friedman MJ, and Fullerton CS. (2013). A systematic review of PTSD prevalence and trajectories in DSM-5 defined trauma exposed populations: intentional and non-intentional traumatic events. *PLoS One*, 8/4: e59236.

Sayed S, Iacoviello BM, and Charney DS. (2015). Risk factors for the development of psychopathology following trauma. *Curr Psychiatry Rep*, 17/8: 612.

Shorter E. (2005). A historical dictionary of psychiatry. New York: Oxford University Press.

Spoont MR, Williams JW, Jr., Kehle-Forbes S, Nieuwsma JA, Mann-Wrobel MC, and Gross R. (2015). Does This Patient Have Posttraumatic Stress Disorder?: Rational Clinical Examination Systematic Review. *JAMA*, 314/5: 501–10.

Stein MB, Kline NA, and Matloff JL. (2002). Adjunctive olanzapine for SSRI-resistant combat-related PTSD: a double-blind, placebo-controlled study. The *Am J Psychiatry*, 159/10: 1777–9.

Stein MB, Kerridge C, Dimsdale JE, and Hoyt DB. (2007). Pharmacotherapy to prevent PTSD: Results from a randomized controlled proof-of-concept trial in physically injured patients. *J Trauma Stress*, 20/6: 923–32.

Trezza V and Campolongo P. (2013). The endocannabinoid system as a possible target to treat both the cognitive and emotional features of post-traumatic stress disorder (PTSD). *Front Behav Neurosci*, 7: 100.

Tsai J, Armour C, Southwick SM, and Pietrzak RH. (2015). Dissociative subtype of DSM-5 posttraumatic stress disorder in U.S. veterans. *J Psychiatr Res*, 66–67: 67–74.

de Vries GJ and Olff M. (2009). The lifetime prevalence of traumatic events and posttraumatic stress disorder in the Netherlands. *J Trauma Stress*, 22/4: 259–67.

Wade D, Howard A, Fletcher S, Cooper J, and Forbes D. (2013). Early response to psychological trauma—what GPs can do. *Aust Fam Physician*, 42/9: 610–4.

Weiss NH, Tull MT, Sullivan TP, Dixon-Gordon KL, and Gratz KL. (2015). Posttraumatic stress disorder symptoms and risky behaviors among trauma-exposed inpatients with substance dependence: The influence of negative and positive urgency. *Drug Alcohol Depend*, 155: 147–53.

Wessely S, Bisson J, and Rose S. (2000). A systematic review of brief psychological interventions (debriefing) for the treatment of post traumatic stress disorder. In: R

Oakley-Browne, D Gill, M Trivedi, and S Wessely, eds., *Depression, Anxiety and Neurosis module of the Cochrane Database of Systematic reviews Oxford*: Issue 3 ed, update Software.

Wittchen HU, Jacobi F, Rehm J, Gustavsson A, Svensson M, Jönsson B, Olesen J, Allgulander C, Alonso J, Faravelli C, Fratiglioni L, Jennum P, Lieb R, Maercker A, van Os J, Preisig M, Salvador-Carulla L, Simon R, and Steinhausen HC. (2011). The size and burden of mental disorders and other disorders of the brain in Europe 2010. *Eur neuropsychopharmacol*, 21/9: 655–79.

World Health Organization. (2013). *Guidelines for the management of conditions specifically related to stress*. Available from: http://apps.who.int/iris/bitstream/10665/85119/1/9789241505406_eng.pdf.

Chapter 10

Depressive disorders

Andrea Fagiolini, Giovanni Amodeo,
and Giuseppe Maina

Introduction

In recent years the delivery of mental health services has changed significantly. Many individuals, especially depressed patients, now receive psychiatric treatment from General Practitioners (GPs), rather than from mental health specialists. For instance, it has been observed that that over a ten-year period, from 1987 to 1997, the percentage of patients who received psychiatric medication from primary care providers (PCPs) increased from 37.3% to 74.5% (Olfson, 2002). Indeed, GPs have a key role in tasks such as: 1) identifying a patient's symptoms early before they intensify into a more serious condition; 2) minimizing adverse outcomes such as suicide or homicide by providing early intervention; 3) reducing drug or alcohol abuse, by providing patients with alternative treatments, such as psychiatric medications and therapy, or an appropriate referral; and 4) improving treatment outcomes by actively collaborating with mental health clinicians in coordinating more comprehensive psychiatric care for patients. The wish of patients to receive treatment from their GP, or at least to have their GPs more involved in their care, has been repeatedly recognized. Hence, improving mental health treatment requires enhancing the ability of GPs to screen, diagnose, treat, and appropriately manage the psychiatric conditions of their patients. These enhancements can happen through 'collaborative care' programmes, i.e. specific interventions incorporating a multiprofessional approach to patient care. These collaborative care programmes include a structured management plan, scheduled patient follow-ups, and enhanced interprofessional communication between GPs and mental health specialists. They are facilitated by appropriate continuing medical education programmes and by the introduction of a care manager (CM). The CM is responsible for delivering care to patients with depression under the supervision of both a GP and a specialist, and, at the same time, is responsible for liaising between GPs and mental health specialists (Richards, 2013).

Depression is a serious illness that has an impact on both body and mental health. The sadness of depression is characterized by a greater intensity and duration and by more severe symptoms and functional impairment than is normal. In addition to depressed mood, individuals with depression experiment a combination of symptoms that interfere with the ability to sleep, concentrate, eat, work, study, or enjoy everyday activities. Depression causes pain for both the person with the disorder and those who care about them. Depression is not a sign of personal weakness, nor is it a condition that can be willed away. Without an appropriate treatment, symptoms can last over long periods, and can stretch to months or years.

According to DSM-5, depressive disorders come in different forms and include major depressive disorder (MDD), persistent depressive disorder (PDD)—also known as dysthymic disorder or dysthymia-, disruptive mood dysregulation disorder (DMDD), premenstrual dysphoric disorder (PMDD), substance-induced depressive disorder (SMDD), and depressive disorder due to another medical condition (DDAM) (American Psychiatric Association, 2013).

Major depressive disorder

Major depressive disorder (MDD) represents the classic condition among depressive disorders and is characterized by the occurrence of one or more depressive episodes in a person that has never experienced a period of abnormal mood elation. A depressive episode involves a period of at least two weeks and the person experiences symptoms such as depressed mood, loss of interest or pleasure in everyday activities, feelings of emptiness, tearfulness, hopelessness, low self-esteem, worthlessness, guilt, insomnia or hypersomnia, changes in appetite, problems concentrating, remembering details or making decisions, and thoughts of, or attempts at, suicide. Individuals may also report feeling less interested in things they used to enjoy, such as sport, hobbies, or other activities that were previously considered pleasurable (American Psychiatric Association, 2013).

Appetite change may involve either an increase or reduction of appetite. Regardless of eating more or less, depressed individuals usually do not enjoy eating. Sleep disturbance may include insomnia or hypersomnia (sleeping excessively). Individuals typically experience middle insomnia (i.e. waking up in the middle of the night and then having difficulty returning to sleep) or late insomnia (i.e. waking up too early in the morning and being unable to return to sleep). However, early insomnia (i.e. difficulty falling asleep) may occur as well. Other depressed individuals present with oversleeping (hypersomnia) and may experience prolonged sleep at night or increased daytime sleep. Regardless of the presence of insomnia or hypersomnia, depressed individuals almost always complain of non-restful sleep.

Psychomotor agitation (e.g. pacing, inability to sit still, pulling the skin) or psychomotor retardation (e.g. slowed thinking, slowed speech, reduced body movements) may also be present. Frequently, depressed subjects also report fatigue, decreased energy, and tiredness. Many individuals complain of a difficulty to concentrate, make even minor decisions, memory difficulties, or distractibility.

Patients with depression may also experience symptoms such as feeling that life is not worth living or that they would be better off dead. Occasionally patients with depression may express a wish for a fatal illness or to die because of an accident. Unfortunately, a number of patients plan, attempt, or complete suicide. One of the most constantly described risk-factors for suicide is a history of suicide attempts or threats. However, many completed suicides are not preceded by previous unsuccessful attempts. Other features associated with an increased risk for suicide include being single or living alone, male sex, and hopelessness.

Common symptoms and signs of depression in *children and teenagers* are similar to those of adults, but younger children may present with refusal to go to school, clinginess, irritability, worry, aches and pains, or reduced appetite and being underweight. In teens, symptoms may include worthlessness, sadness, irritability, anger, self-harm, poor performance at school, avoidance of social interactions, being very sensitive and feeling misunderstood, loss of interest, using drugs or alcohol, and eating or sleeping too much.

In *older adults*, symptoms may be less obvious and different than those that manifest in younger adults. Elderly patients with depression often complain of memory problems, physical aches or pain, fatigue, loss of appetite, sleep problems, the inability to leave the house, socialize or doing new things, and suicidal thoughts or feelings. Memory difficulties may be mistaken for early signs of a dementia ('pseudo-dementia'). Yet, a major depressive episode may be still the initial presentation of an irreversible dementia.

Patients with *bipolar disorder* may present with episodes of depression identical to the episodes observed in patients with MDD. However, a history of manic or hypomanic episodes is never recorded in MDD patients and the treatment of bipolar depression is very different. In fact, it is paramount that patients with BPD never be treated with an antidepressant before a treatment with an anti-manic agent (i.e. a mood stabilizer or an atypical antipsychotic) has been established.

Persistent depressive disorder

Persistent depressive disorder (PDD), also known as dysthymic disorder or dysthymia, involves long-term (two years or longer) symptoms, which are usually less severe than MDD symptoms and do not severely disable the patient. However, usually the patient complains of not feeling well and/or not functioning normally.

People with dysthymia experience a depressed mood for at least 2 years, accompanied by other symptoms such as reduced/increased appetite, reduced/increased sleep, low energy or fatigue, low self-esteem, and poor concentration or difficulty making decisions. Many people with dysthymia may also experience superimposed major depressive episodes at some time in their lives (American Psychiatric Association, 2013).

Premenstrual dysphoric disorder

Premenstrual dysphoric disorder (PDD) is characterized by mood lability (e.g. mood swings, feeling suddenly tearful or sad, or increased sensitivity to rejection or increased interpersonal conflicts), irritability, dysphoria, and anxiety symptoms that occur repeatedly during the premenstrual phase and remit around the onset of menses or shortly thereafter. These symptoms may be accompanied by feelings of hopelessness, tension, feelings of being 'keyed up', decreased interest in usual activities, difficulty in concentration, lack of energy, fatigability, change in appetite, overeating, hypersomnia or insomnia, and feeling overwhelmed or out of control.

Additionally, there may also be a presence of physical symptoms, such as breast tenderness or swelling, joint or muscle pain, a sensation of 'bloating', or weight gain (American Psychiatric Association, 2013).

Substance-induced depressive disorder

The diagnostic features of Substance-induced depressive disorder (SIDD) includes symptoms such depressed mood or diminished interest in everyday activities and which developed during or soon after substance intoxication or withdrawal or after exposure to a medication. A SIDD is distinguished from a primary depressive disorder by considering the onset, course as well as other factors associated with the substance use. Of course, to make this diagnosis, there must be evidence of substance use, abuse, intoxication, or withdrawal prior to the onset of the depressive disorder. Also, the diagnosis should not be better explained by an independent depressive disorder, such as in those cases when the depressive disorder preceded the onset of ingestion or withdrawal from the substance (American Psychiatric Association, 2013).

Depressive disorder due to another medical condition

Depressive disorder due to another medical condition (DDAMC) may be diagnosed when there is evidence from the history, physical examination, or laboratory findings that a depressive disorder is the direct pathophysiological consequence of another medical condition (American Psychiatric Association, 2013). Hence, the clinician should establish that the mood disturbance is etiologically related to the general medical condition.

Disruptive mood dysregulation disorder

Disruptive mood dysregulation disorder (DMDD) refers to the presentation of children with persistent irritability and severe recurrent temper outbursts. Recurrent episodes of severe behavioural dyscontrol usually include verbal rages and physical aggression toward people or property. The mood is persistently angry and irritable even between temper outbursts.

According to DSM, onset must be before the age of ten years, and the diagnosis should not be applied to children that are less than six years, nor should it be made for the first time after 18 years of age. DMDD cannot coexist with oppositional defiant disorder (ODD), intermittent explosive disorder (IED), MDD, attention-deficit/hyperactivity disorder (ADHD), conduct disorder (CD), and substance use disorders (SUD) (American Psychiatric Association, 2013).

Treatment of major depressive disorder

Multiple drug classes are available for the treatment of MDD. While newer classes of medications are usually the first line of treatment, older medications might still be chosen, depending on the subtype of MDD, the age of the patient, cost considerations, and the practitioner's preferences. Before starting a treatment, a careful evaluation of suicide risk is necessary, including specific inquiries about suicidal thoughts, plans, means, intent, and behaviours; evaluation of current or past presence of symptoms and conditions such as psychosis, substance use, bipolar symptoms, and severe anxiety, all of which may increase the likelihood of acting on suicidal thoughts. Past and recent suicidal behaviour should be evaluated along with the current stressors and potential protective factors (e.g. presence of children at home, religious/spiritual beliefs, positive reasons for living, and a high level of social support). Family history of suicide should be carefully evaluated and given appropriate weight in treatment decisions. Impulsivity and potential for risk to others should also be assessed, including any history of violence or homicidal ideas, plans, or intentions. The patient's risk of self-harm or harm to others should also be monitored as treatment proceeds (American Psychiatric Association, 2010).

Most antidepressants have similar rates of efficacy overall but differ in terms of side-effect profiles. Usually, the initial selection of an antidepressant medication is based on the safety, anticipated side effects, and their tolerability for the individual patient. Pharmacological properties of the medication (e.g. half-life, actions on cytochrome P450 enzymes, other drug interactions, efficacy on sleep, efficacy on anxiety), and additional factors such history of response in prior episodes, cost, and patient preference must be considered as well. For most patients, the first-line treatment is usually a selective serotonin-reuptake inhibitor, psychotherapy, or a combination of pharmacotherapy and psychotherapy (Gelenberg, 2010).

Selective serotonin reuptake inhibitors currently available include fluoxetine, sertraline, paroxetine, fluvoxamine, citalopram, and escitalopram. A large body of literature supports the superiority of SSRIs compared with placebo, including trials conducted in primary care settings (Arroll et al., 2005). Also, in several trials, SSRIs have demonstrated comparable efficacy to the TCAs (Cipriani, 2005; Anderson, 2000; Montgomery, 2001).

Serotonin norepinephrine reuptake inhibitors (SNRIs) mirtazapine or bupropion are good choices as well. Next-step treatment recommendations are switching or augmentation, depending on patient response to the initial treatment. In general, the use of nonselective monoamine oxidase inhibitors (MAOIs) should be restricted to patients who do not respond to other treatments, given the potential for deleterious drug-drug interactions (DDIs) and the necessity for dietary restrictions (American Psychiatric Association, 2010).

Electroconvulsive therapy (ECT) should be considered as a treatment option for individuals with major depressive disorder who experience psychotic features or catatonia. Also, ECT is a first line choice for patients with an urgent need for response, such as patients at high suicide risk or those who refuse to eat. Other situations favouring ECT include the presence of co-occurring general medical conditions that preclude the use of antidepressant medications, a prior history of positive response to ECT, and patient preference (American Psychiatric Association, 2010).

Once an antidepressant medication has been initiated, the titration rate to a full therapeutic dose usually depends upon tolerability, patient's age, co-occurring illnesses, and concomitant medications. During the acute phase of treatment, patients should be evaluated on a regular basis to assess their response and patient safety, and to identify the emergence of side effects (e.g. dizziness, blurred vision, gastrointestinal symptoms, sedation, insomnia, activation, changes in weight, and cardiovascular, neurological, anticholinergic, sexual side effects, etc.).

The starting and usual doses of the most commonly used antidepressants are reported in Table 10.1. Links to the FDA-approved prescribing information are reported in Box 10.1.

SSRIs undergo hepatic oxidative metabolism before their elimination from the body; therefore, genetic differences in oxidative metabolism can significantly impact the levels of an active drug circulating in a patient. Also, SSRIs have variable effects on hepatic microsomal enzymes and may increase or decrease the blood levels of other medications. For instance, SSRIs that strongly inhibit the CYP 2D6 isoenzyme (e.g.

Table 10.1 Doses of most commonly used antidepressants

Initial Dose (mg)		Range (mg)
SSRIs		
Citalopram	20	20–40*
Escitalopram	10	10–20**
Fluoxetine	20	20–80
Paroxetine	20	10–50
Paroxetine extended release	25	25–62.5
Sertraline	50	50–200
SNRIs		
Duloxetine	40–60	40–60
Venlafaxine extended release	37.5–75	75–225
Desvenlafaxine	50	50
Atypical		
Bupropion	100 twice a day	100–400***
Bupropion extended release (XL)	150	150–450
Mirtazapine	37.5–75	15–45
Trazodone Contramid COAD	150	150–300

*20 mg/day is the citalopram recommended dose for most elderly patients and patients with hepatic impairment

**10 mg/day is the escitalopram recommended dose for most elderly patients and patients with hepatic impairment

***The limit of 150 mg in a single dose of non-XL bupropion should never be exceeded

Box 10.1 FDA-approved prescribing information

Bupropion, FDA-approved prescribing information. Accessed on January 2016 at:
http://www.fda.gov/ohrms/dockets/ac/04/briefing/2004-4065b1-20-tab11A-Wellbutrin-Tabs-SLR028.pdf

Buproprion extended release (wellbutrin XL), FDA-approved prescribing information. Accessed on January 2016 at:
http://www.accessdata.fda.gov/drugsatfda_docs/label/2009/021515s023s024lbl.pdf

Citalopram, FDA-approved prescribing information. Accessed on January 2016 at:
http://www.accessdata.fda.gov/drugsatfda_docs/label/2009/020822s037, 021046s015lbl.pdf

Desvenlafaxine, FDA approved prescribing information. Accessed on January 2016 at:
http://labeling.pfizer.com/showlabeling.aspx?id=497%20

Duloxetine, FDA approved prescribing information. Accessed on January 2016 at:
http://pi.lilly.com/us/cymbalta-pi.pdf

Escitalopram, FDA approved prescribing information. Accessed on January 2016 at:
http://pi.actavis.com/data_stream.asp?product_group=1907&p=pi&language=E

Fluoxetine, FDA approved prescribing information. Accessed on January 2016 at:
http://www.accessdata.fda.gov/drugsatfda_docs/label/2011/018936s091lbl.pdf

Mirtazapine, FDA approved prescribing information. Accessed on January 2016 at:
https://www.merck.com/product/usa/pi_circulars/r/remeron/remerontablets_pi.pdf

Paroxetine, FDA approved prescribing information. Accessed on January 2016 at:
https://www.apotex.com/us/en/products/downloads/pil/paxil_irtb_ins.pdf

Paroxetine extended release, FDA approved prescribing information. Accessed on January 2016 at:
http://www.fda.gov/ohrms/dockets/ac/04/briefing/4006b1_08_paxil-label.pdf

Sertraline, FDA approved prescribing information. Accessed on January 2016 at:
http://www.accessdata.fda.gov/drugsatfda_docs/label/2009/019839s070, 020990s032lbl.pdf

Trazodone OAD Contramid, FDA approved prescribing information. Accessed on January 2016 at:
http://www.accessdata.fda.gov/drugsatfda_docs/label/2010/022411lbl.pdf

Venlafaxine, FDA approved prescribing information. Accessed on January 2016 at:
http://labeling.pfizer.com/showlabeling.aspx?ID=100

paroxetine, fluoxetine) may reduce the metabolism of tamoxifen to its active metabolite is reduced, resulting in a decrease in its efficacy in preventing breast cancer relapse (Stearns, 2003; Jin, 2005; Desmarais, 2009). This effect is also observed for other antidepressants, such as bupropion (Desmarais, 2009).

Serotonin norepinephrine reuptake inhibitors

The serotonin norepinephrine reuptake inhibitors currently available are venlafaxine, desvenlafaxine (the primary metabolite of venlafaxine), and duloxetine. For venlafaxine and most likely desvenlafaxine, norepinephrine reuptake inhibition may not be achieved at lower therapeutic doses. Venlafaxine and duloxetine are generally as effective as SSRIs (Nemeroff, 2008; Thase, 2007). Analyses of pooled data sets have found small advantage for SNRIs over SSRIs, which might suggest a benefit for patients with more severe depression or for individuals who have not responded to SSRIs (Thase, 2007; Papakostas, 2008a). However, equivalent efficacy for SSRIs and SNRIs has been suggested by other meta-analyses (Gartlehner, 2008).

Other antidepressant medications

Bupropion is often classified as a norepinephrine and dopamine reuptake inhibitor. However, its mechanism of action remains unclear and the dopamine reuptake inhibitor effect is relatively weak (Fava, 2005). Bupropion may be less well-tolerated than other antidepressants among patients with significant anxiety For instance, a meta-analysis showed that SSRIs were superior to bupropion for patients with MDD and anxiety. (Papakostas, 2008b). However, another meta-analysis suggested that bupropion may be more likely to improve symptoms of fatigue and sleepiness than some of the SSRIs (Papakostas, 2006).

Mirtazapine has comparable efficacy to SSRIs (Papakostas, 2008c).

Evidence gathered in preclinical studies suggests that mirtazapine enhances central noradrenergic and serotonergic activity. These studies have shown that mirtazapine acts as an antagonist at central presynaptic α2-adrenergic inhibitory autoreceptors and heteroreceptors, an action that is postulated to result in an increase in central noradrenergic and serotonergic activity.

Trazodone is a triazolopyridine derivative that belongs to the class of serotonin receptor antagonists and reuptake inhibitors (SARIs). In clinical studies, trazodone has demonstrated comparable antidepressant activity to other drug classes, including TCAs, SSRIs, and SNRIs. A novel, prolonged-release, once-a-day formulation of trazodone (TCOAD) utilizing Contramid drug-delivery technology (trazodone Contramid) has been recently developed in an attempt to enhance patient adherence to treatment and to improve tolerability by avoiding the early high-peak plasma concentration seen with conventional immediate release formulations.

Table 10.1 reports the usual starting and target doses of the medications described here.

Tricyclic and monoamine oxidase inhibitor antidepressants

Tricyclic antidepressants (amitriptyline, clomipramine, desipramine, doxepin, imipramine, nortriptyline, protriptyline, and trimipramine) have shown comparable efficacy to other classes of antidepressants, including SSRIs, SNRIs, and MAOIs but may be particularly effective in certain populations, such as in hospitalized and/or severe patients or patients with melancholia (Anderson, 2000; Barbui, 2001).

MAOIs include phenelzine, tranylcypromine, isocarboxazid, moclobemide, and the transdermally delivered formulation of selegiline. MAOIs have shown comparable efficacy to other antidepressants for outpatients with MDD and may be appropriate for patients with MDD who have not responded to safer and more easily used treatments (Thase, 1995; Quitkin, 1979). Of interest, MAOIs have been shown to be particularly effective for patients with atypical features, such as reactive moods, reverse neurovegetative symptoms, and sensitivity to rejection (Thase, 1995; Quitkin, 1979; Henkel, 2006). MAOIs can cause dangerous interactions with certain foods and beverages, and therefore patients on MAOIs need to avoid foods containing high levels of tyramine, such as aged cheeses, sauerkraut, cured meats, draft beer and fermented soy products like soy sauce, miso, or tofu. The interaction of tyramine with MAOIs can cause dangerously high blood pressure.

Serotonin syndrome is a potentially lethal interaction between SSRIs or other serotonergic drugs and MAOIs. It most often occurs when two medications that raise serotonin are combined. These include other antidepressants, certain pain or headache medications, and the herbal supplement St John's wort. Signs and symptoms of serotonin syndrome include anxiety, agitation, sweating, confusion, tremors, restlessness, lack of coordination, and rapid heart rate. For the reasons above, a minimum of five half-lives should elapse between the time an SSRI is stopped and an MAOI is started. When an MAOI is discontinued, at least two weeks should pass before starting an SSRI or another MAOI.

Maintenance treatment

The evidence suggests that many patients with recurrent depressive disorders who have responded well to acute phase treatment would benefit from continued treatment with antidepressants. The treatment benefit for an individual patient will depend on their underlying risk of relapse. Specific recommendations about which patients should or should not be offered long-term treatment with antidepressants is difficult to make, because treatment will depend on an individual patient's baseline risk, a patient's treatment preferences, and the clinician's prior beliefs. However, it has been clearly established that for patients who are still at appreciable risk of recurrence after four to six months of treatment with antidepressants, another year (and probably more) of continuation treatment will approximately halve their risk (Geddes, 2003).

Psychotherapy

Psychotherapy helps people with depression understand the thoughts, behaviours, events, and emotions that contribute to their depression. It helps patients restructure ways of thinking and reverse negative attitudes and ways in which faulty thinking may perpetuate depression. Psychotherapy can be given in different formats, including:

+ Individual: A therapy that involves only the patient and the therapist.
+ Group: A therapy that involves more than 1 patient and the therapist.
+ Marital/couples: A therapy that involves both partners to help them understand why one of them has depression and to identify changes in thinking and communication and behaviours that may help.
+ Family: A therapy that involves the entire family to help family members understand what one of them is going through, which conflicts may contribute to depression, and what they can do to help.

One of the most studied form of psychotherapy for depression is cognitive-behavioural therapy (CBT), thought to work by teaching patients to learn a set of cognitive and behavioural skills that they can employ on their own. Another example of psychotherapy is Interpersonal psychotherapy, which focuses on the social and interpersonal triggers that may cause depression. There is evidence that it is an effective treatment for depression (Weissman, 2000).

Treatment of other depressive disorders

Psychotherapy and medication management are effective treatment modalities also for depressive disorders other than MDD.

SSRIs appear to be a viable treatment option for patients with dysthymia, although there are few documented systematic studies of the use of these agents in patients with this disease (Ravindran, 1994; De Lima, 2003; Invernizzi, 1997). A meta-analytic study from 2005 found that both SSRIs and TCAs are effective in treating PDD (dysthymia). It also found that MAOIs have a slight advantage over the use of other medications in treating this disorder, but cautioned that MAOIs should not necessarily be the first line in the treatment of dysthymia, as they are often less tolerable than other antidepressants (Ballesteros, 2005).

Psychotherapy research on dysthymia has been primarily confined to small and often uncontrolled studies. Cognitive approaches have been most frequently studied and the results suggest that some dysthymic patients respond to brief cognitive therapies (Markowitz, 1994). A prospective randomized 36-week study of dysthymic patients, comparing continued treatment with antidepressant medication (fluoxetine) alone and medication with the addition of group therapy treatment, suggested that group therapy may provide additional benefit to medication-responding dysthymic patients, particularly in interpersonal and psychosocial functioning (Hellerstein, 2001).

SSRIs have been established as the first-line treatment for PMDD. However, more research is needed to evaluate the efficacy and differential symptom response of continuous, semi-intermittent, luteal phase, and symptoms-onset dosing. Medications such as venlafaxine, duloxetine, alprazolam, and buspirone have also been found to be useful for PMDD. A variety of supplement and herbal-related treatments have been proposed, but only calcium supplementation has demonstrated a consistent therapeutic benefit (Maharaj, 2015).

Currently there are no established guidelines or thorough reviews summarizing the treatment of DMDD. However, pharmacological treatment options of both aggression and chronic irritability include selective norepinephrine reuptake inhibitors, mood stabilizers, psychostimulants, antipsychotics, and alpha-2 agonists. Further studies and clinical trials are warranted to determine efficacious and safe treatment modalities (Renaud, 2015; Maharaj, 2015).

Conclusion

Depression occurs commonly, causing suffering, functional impairment, an increased risk of suicide, added health care costs, and productivity losses. While psychiatric professionals are an essential element of the total health care continuum, the majority of patients with mental health issues will continue to access the health care system through GPs, who are major providers of psychiatric care. Many cases of depression seen in general medical settings are suitable for treatment within those settings, especially when GPs are adequately supported with continuing medical education programs for the recognition, diagnosis, and optimal management of depression in general medical settings. Consultation with a psychiatrist is recommended when it is difficult to rule out bipolar disorder, psychotic symptoms and/or a substance use disorder, where there is a high risk of suicide or harm to others, in the presence of severe co-morbid psychiatric illness, in cases with treatment resistance, or when an unclear diagnosis that needs a more comprehensive evaluation. Even in those cases, GPs may serve a key role in the collaborative care of their depressed patients.

References

American Psychiatric Association. (2010). *Practice Guideline for the Treatment of Patients with Major Depressive Disorder*, 3rd edn Washington, DC: American Psychiatric Association. Accessed Jan 2, 2016. https://psychiatryonline.org/pb/assets/raw/sitewide/practice_guidelines/guidelines/mdd.pdf

American Psychiatric Association. (2013). *Diagnostic and Statistical Manual of Mental Disorders*, 5th edn. Washington, DC: American Psychiatric Association.

Anderson IM. (2000). Selective serotonin reuptake inhibitors versus tricyclic antidepressants: a meta-analysis of efficacy and tolerability. *J Affect Disord*, **58**: 19–36

Arroll B, Macgillivray S, Ogston S, Reid I, Sullivan F, Williams B, and **Crombie I**. (2005). Efficacy and tolerability of tricyclic antidepressants and ssris compared with placebo for treatment of depression in primary care: a meta-analysis. *Ann Fam Med*, 3/5: 449–56.

Ballesteros J. (2005). Orphan comparisons and indirect meta-analysis: A case study on antidepressant efficacy in dysthymia comparing tricyclic antidepressants, selective serotonin reuptake inhibitors, and monoamine oxidase inhibitors by using general linear models. *J Clin Psychopharmacol*, 25/2: 127–31.

Barbui C and **Hotopf M**. (2001). Amitriptyline v the rest: still the leading antidepressant after 40 years of randomised controlled trials. *Br J Psychiatry*, **178**: 129–44.

Cipriani A, Brambilla P, Furukawa T, Geddes J, Gregis M, Hotopf M, Malvini L, and **Barbui C**. (2005). Fluoxetine versus other types of pharmacotherapy for depression. *Cochrane Database Syst Rev*, **4**: CD004185.

De Lima MS and Hotopf M. (2003). Benefits and risks of pharmacotherapy for dysthymia: a systematic appraisal of the evidence. *Drug Saf,* **26**/1: 55–64.

Desmarais JE and Looper KJ. (2009). Interactions between tamoxifen and antidepressants via cytochrome P450 2D6. *J Clin Psychiatry,* **70**: 1688–97.

Fava M, Rush AJ, Thase ME, Clayton A, Stahl SM, Pradko JF, and Johnston JA. (2005). 15 years of clinical ex-perience with bupropion HCl: from bupropion to bupropion SR to bupropion XL. *Prim Care Companion. J Clin Psychiatry,* **7**: 106–13.

Gartlehner G, Gaynes BN, Hansen RA, Thieda P, DeVeaugh-Geiss A, Krebs EE, Moore CG, Morgan L, and Lohr KN. (2008). Comparative benefits and harms of second-generation antidepressants: background paper for the American College of Physicians. *Ann Intern Med,* **149**: 734–50.

Geddes JR, Carney SM, Davies C, Furukawa TA, Kupfer DJ, Frank E, and Goodwin GM. (2003). Relapse prevention with antidepressant drug treatment in depressive disorders: a systematic review. *Lancet,* **361**/9358: 653–61.

Gelenberg AJ. (2010). A review of the current guidelines for depression treatment. *J Clin Psychiatry,* **71**/7: e15.

Henkel V, Mergl R, Allgaier AK, Kohnen R, Moller HJ, and Hegerl U. (2006). Treatment of depression with atypical features: a meta-analytic approach. *Psychiatry Res,* **141**: 89–101

Invernizzi G, Mauri MC, and Waintraub L. (1997). Antidepressant efficacy in the treatment of dysthymia. *Eur Neuropsychopharmacol,* **7**/Suppl 3: S329–36.

Jin Y, Desta Z, Stearns V, Ward B, Ho H, Lee KH, Skaar T, Storniolo AM, Li L, Araba A, Blanchard R, Nguyen A, Ullmer L, Hayden J, Lemler S, Weinshilboum RM, Rae JM, Hayes DF, and Flockhart DA. (2005). CYP2D6 genotype, antidepressant use, and tamoxifen metabolism during adjuvant breast cancer treatment. *J Natl Cancer Inst,* **97**: 30–9.

Maharaj S and Trevino K. (2015). A Comprehensive Review of Treatment Options for Premenstrual Syndrome and Premenstrual Dysphoric Disorder. *J Psychiatr Pract,* **21**/5: 334–50.

Markowitz JC. (1994). Psychotherapy of dysthymia. *Am J Psychiatry,* **151**/8: 1114–21.

Montgomery SA. (2001): A meta-analysis of the efficacy and tolerability of paroxetine versus tricyclic antidepressants in the treatment of major depression. *Int Clin Psychopharmacol,* **16**: 169–78.

Nemeroff CB, Entsuah R, Benattia I, Demitrack M, Sloan DM, and Thase ME. (2008). Comprehensive analysis of remission (COMPARE) with venlafaxine versus SSRIs. *Biol Psychiatry,* **63**: 424–34.

Olfson M, Marcus SC, Druss B, Elinson L, Tanielian T, and Pincus HA. National trends in the outpatient treatment of depression. *JAMA,* **287**/2: 203–9.

Papakostas GI, Fava M, and Thase ME. (2008a). Treatment of SSRI-resistant depression: a meta-analysis comparing within- versus across-class switches. *Biol Psychiatry,* **63**: 699–704.

Papakostas GI, Stahl SM, Krishen A, Seifert CA, Tucker VL, Goodale EP, and Fava M. (2008b). Efficacy of bupropion and the selective serotonin reuptake inhibitors in the treatment of major depressive disorder with high levels of anxiety (anxious depression): a pooled analysis of 10 studies. *J Clin Psychiatry,* **69**: 1287–92.

Papakostas GI, Homberger CH, and Fava M. (2008c). A meta- analysis of clinical trials comparing mirtazapine with selective serotonin reuptake inhibitors for the treatment of major depressive disorder. *J Psychopharmacol,* **22**: 843–8.

Papakostas GI, Nutt DJ, Hallett LA, Tucker VL, Krishen A, and Fava M. (2006). Resolution of sleepiness and fatigue in major depressive disorder: a comparison of bupropion and the selective serotonin reuptake inhibitors. *Biol Psychiatry,* **60**: 1350–5.

Quitkin F, Rifkin A, and Klein DF. (1979). Monoamine oxidase inhibitors: a review of antidepressant effectiveness. *Arch Gen Psychiatry*. 36: 749–60.

Ravindran AV, Bialik RJ, and Lapierre YD. (1994). Therapeutic efficacy of specific serotonin reuptake inhibitors (SSRIs) in dysthymia. *Can J Psychiatry*, 39/1: 21–6.

Richards DA, Hill JJ, Gask L, Lovell K, Chew-Graham C, Bower P, Cape J, Pilling S, Araya R, Kessler D, Bland JM, Green C, Gilbody S, Lewis G, Manning C, Hughes-Morley A, and Barkham M. Clinical effectiveness of collaborative care for depression in UK primary care (CADET): cluster randomised controlled trial. *BMJ*, 19/347: f4913.

Stearns V, Johnson MD, Rae JM, Morocho A, Novielli A, Bhargava P, Hayes DF, Desta Z, and Flockhart DA. (2003). Active tamoxifen metabolite plasma concentrations after coadministration of tamoxifen and the selective serotonin reuptake inhibitor paroxetine. *J Natl Cancer Inst*, 95: 1758–64.

Thase ME, Pritchett YL, Ossanna MJ, Swindle RW, Xu J, and Detke MJ. (2007). Efficacy of duloxetine and selective serotonin reuptake inhibitors: comparisons as assessed by remission rates in patients with major depressive disorder. *J Clin Psychopharmacol*, 27: 672–6.

Thase ME, Trivedi MH, and Rush AJ. (1995). MAOIs in the contemporary treatment of depression. *Neuropsychopharmacology*, 12: 185–219.

Tourian L, LeBoeuf A, Breton JJ, Cohen D, Gignac M, Labelle R, Guile JM, and Renaud J. (2015). Treatment options for the cardinal symptoms of disruptive mood dysregulation disorder. *J Can Acad Child Adolesc Psychiatry*, 24/1: 41–54.

Weissman MM, Markowitz JC, and Klerman GL. (2000). *Comprehensive guide to interpersonal psychotherapy*. New York: Basic Books.

Chapter 11

Bipolar disorder

Paulo R. Nunes Neto, Cristiano A. Köhler,
Michael Berk, and André F. Carvalho

Introduction

Bipolar Disorder (BD) is a highly disabling and chronic disorder characterized by recurring (hypo) manic and depressive episodes, as well as mixed states (American Psychiatric Association. (2013). Bipolar spectrum disorders may affect up to 2.4% of the general population worldwide (Merikangas et al., 2011). While a diagnosis of BD requires that patients fulfil criteria for (hypo) mania, evidence indicates that patients with BD spend significantly more time with depressive symptoms and/or episodes (Kupka et al., 2007). Consequently, the assessment of past manic symptoms is a necessary step for the establishment of a diagnosis of BD. Bipolar disorder commonly goes unrecognized or misdiagnosed (i.e. it is frequently diagnosed as unipolar depression) for several years (Cerimele et al., 2013; Lewis et al., 2004), although other disorders equally can masquerade with bipolar symptoms.

The early recognition of BD is a clear unmet priority—a delay in diagnosis and treatment may activate neuroprogressive mechanisms, which may lead to cognitive deterioration and treatment resistance (Berk et al., 2011; Cardoso et al., 2015). On the other hand, a significant proportion of bipolar patients may be exposed to antidepressant monotherapy with possible deleterious consequences in a subgroup, including but not limited to the emergence of suicidality, the induction of mixed states, treatment-emergent affective switches, and cycle acceleration (Wang et al., 2009, McElroy et al., 2006).

Bipolar disorder is frequently associated with psychiatric (e.g. anxiety, personality, and substance use disorders) and somatic comorbidities (e.g. cardio-metabolic disturbances), which may significantly contribute to morbidity and mortality (McIntyre et al., 2007). Furthermore, patients with BD often seek treatment in primary care (PC), and evidence suggests that some cases of BD go unrecognized in these settings (Bhugra and Flick, 2012; Das et al., 2005).

Emerging evidence indicates that collaborative care models for BD in primary care settings may lead to better outcomes compared to treatment as usual, including not only an amelioration of affective, but also improvements in functioning and quality of life (Miller et al., 2013; van der Voort et al., 2015).

The proper training of general practitioners (GPs) and a better organization of PC services and adoption of collaborative care models with bidirectional permeable boundaries are thus necessary steps for the management of BD (Hodges et al., 2001; Kilbourne et al., 2012). Furthermore, patients with severe mental disorders often face stigma when seeking treatment (e.g. follow-up appointments are scheduled less frequently when compared to patients without severe mental illnesses) (Küey, 2008). This chapter provides an overview of the epidemiology, diagnosis, and treatment of BD, primarily focusing on the main issues related to the management of this disorder in PC services.

Epidemiology

Evidence indicates that bipolar spectrum disorders are highly prevalent in PC settings. For example, Olfon et al. found a 9.8% (n = 112) prevalence for a positive screening for BD in a US low-income PC centre, while only 8.4% of those with a positive screen for BD received a diagnosis of BD (Das et al., 2005). Other recent PC studies have replicated these findings (Castelo et al., 2012).

BD is frequently misdiagnosed as unipolar depression (also known as major depressive disorder, or MDD) and sometimes as schizophrenia. In saying this, it needs to be emphasized that the phenomenology evolves over time, and as an exemplar, the Dutch Bipolar offspring study found considerable diagnostic instability in the early stages of the disorder. For instance, approximately 25% of patients with a current major depressive episode had a lifetime history of BD in a low-income primary care service (Olfson et al., 2005). In addition, nearly one-half of depressive patients who screened positive for BD took an antidepressant in past month, and most of them were not using a mood stabilizer or an antipsychotic. However, extensive antidepressant use remains the case even in documented bipolar disorder. It also was observed that patients with bipolar depression reported more hallucinations, suicidal ideation, and low self-esteem than subjects with a positive screen for unipolar depression (Olfson et al., 2005).

Patients with BD are about eight times more likely to have a first-degree relative with BD than healthy controls (OR = 7.92, 95% CI 2.45–25.61) (Wilde et al., 2014). Furthermore, a recent study indicates that a multigenerational family history of psychiatric disorders may be associated with seven factors related to a poor prognosis among patients with BD, namely childhood abuse, an earlier age of illness onset, comorbid anxiety and substance use disorder, rapid cycling, multiple episodes, and worsening of severity or frequency of episodes (Post et al., 2015).

Furthermore, the presence of medical and psychiatric comorbidities is more a rule than an exception among patients with BD. Hence anxiety disorders, substance use disorders, and borderline personality disorder frequently accompany BD, while other medical conditions (e.g. cardiovascular, respiratory, and endocrine-metabolic diseases) are also more frequent in patients with BD compared to the general population (Krishnan, 2005; Kilbourne et al., 2004). Table 11.1 summarizes the rates of medical and psychiatry comorbidities in BD.

Table 11.1 Rates of comorbid psychiatric and other medical conditions with bipolar disorder

Psychiatric condition[22]	Rate (%)	Other medical condition[23]	Rate (%)
Substance use disorder	56.0	Hypertension	34.8
Alcohol abuse	49.0	Ischemic heart disease	10.6
Other drug abuse	44.0	Hyperlipidemia	226
Anxiety disorder	71.0	Diabetes	17.2
Social phobia	47.0	Thyroid disorders	7.0
Posttraumatic stress disorder	39.0	COPD	10.6
Panic disorder	11.0	Asthma	3.0
Obsessive-compulsive disorder	10.0	Headache	4.2
Binge-eating disorder	13.0	Dementia	1.8
Any DSM-IV axis I disorder	65.0	Hepatitis C	5.9
Any DSM-IV axis II disorder	36.0	HIV infection	0.8

Data from Krishnan K.R, 2005, 67, 'Psychiatric and medical comorbidities of bipolar disorder', *Psychosomatic medicine*, pp. 1–8; data from Kilbourne A.M et al, 2004, 6, 'Burden of general medical conditions among individuals with bipolar disorder', *Bipolar disorders*, pp. 368–73.

Diagnosis

The DSM-5 incorporated five main changes in the diagnostic criteria for bipolar disorders (American Psychiatric Association. (2013). First, 'Bipolar and Related Disorders' was included as a new section that was separated from 'Depressive Disorders'. Second, 'increased goal-directed activity or energy' was includes as a core manifestation of mania. Third, the DSM-IV-TR used stringent diagnostic criteria for mixed episodes, i.e. required the simultaneous fulfilment of criteria for both mania and depressive episode. Conversely, the DSM-5 removed the need for threshold criteria for mixed episodes, and introduced the mixed feature specifier, in which the criteria for a mood episode (i.e. manic, hypomanic, or depressive) should be met, along with at least three concomitant symptoms of the opposite mood polarity. Fourth, an 'anxious distress' specifier was included for patients with at least two concomitant anxiety symptoms, including tension, restlessness, difficulty of concentration, fear that something happened, or feeling of loss of control during a current mood episode. Fifth, an 'Other Unspecified Bipolar and Related Disorders' was included, which includes individuals with a past history of major depressive disorder who meet the criteria for hypomania except for the duration (hypomania requires at least four consecutive days of symptoms) or individuals with insufficient hypomanic symptoms to establish a diagnosis of type II BD. See Table 11.2 for a general view of DSM-5 categories of bipolar and related disorders, as well as the main specifiers for bipolar disorders.

Table 11.2 Nosologic categories of bipolar and related disorders in DSM-5

DSM 5	Key features
Bipolar I disorder	At least one lifetime manic episode; the manic episode may have been preceded by hypomanic or depressive episodes.
Bipolar II disorder	At least one lifetime major depressive episode accompanied by at least one hypomanic episode; no previous manic episode.
Cyclothymic disorder	At least two years (for children, a full year) of manic and depressive symptoms; do not meet criteria for hypomanic or depressive episode.
Unspecified bipolar and related disorders	History of MDD and fulfilment of criteria for hypomania (except duration is < 4 consecutive days) History of MDD and hypomanic episodes with insufficient symptoms to meet criteria for bipolar II disorder (notwithstanding duration is ≥ 4 days) Hypomanic episode without MDD Short-duration cyclothymia
Specifiers for bipolar disorders	
Rapid cycling	≥ 4 mood episodes during a 12-month period
Anxious distress	At least two of the following symptoms on most days during most recent mood episode: (1) Feeling keyed up or tense; (2) Feeling unusually restless; (3) Difficulty concentrating because of worry; (4) Fear that something awful may happen; (5) Feeling that individual might lose control
Mixed features	*Manic or hypomanic episode with mixed features* Full criteria for a manic or hypomanic episode, with at least 3 of the following depressive symptoms: (1) Prominent dysphoria or depressed mood; (2) Diminished interest or pleasure in activities; (3) Psychomotor retardation; (4) Fatigue or loss of energy; (5) Feeling of worthlessness or excessive or inappropriate guilt; (6) Recurrent thoughts of death *Depressive episode, with mixed features* Full criteria for a depressive episode, with at least 3 of the following manic/hypomanic symptoms: (1) Elevated expansive mood; (2) Inflated self-esteem or grandiosity; (3) More talkative than usual or pressure to keep talking; (4) Flight of ideas or experience that thoughts are racing; (5) Increase in energy or goal-directed behaviour; (6) Increased or excessive involvement in activities that have high potential for painful consequences; (7) Decreased need for sleep

Data from *Diagnostic and statistical manual of mental disorder*, 5th ed., 2013, American Psychiatric Association.

A GP should obtain a careful medical and psychiatric history. In addition a succinct medical and psychiatric examination is a necessary step to establish a proper diagnosis (Brenner and Shyn, 2014). Furthermore, other relevant topics should be thoroughly investigated, including: a lifetime history of mood episodes; the duration and severity of past affective episodes; presence of psychiatric (e.g. substance use disorders, anxiety disorders, personality disorders) and medical (e.g. cardio-metabolic disturbances) comorbidities; past therapeutic response; an assessment of suicidality/past suicidal acts); somatic symptoms (e.g. pain); and a family history for mood disorders (Brenner and Shyn, 2014; Culpepper, 2014). The GP should seek collateral information from close relatives and other sources (e.g. charts). It is worth noting that the primary care setting is a privileged setting for the early detection and treatment of BD (Culpepper, 2014).

In addition, physical and laboratory exams may aid in the diagnostic evaluation process. The identification of chronic medical and psychiatric comorbidities (e.g. substance use disorders) are also necessary steps. Thus, some exams may be relevant in the first medical evaluation of BD, including: complete blood count, fasting glucose, oral glucose tolerance tests, serum electrolytes, liver function tests, kidney function tests, lipid profile, thyroid hormones, serum prolactin, blood lipids, vitamin D, folate and B12, toxicological screening, urinalysis, serology for sexually transmitted diseases, electrocardiogram, polysomnography, and actigraphy (Krishnan, 2005). It needs to be stressed that the yield from routine screening, without clinical indicators, is very low.

As aforementioned, BD is often erroneously diagnosed as MDD. There are no straightforward psychopathological distinctions between a unipolar depressive episode and bipolar depression, and objective biomarkers are not yet available to aid in the differential diagnosis. See Table 11.3 for clinical characteristics associated with unipolar and bipolar depression (Mitchell et al., 2008).

Case-finding tools

Case-finding tools may aid in the identification of bipolar spectrum disorders, although few investigations have examined their psychometric properties in primary care settings (Carvalho et al., 2014). In addition, the use of these instruments do not preclude a clinical diagnostic evaluation. These instruments include the MDQ (*Mood Disorder Questionnaire*), the BSDS (Bipolar Spectrum Disorders Scale), the HCL-32 (*Hypomania Check-list-32 items*), and the Composite International Diagnostic Interview (CIDI) Version 3.0. A positive screen for BD indicates a higher probability of having the disorder. However, it needs to be stressed that while the sensitivity and specificity of these tools may be adequate in clinical settings, it is very poor in community settings.

The MDQ is a self-report tool which includes 13 items to establish the presence of a bipolar spectrum disorder, an item that determines whether the (hypo) manic symptoms seem to cluster in the same period of time, and a final question that rates the degree of functional impairment. If the patient endorses having had seven out of 13 hypo (manic) symptoms, confirms that two or more symptoms occurred at the same time, and rates the functional impairment as moderate to severe, the MDQ is

Table 11.3 Clinical features associated with bipolar and unipolar depression

Higher probability of bipolar depression in BD I	Higher probability of unipolar depression
Signs and symptoms	
Hypersomnia	Initial insomnia/reduced sleep
Hyperphagia (or gain weight)	Loss of appetite/lost weight
Other atypical symptoms	Normal or increased psychomotor
Psychomotor retardation	activity
Psychotic features	
Pathologic guilt	
Mood fluctuations	
Course profiles	
Early onset of the first depressive episode (less than 25 years)	Late onset of the first depressive episode (more than 25 years)
Multiple prior depressive episodes (more than five episodes)	Long duration of the index episode (more than six months)
Family history	
History of BD cases in family	Absence of history of BD cases in family
Treatment response to antidepressants	
Lower probability	Higher probability

considered positive. The BSDS and the HCL-32 are alternative self-report screening instruments. Evidence indicates that the MDQ, BSDS and HCL-32 do not significantly differ in their diagnostic accuracy (Carvalho et al., 2014).

The CIDI is a structured interview performed by the clinician (Kessler et al., 2006). A positive response to one of two core questions leads to 12 questions that are designed to identify manic symptoms. The higher the endorsement of symptoms, the greater the likelihood is of having BD.

Notwithstanding that screening for BD (with the MDQ) in primary care attendees with a major depressive episode may be cost-effective (Menzin et al., 2009), no randomized controlled trial has evaluated the sensitivity, specificity, or impact of routine screening for BD in disease-related outcomes in primary care settings.

Long-term course and prognosis

Follow-up studies indicate that highly recurring episodes of mania, depression, and mixed states alternating with asymptomatic periods (euthymia) are hallmarks of the disorder, with clear a tendency towards progressive shortening inter-episode intervals over time (Angst and Sellaro, 2000). Evidence indicates that individuals with both BD I and II may spend approximately half of their lifetime with affective symptomatology, with the remaining lifetime in euthymia. Hypomanic or manic episodes account for 8.9% of follow-up weeks, while depression is present in BD I and II on 31.9% and 53.9% weeks respectively (Judd et al., 2002; Judd et al., 2003).

An international multicentre study found relapse and recurrence rates of 18.2% and 40% respectively (N = 2896) in bipolar patients followed-up for nine months (Vieta et al., 2013). In addition, residual symptoms affected approximately 29.6% of recovered participants with BD I and II , and are associated with higher risk of recurrences (hazard ratio, 3.36; 95% confidence interval, 2.25–4.98; P < .001) (Judd et al., 2008).

Some clinical features may be associated with worse outcomes in BD. For example, mixed mood episodes, shortening of cycles, rapid cycling, and history of multiple episodes may indicate higher severity. In addition, the presence of residual symptoms, an earlier age of illness onset, a delayed diagnosis, more impaired functioning and cognition, and non-adherence to therapy seem related to a worse prognosis (Judd et al., 2008; Treuer and Tohen, 2010). Lastly, psychiatric and other medical comorbidities, such as comorbid personality disorder, a history of trauma, substance use disorders, obesity, anxiety, smoking, an anxiety disorder, and medical comorbidity may further aggravate the course of BD (Forty et al., 2014; McIntyre et al., 2006).

Treatment

Treatment of acute mania

The pharmacologic armamentarium for mania incorporates a few groups of drugs. Lithium, anticonvulsants, and antipsychotics are the main choices still to date, and other kinds of drugs have been tested to control manic symptoms. Treatment guidelines are available for the acute and maintenance treatment of BD (Jeong et al., 2015; Yatham et al., 2013; Fountoulakis et al., 2012). Here we provide a brief clinical overview.

Table 11.4 provides a list of agents classified according to the level of evidence and treatment/regimen of use (monotherapy and/or combined pharmacotherapy), providing support for the clinical judgement in the various steps of management of BD (Yatham et al., 2013). First-line agents have a more consistent efficacy and safety profile for the treatment of acute mania (e.g. a mood stabilizer, atypical antipsychotic, or a combination of these options). Ideally, remission should be achievable with monotherapy, but in the 'real-world' of clinical work, the use of combined treatments is necessary for a substantial proportion of patients. When an unsatisfactory response ensues, it is possible to either change therapy to another first-line agent or to combine different dugs. There are alternatives provided as second- and third-line options to be chosen as either monotherapy or combined therapy (Yatham et al., 2013).

Classical mood stabilizers are the foundation in all phases of the treatment of BD, and could be defined as agents that treat at least one phase (depression or mania) without promoting a higher risk of switching to an episode of opposing polarity (Keck and McElroy, 2003). Lithium is effective for the treatment of acute mania. However, a careful titration of dosage is required, with a proper monitoring of serum levels (every three to six months once stable levels are accomplished) due to concerns of troublesome toxicity (reference values: 0.6–0.8 for maintenance with a maximum of 1.2mEq/L in acute mania). In addition, valproate (and divalproex) and carbamazepine may be effective for the treatment of acute mania, and these drugs may occasionally

Table 11.4 Level of evidence, regimen of treatment, usual dosage, adverse effects and pregnancy safety categories (PSC) of medications for BD

Drug	Mania	Depression	Maintenance	Usual dDosage (mg/day)	Common side effects	PSC
Lithium	+++[a,b,c]	++[a,bc]	+++[a,b,c]	900–1200	Nausea, diarrhoea, tremor, hypothyroidism, polydipsia, polyuria	D
Valproate	+++[a,b,c]	±[b,c]	+++[a,b,c]	500–2500	Nausea, alopecia, weight gain, diarrhoea, sedation, tremor, elevation liver transaminase, polycystic ovary syndrome	D
Carbamazepine	++[a,b]	±[b,c]	±[a,b]	200–1600	Nausea, epigastric pain, sedation, ataxia, diplopia, itch, skin rash, hyponatremia, dizziness	D
Oxcarbazepine	+[a]	±[e]	+[***]	600–1200	Fatigue, sedation, dizziness, hyponatremia, skin rash	C
Lamotrigine	±[e]	++[a,b]	++[a]	50–200	Nausea, headache, diplopia, sedation, dizziness, skin rash	C
Topiramate	±[e]	±[e]	±[e]	50–200	Nausea, diarrhoea, dyspepsia, weight loss, insomnia, headache, concentration and memory impairment, fatigue, dizziness, tremor, paraesthesia	D
Haloperidol	++[a,b]	±[e]	±[e]	0.5–10	Akathisia, dystonia, rigidity, tardive dyskinesia, extrapyramidal syndrome, tremor, sedation, hyperprolactinemia	C
Chlorpromazine	+[a]	±[e]	±[e]	400–800	Dry mouth, weight gain, akathisia, dystonia, rigidity, tardive dyskinesia, extrapyramidal syndrome, tremor, sedation, urinary retention, hyperprolactinemia	C
Risperidone	+++[a,b]	±[e]	++[a,c]	2–8	Weight gain, akathisia, agitation, anxious, tremor, extrapyramidal syndrome, sedation, headache, retrograde ejaculation	C

				Dosage		
Quetiapine	+++[a,b]	+++[a,c,d]	+++[a,c]	300–800	weight gain, sedation, dizziness, hypotension, dry mouth	C
Olanzapine	+++[a,b]	++[c,d*]	+++[a,c,d]	10–30	Sedation, weight gain, glucose elevation, dyslipidaemia, transitory transaminase elevation	C
Ziprazidone	+++[a]	+[b]	++[c]	120–200	Nausea, constipation, runny nose, asthenia, skin rash, extension of QT interval	C
Aripiprazole	+++[a,b]	±[e]	+++[a,c*****]	10–30	Nausea, vomiting, constipation, orthostatic hypotension, anxious, akathisia, sedation, dizziness.	C
Clozapine	+[a]	±[e]	+[***]	200–900	Nausea, drooling, dry mouth, increasing appetite, constipation, increased risk of agranulocytosis	C
Paliperidone	++[a]	±[e]	++[a]	6–12	Restlessness, tremor, rigidity, dystonia, shuffling walk, uncontrolled involuntary movements (especially of face, neck, and back), fast heartbeat	C
Asenapine	+++[a]	±[e]	+[a]	5–10	Nausea, increased appetite, weight gain, numbing of the mouth, strange sense of taste, sedation, agitation, dizziness, extrapyramidal symptoms, muscle weakness, transitory transaminase elevation	C
Lurasidone	±[e]	+++[e**]	±[e]	20–120	Nausea, tremor, akathisia, difficulty moving, slow movements, muscle stiffness, sleepiness or drowsiness	B
SSRI	±[e]	++[c,d]	±[e]	Different dosages	Nausea, dyspepsia, constipation, diarrhoea, anorexia, increasing of appetite, weight gain, sedation, insomnia, akathisia, ejaculation retardation, diminished libido	C/D

(continued)

Table 11.4 Continued

Drug	Mania	Depression	Maintenance	Usual dDosage (mg/day)	Common side effects	PSC
Bupropion	±[e]	+[b]	±[e]	150–300	Nausea, dry mouth, loss of appetite, weight loss, difficult sleeping, agitation, anxiety, dizziness, sweating, sore throat, skin rash, ringing in the ears, tremor, stomach pain, muscle pain, fast heartbeat, and more frequent urination.	C
Venlafaxine	±[e]	+[b]	±[e]	75–225	Nausea, vomiting, dry mouth, diarrhoea, appetite loss, blurred vision, dizziness, unusual dreams, anxious, sweating, tremor, fatigue, tachycardia, ejaculation retardation, diminished libido	C
Tryciclic Antidepressants	±[e]	+[c,d]	±[e]	Different dosages	Dry mouth, visual blurring, constipation, urinary retention, increasing of appetite, weight gain, dizziness, sedation, tremor, tachycardia, quinidine-like effect, hypotension, ejaculation retardation, diminished libido.	B/C

Evidence level criteria (E): +++ Meta-analysis or replicated double-blinded randomized controlled trial (DB-RCT); ++ ≥1 DB-RCT or active comparison; + Prospective uncontrolled trial; ± Minimal or inadequate evidence. Regimen: a: monotherapy; b: mood stabilizer combination; c: mood stabilizer plus antipsychotic or antidepressant; d: antipsychotic plus antidepressant; e: not recommended. DD: different dosages. Pregnancy Safety Categories (PSC) according FDA: A: adequate and well-controlled studies have failed to demonstrate a risk of the fetus in the first trimester and there is no evidence of risk in the later trimesters; B: animal reproduction studies have failed to demonstrate a risk to the fetus and there are no adequate well-controlled studies in humans; C: animal reproduction studies have shown an adverse effect on the fetus and there are no adequate well-controlled studies in humans, but potential benefits may warrant use in pregnant women despite potential risks; D: there is positive evidence of of human fetal risk based on adverse reaction data from investigational or marketing experience, but potential benefits may warrant use in pregnant women despite potential risks; X: studies in animals or humans have demonstrated fetal abnormalities and/or there is positive evidence of human fetal risk based on adverse reaction data from investigational or marketing experience, and the risks involved in ue of the drug in pregnant women clearly outweigh potential benefits.

Notes: *Olanzapine only with SSRI, **Received FDA approval for use in monotherapy or combined with lithium or valproate, ***adjunctive use, ****mainly for the prevention of mania, but not for the depression.

need to have serum levels monitored. Oxcarbazepine have fewer side effects and pharmacokinetic interactions than carbamazepine and may be useful in mania either as monotherapy or combined with lithium. However, evidence thus far for oxcarbazepine remains limited and contradictory. Other anticonvulsants (e.g. topiramate or gabapentin) have little evidence to support its use in mania, and should be avoided (Yatham et al., 2013; Gitlin and Frye, 2012).

Antipsychotics have accumulated a consistent evidence base over the years for the treatment of mania. Atypical antipsychotics have gained widespread acceptance because of their rapid effects compared to lithium and anticonvulsivants and a lower tendency (compared to typical neuroleptics) to cause extrapyramidal side effects (EPS) (Yildiz et al., 2011). On the other hand, first-generation antipsychotics (e.g. haloperidol and chlorpromazine) should not be discarded as effective treatment options for mania (Cipriani et al., 2011). However, a meta-analysis suggests that typical antipsychotics may be more likely to induce a depressive switch compared to atypical agents (Goikolea et al., 2013), and those with bipolar disorder are more vulnerable to EPS than those with schizophrenia. Following a treatment failure, a mood stabilizer may be combined with an antipsychotic (Yatham et al., 2013).

Research findings have associated mixed symptoms with a worse prognosis, both in mania and bipolar depression (Treuer and Tohen, 2010). Following the DSM-5, there are no guidelines to the treatment of BD using a mixed feature specifier. The presence of mixed features may point to a more severe illness, and also to possible therapeutic choices (Hu et al., 2014). Thus, some agents have a more robust evidence for the treatment of a mania (or depression) episode with symptoms of the opposite pole. For mixed features, valproate, carbamazepine, and atypical antipsychotics (i.e. aripiprazole, asenapine, olanzapine, quetiapine, risperidone, ziprasidone) have more evidence to date, especially when combined (McIntyre and Yoon, 2012). Nevertheless, a very limited evidence base is available to guide the acute treatment of mixed states in BD.

The treatment of bipolar depression

Depressive episodes occur more frequently in most patients with BD, and may account for a significant proportion of functional impairment attributed to this illness. Even in euthymia, residual depressive symptoms are common leading to a significant reduction in quality of life and functioning. Currently, the treatment of bipolar depression is a clinical challenge because available options are relatively limited (Citrome, 2014).

The US Food and Drug Administration (FDA) has approved new strategies for the treatment bipolar depression in the last ten years. The FDA approved quetiapine (immediate or extended release), a olanzapine-fluoxetine combination (OFC), and more recently, lurasidone for the acute treatment of bipolar depression (McIntyre et al., 2013). Quetiapine is indicated both for mania and depression in BD and its extended-release formulation enables a single daily administration, although residual sedation may be burdensome for some patients. Some studies suggest the efficacy of the OFC in bipolar depression. Side effects of OFC include sedation, weight gain, and metabolic disturbances. The new atypical antipsychotic lurasidone was approved for use in monotherapy or adjunctively to lithium or valproate in bipolar I depression, and EPS/akathisia may be frequent, but this agent seems to have a relatively safe profile regarding metabolic disturbances (Yatham et al., 2013; McIntyre et al., 2013). These findings indicate that lurasidone could be included as a first-line treatment for bipolar depression in future guidelines (Yatham et al., 2013; Franklin et al., 2015).

Lithium has a prominent role in the prophylaxis of new episodes and in the reduction of suicidal behaviour, although there are few trials that have had evaluated its role in bipolar depression in monotherapy (Selle et al., 2014; Cipriani et al., 2013a). However, lithium either in monotherapy or in combination remains a first-line option for the treatment of bipolar depression. When lithium alone fails, it is possible to combine it with other drugs, especially valproate, atypical antipsychotics (e.g. quetiapine or lurasidone), antidepressants (SSRI and bupropion as first-choice, and venlafaxine and tricyclic as third-line choices), carbamazepine, and lamotrigine (Jeong et al., 2015; Yatham et al., 2013; Grunze et al., 2010).

Anticonvulsants have a limited role in the acute treatment of bipolar depression. There are two positive double-blind studies of lamotrigine in BD and a positive meta-analysis (Geddes et al., 2009), although a recent network meta-analysis found no evidence of efficacy for lamotrigine (McIntyre et al., 2013; Taylor et al., 2014). Lamotrigine studies are hamstrung by the need for a six-week titration phase in eight-week studies, leaving only two weeks to display efficacy. Valproate seems to have efficacy for the treatment of bipolar depression based on a small number of studies. Evidence does not support the use of carbamazepine and topiramate for bipolar depression (Selle et al., 2014, Vieta et al., 2002).

Significant controversy remains regarding the use of antidepressants for the acute treatment of bipolar depression. There are significant concerns relative to the propensity of these agents to promote affective switches, cycle acceleration, and even the emergence of suicidality (McElroy et al., 2006; Vázquez et al., 2013). Thus, most guidelines recommend the use of antidepressants for the treatment of BD when associated with a classic mood stabilizer or an antipsychotic. Among antidepressants, tricyclic agents and venlafaxine seem to carry a greater risk of treatment emergent affective switches, while bupropion and SSRIs have the lowest (except paroxetine) (Yatham et al., 2013; Vázquez et al., 2013). The patient must be advised to notify his/her clinician of any abrupt changes in mood during the use of an antidepressant (Vázquez et al., 2013).

Maintenance pharmacotherapy

The main goal of this treatment phase is to achieve long-term stabilization of the disorder with the prophylaxis of acute mood episodes, while incapacitating sub-syndromal symptoms should also be addressed. Therefore, some clinical principles should be followed (Gitlin and Frye, 2012 Yatham et al., 2005):

+ Review the clinical history, searching for correlates related to worse outcome;
+ Keep on the index medication administered for the acute treatment phase if the patient responds to a treatment with established efficacy for the long-term management of BD;
+ Aggressively treat depressive symptoms;
+ Monitor depressive/manic symptoms through the use of standard rating scales;

+ Monitor pharmacological side effects and treatment adherence;
+ Determine the predominant polarity of the illness (manic versus depressive); it may aid in treatment selection (Carvalho et al., 2015);
+ Provide psychotherapy and/or psychoeducation as it may promote treatment adherence and aid in the early identification of relapses and/or recurrences.

There is a wide range of the efficacy and tolerability of diverse agents used in the maintenance treatment of BD. A recent network meta-analysis of maintenance treatments for BD indicates that lithium remains the mainstay of treatment (Miura et al., 2014), because it decreases manic and depressive recurrences, and, in addition, prevents suicidal behaviour (Cipriani et al., 2013a; Vazquez et al., 2015). Anticonvulsants are effective agents for the maintenance treatment of BD. Valproate had lower efficacy compared to lithium, and the combination of lithium-valproate was more likely to prevent recurrences than valproate monotherapy (Cipriani et al., 2013b). Lamotrigine has replicated positive findings for the prevention of bipolar depression, but appears to have limited or no efficacy for the prevention of mania (McIntyre et al., 2013). Other anticonvulsants (e.g. carbamazepine) have shown little evidence for the prevention of recurrences and are currently regarded as second- or third-line options (Yatham et al., 2013).

Atypical antipsychotics have also gained an important role in the maintenance treatment of BD. Some agents have been recommended as first-line treatment options, including quetiapine, olanzapine, risperidone, and aripiprazole in monotherapy or combined with lithium or valproate, and ziprasidone in combination with a mood stabilizer. Aripiprazole, ziprasidone, and risperidone are effective for the prevention of manic, but not of depressive, episodes. Quetiapine and lurasidone show efficacy in depression. The emergence of weight gain and metabolic disturbances (e.g. type 2 diabetes, dyslipidemia, or the metabolic syndrome) are significant adverse effects of atypical antipsychotics, especially olanzapine and quetiapine. Therefore, clinicians should routinely monitor their patients for adverse effects.

Psychosocial approaches

Psychosocial factors, non-adherence to treatment, as well as medical and psychiatric comorbidities influence clinical outcomes, and should be considered in the long-term treatment of BD. Thus, the GP and the health team as whole should consider all these in order to avoid relapses and recurrences in BD (Treuer and Tohen, 2010; Miziou et al., 2015).

Psychosocial approaches have an established place in the treatment of BD (Lauder et al., 2010). A meta-analysis showed that cognitive-behavioural therapy (CBT) may improve symptoms and enhance treatment adherence; however, few significant effects in the prevention of mood episodes were observed (Szentagotai and David, 2010). In addition, psychoeducation may improve adherence and prevent recurrences in BD (Yatham et al., 2005). Interpersonal therapy and social rhythm therapy may improve acute symptoms, but the evidence for these is small (Miklowitz and Scott, 2009). Web-based psychotherapy approaches show promise, although mode studies are necessary

(Hidalgo-Mazzei et al., 2015). The advent of well-designed trials of these various options is an unmet need in the treatment of BD (Miziou et al., 2015).

Clinical monitoring

Clinical monitoring is an essential ingredient in the treatment of BD. Common side effects, comorbidities, and clinical response should be regularly assessed (Culpepper, 2014; Gitlin and Frye, 2012; Yatham et al., 2005).

It is particularly important to assess the more common side effects associated with psychotropic drugs, including lithium (e.g. nephrotoxicity) or valproate (e.g. elevation of liver enzymes and hepatic failure), weight gain, metabolic disturbances, and endocrine dysfunctions (e.g. lithium-induced hypothyroidism). Moreover, the use of antipsychotics carries a risk of EPS (for example, akathisia, parkinsonism and dystonia) and hyperprolactinemia. Side effects commonly drive non-adherence to treatment, leading to a suboptimal response to pharmacological treatment (Mago et al, 2014).

Psychiatric and medical comorbidities may also complicate the clinical course of BD. Thus, it is necessary to establish and treat comorbid long-term conditions at baseline and at follow-up visits. In addition, pregnancy in bipolar patients is often a source of significant concern, and there is often a clinical need to make difficult decisions weighing risks and benefits of available treatments. In general, psychosocial treatments should always be preferred. Notwithstanding, lithium was once thought to be associated with a significant risk for cardiac malformations in the newborn, mainly Ebstein's anomaly, but recent evidence indicates that lithium may be relatively safe in pregnancy. Preliminary evidence also suggests that atypical antipsychotics may be relatively safe. However, it is important to note that valproate is a known teratogen. A recent narrative review underscores the basic principles of the management of perinatal mood disorders (Meltzer-Brody and Jones, 2015).

Lastly, manic and depressive symptoms should be routinely monitored with standard measure, e.g. the Hamilton Depression Scale (HAM-D) for depression and the Young Mania Rating Scale (YMRS) for mania (Picardi, 2009).

Collaborative care models

Collaborative care is an intervention model based on team work aiming to provide integrated care for chronic conditions (Bodenheimer et al., 2002; Goodrich et al., 2013). This model has accumulated significant evidence of effectiveness for the delivery of care for mental disorders in PC. A meta-analysis indicates a significant improvement in clinical outcomes in people with severe mental disorders, including BD (Woltmann et al., 2012). Six basic elements comprise collaborative care models (Kilbourne et al., 2012; Woltmann et al., 2012):

- clinical information system (for screening and monitoring);
- delivery system redesign (i.e. defining a work plan to preventive and management actions, including access to specialized support when necessary);
- decision support by a mental health specialist;

- the promotion of self-management strategies by the patient through psychoeducation and/or other psychosocial approaches;
- a link with community resources;
- leadership support to achieve goals by the team.

In the primary care setting, the GP plays a critical role in detection, diagnosis, and management of BD (Brenner and Shyn, 2014; Culpepper, 2014). Basic training in mental health, guidelines for BD, available scales to aid in the recognition of BD as well as in the measurement of symptoms, are important to integrate the GP in a set of actions aiming to improve the overall diagnosis and management of BD. In addition, refractory cases usually require specialist support. The complexity of BD requires an interdisciplinary dialogue and integration between nurses, psychologists, nutritionists, social workers, and caregivers throughout treatment.

Conclusion

It has been increasingly recognized that a substantial majority of individuals with BD need treatment in PC settings. In addition, PC has a strategic position in health care systems to aid in the prompt recognition of BD at its early stages and in its integrated management. Several pharmacological agents are effective for the acute and maintenance treatment of BD. Furthermore, evidence indicates that psychosocial approaches are also effective. Patients with BD often present in PC with complex medical and psychiatric comorbidities. In addition, available treatments for BD can be associated with significant adverse effects. Therefore, GPs should regularly monitor their bipolar patients not only for affective symptoms, but also for burdensome medical (e.g. obesity and metabolic syndrome) and psychiatric (e.g. substance use disorder) comorbidities.

Notwithstanding the fact that collaborative care models are still an area in active development, evidence thus far points to this treatment strategy significantly improving outcomes in BD, when implemented in primary care.

Acknowledgements

AF is supported by a research fellowship award from the Conselho de Desenvolvimento Científico e Tecnológico (CNPq, Brazil). MB is supported by a NHMRC Senior Principal Research Fellowship 1059660.

References

American Psychiatric Association. (2013). *Diagnostic and Statistical Manual of Mental Disorders*, 5th edn. Arlington, VA: American Psychiatric Association.

Angst J and Sellaro R. (2000). Historical perspectives and natural history of bipolar disorder. *Biol Psychiatry*, 48/6: 445–57.

Berk M, Kapczinski F, Andreazza AC, Dean OM, Giorlando F, Maes M, Yücel M, Gama CS, Dodd S, Dean B, Magalhães PV, Amminger P, McGorry P, and Malhi GS. (2011). Pathways underlying neuroprogression in bipolar disorder: focus on inflammation, oxidative stress and neurotrophic factors. *Neurosci Biobehav Rev*, 35/3: 804–17.

Bhugra D and Flick GR. (2005). Pathways to care for patients with bipolar disorder. *Bipolar Disord*, 7/3: 236–45.

Bodenheimer T, Wagner EH, and Grumbach K. (2002). Improving primary care for patients with chronic illness: the chronic care model, Part 2. *JAMA*, **288**/15: 1909–14.

Brenner CJ and Shyn SI. (2014). Diagnosis and management of bipolar disorder in primary care: a DSM-5 update. *Med Clin North Am*, **98**/5: 1025–48.

Cardoso T, Bauer IE, Meyer TD, Kapczinski F, and Soares JC. (2015). Neuroprogression and Cognitive Functioning in Bipolar Disorder: A Systematic Review. Curr Psychiatry Rep, 17/9:605.

Carvalho AF, Takwoingi Y, Sales PMG, Soczynska JK, Köhler CA, Freitas TH, Quevedo J, Hyphantis TN, McIntyre RS, and Vieta E. (2014). Screening for bipolar spectrum disorders: A comprehensive meta-analysis of accuracy studies. *J Affect Disord*, **172**: 337–46.

Carvalho AF, Quevedo J, McIntyre RS, Soeiro-de-Souza MG, Fountoulakis KN, Berk M, Hyphantis TN, and Vieta E. (2015). Treatment implications of predominant polarity and the polarity index: a comprehensive review. *Int J Neuropsychopharmacol*, **18**/2: doi: 10.1093/ijnp/pyu079

Castelo MS, Hyphantis TN, Macedo DS, Lemos GO, Machado YO, Kapczinski F, McIntyre RS, and Carvalho AF. (2012). Screening for bipolar disorder in the primary care: a Brazilian survey. *J Affect Disord*, **143**/1–3: 118–24.

Cerimele JM, Chwastiak LA, Chan Y-F, Harrison DA, and Unützer J. (2013). The Presentation, Recognition and Management of Bipolar Depression in Primary Care. *J Gen Intern Med*, **28**/12: 1648–56.

Cipriani A, Barbui C, Salanti G, Rendell J, Brown R, Stockton S, Purgato M, Spineli LM, Goodwin GM, and Geddes JR. (2011). Comparative efficacy and acceptability of antimanic drugs in acute mania: a multiple-treatments meta-analysis. *Lancet*, **378**/9799: 1306–15.

Cipriani A, Hawton K, Stockton S, and Geddes JR. (2013a). Lithium in the prevention of suicide in mood disorders: updated systematic review and meta-analysis. *BMJ*, 27/346: f3646.

Cipriani A, Reid K, Young AH, Macritchie K, and Geddes J. (2013b). Valproic acid, valproate and divalproex in the maintenance treatment of bipolar disorder. *Cochrane Database Syst Rev*, **10**: CD003196.

Citrome L. (2014). Treatment of bipolar depression: making sensible decisions. *CNS Spectr*, 19/Suppl 1: 4–11.

Culpepper L. (2014). The diagnosis and treatment of bipolar disorder: decision-making in primary care. *Prim Care Companion CNS Disord*, 16/3: doi: 10.4088/PCC.13r01609

Das AK, Olfson M, Gameroff MJ, Pilowsky DJ, Blanco C, Feder A, Gross R, Neria Y, Lantigua R, Shea S, and Weissman MM. (2005). Screening for bipolar disorder in a primary care practice. *JAMA*, **293**/8: 956–63.

Forty L, Ulanova A, Jones L, Jones I, Gordon-Smith K, Fraser C, Farmer A, McGuffin P, Lewis CM, Hosang GM, Rivera M, and Craddock N. (2014). Comorbid medical illness in bipolar disorder. *Br J Psychiatry*, **205**/6: 465–72 p.

Fountoulakis KN, Kasper S, Andreassen O, Blier P, Okasha A, Severus E, Versiani M, Tandon R, Möller HJ, and Vieta E. (2012). Efficacy of pharmacotherapy in bipolar disorder: a report by the WPA section on pharmacopsychiatry. *Eur Arch Psychiatry Clin Neurosci*, **262**/Suppl 1: 1–48.

Franklin R, Zorowitz S, Corse AK, Widge AS, and Deckersbach T. (2015). Lurasidone for the treatment of bipolar depression: an evidence-based review. *Neuropsychiatr Dis Treat*, 11: 2143–52.

Geddes JR, Calabrese JR, and Goodwin GM. (2009). Lamotrigine for treatment of bipolar depression: independent meta-analysis and meta-regression of individual patient data from five randomised trials. *Br J Psychiatry*, 194/1: 4–9.

Gitlin M and Frye MA. (2012). Maintenance therapies in bipolar disorders. *Bipolar disord*, 14: 51–65.

Goikolea JM, Colom F, Torres I, Capapey J, Valenti M, Undurraga J, Grande I, Sanchez-Moreno J, and Vieta E. (2013). Lower rate of depressive switch following antimanic treatment with second-generation antipsychotics versus haloperidol. *J Affect Disord*, 144/3: 191–8.

Goodrich DE, Kilbourne AM, Nord KM, and Bauer MS. (2013). Mental Health Collaborative Care and Its Role in Primary Care Settings. *Curr Psychiatry Rep*, 15/8: doi: 10.1007/s11920-013-0383-2

Grunze H, Vieta E, Goodwin GM, Bowden C, Licht RW, Moller HJ, Kasper S; WFSBP Task Force On Treatment Guidelines For Bipolar Disorders. (2010). The World Federation of Societies of Biological Psychiatry (WFSBP) Guidelines for the biological treatment of bipolar disorders: update 2010 on the treatment of acute bipolar depression. *World J Biol Psychiatry*, 11/2: 81–109.

Hidalgo-Mazzei D, Mateu A, Reinares M, Matic A, Vieta E, and Colom F. (2015). Internet-based psychological interventions for bipolar disorder: Review of the present and insights into the future. *J Affect Disord*, 188: 1–13.

Hodges B, Inch C, and Silver I. (2001). Improving the psychiatric knowledge, skills, and attitudes of primary care physicians, 1950–2000: a review. *Am J Psychiatry*. 158/10: 1579–86.

Hu J, Mansur R, and McIntyre RS. (2014). Mixed Specifier for Bipolar Mania and Depression: Highlights of DSM-5 Changes and Implications for Diagnosis and Treatment in Primary Care. *Prim Care Companion CNS Disord*, 16/2: 17.

Jeong JH, Lee JG, Kim MD, Sohn I, Shim SH, Wang HR, Woo YS, Jon DI, Seo JS, Shin YC, Min KJ, Yoon BH, and Bahk WM. (2015). Korean Medication Algorithm for Bipolar Disorder 2014: comparisons with other treatment guidelines. *Neuropsychiatr Dis Treat*, 11: 1561–71.

Judd LL, Akiskal HS, Schettler PJ, Endicott J, Maser J, Solomon DA, Leon AC, Rice JA, and Keller MB. (2002). The long-term natural history of the weekly symptomatic status of bipolar I disorder. *Arch Gen Psychiatry*, 59/6: 530–7.

Judd LL, Akiskal HS, Schettler PJ, Coryell W, Endicott J, Maser JD, Solomon DA, Leon AC, and Keller MB. (2003). A prospective investigation of the natural history of the long-term weekly symptomatic status of bipolar II disorder. *Arch Gen Psychiatry*, 60/3: 261–9.

Judd LL, Schettler PJ, Akiskal HS, Coryell W, Leon AC, Maser JD, and Solomon DA. (2008). Residual symptom recovery from major affective episodes in bipolar disorders and rapid episode relapse/recurrence. *Arch Gen Psychiatry*, 65/4: 386–94.

Keck PE Jr and McElroy SL. (2003). Redefining mood stabilization. *J Affect Disord*, 73/1–2: 163–9.

Kessler RC, Akiskal HS, Angst J, Guyer M, Hirschfeld RM, Merikangas KR, and Stang PE. (2006). Validity of the assessment of bipolar spectrum disorders in the WHO CIDI 3.0. *J Affect Disord*, 96/3: 259–69.

Kilbourne AM, Cornelius JR, Han X, Pincus HA, Shad M, Salloum I, Conigliaro J, Haas GL. (2004). Burden of general medical conditions among individuals with bipolar disorder. *Bipolar Disord*, 6/5: 368–73.

Kilbourne AM, Goodrich DE, O'Donnell AN, and Miller CJ. (2012). Integrating bipolar disorder management in primary care. *Curr Psychiatry Rep*, 14/6: 687–95.

Krishnan KR. Psychiatric and medical comorbidities of bipolar disorder. (2005). *Psychosom Med*, 67/1: 1–8.

Küey L. The impact of stigma on somatic treatment and care for people with comorbid mental and somatic disorders. (2008). Curr Opin Psychiatry. 21/4: 403–11.

Kupka RW, Altshuler LL, Nolen WA, Suppes T, Luckenbaugh DA, Leverich GS, Frye MA, Keck PE Jr, McElroy SL, Grunze H, and Post RM. (2007). Three times more days depressed than manic or hypomanic in both bipolar I and bipolar II disorder. Bipolar Disord, 9/5: 531–5.

Lauder SD, Berk M, Castle DJ, Dodd S, and Berk L. (2010). The role of psychotherapy in bipolar disorder. *Med J Aust*, 193/4 Suppl: S31–5.

Lewis FT, Kass E, and Klein RM. (2004). An overview of primary care assessment and management of bipolar disorder. *J Am Osteopath Assoc*, 104/6 Suppl: S2–8.

Mago R, Borra D, and Mahajan R. (2014). Role of adverse effects in medication nonadherence in bipolar disorder. *Harv Rev Psychiatry*, 22/6: 363–6.

McElroy SL, Kotwal R, Kaneria R, and Keck PE, Jr. (2006). Antidepressants and suicidal behavior in bipolar disorder. Bipolar Disord, 8/5, Pt 2:596–617.

McIntyre RS, Konarski JZ, Soczynska JK, Wilkins K, Panjwani G, Bouffard B, Bottas A, and Kennedy SH. (2006). Medical comorbidity in bipolar disorder: implications for functional outcomes and health service utilization. *Psychiatr Serv*, 57/8: 1140–4.

McIntyre RS, Soczynska JK, Beyer JL, Woldeyohannes HO, Law CW, Miranda A, Konarski JZ, and Kennedy SH. (2007). Medical comorbidity in bipolar disorder: re-prioritizing unmet needs. *Curr Opin Psychiatry*, 20/4: 406–16.

McIntyre RS and Yoon J. (2012). Efficacy of antimanic treatments in mixed states. *Bipolar Disord*, 2: 22–36.

McIntyre RS, Cha DS, Kim RD, and Mansur RB. (2013). A review of FDA-approved treatment options in bipolar depression. *CNS Spectr*, 18/ Suppl 1:4–20.

Meltzer-Brody S and Jones I. (2015). Optimizing the treatment of mood disorders in the perinatal period. *Dialogues Clin Neurosci*, 17/2: 207–18.

Menzin J, Sussman M, Tafesse E, Duczakowski C, Neumann P, and Friedman M. (2009). A model of the economic impact of a bipolar disorder screening program in primary care. *J Clin Psychiatry*, 70/9: 1230–6.

Merikangas KR, Jin R, He JP, Kessler RC, Lee S, Sampson NA, Viana MC, Andrade LH, Hu C, Karam EG, Ladea M, Medina-Mora ME, Ono Y, Posada-Villa J, Sagar R, Wells JE, and Zarkov Z. (2011). Prevalence and correlates of bipolar spectrum disorder in the world mental health survey initiative. *Arch Gen Psychiatry*, 68/3: 241–51.

Miklowitz DJ and Scott J. (2009). Psychosocial treatments for bipolar disorder: cost-effectiveness, mediating mechanisms, and future directions. *Bipolar Disord*, 2: 110–22.

Miller CJ, Grogan-Kaylor A, Perron BE, Kilbourne AM, Woltmann E, and Bauer MS. (2013). Collaborative chronic care models for mental health conditions: cumulative meta-analysis and metaregression to guide future research and implementation. *Med Care*, 51/10: 922–30.

Mitchell PB, Goodwin GM, Johnson GF, and Hirschfeld RMA. (2008). Diagnostic guidelines for bipolar depression: a probabilistic approach. *Bipolar disord*, 10/1p2: 144–52.

Miura T, Noma H, Furukawa TA, Mitsuyasu H, Tanaka S, Stockton S, Salanti G, Motomura K, Shimano-Katsuki S, Leucht S, Cipriani A, Geddes JR, Kanba S. (2014). Comparative efficacy and tolerability of pharmacological treatments in the maintenance treatment of bipolar disorder: a systematic review and network meta-analysis. *Lancet Psychiatry*, 1/5: 351–9.

Miziou S, Tsitsipa E, Moysidou S, Karavelas V, Dimelis D, Polyzoidou V, et al. (2015). Psychosocial treatment and interventions for bipolar disorder: a systematic review. *Ann Gen Psychiatry*, 14:19: doi: 10.1186/s12991-015-0057-z

Olfson M, Das AK, Gameroff MJ, Pilowsky D, Feder A, Gross R, Lantigua R, Shea S, and Weissman MM. (2005). Bipolar depression in a low-income primary care clinic. *Am J Psychiatry*, 162/11: 2146–51.

Picardi A. (2009). Rating scales in bipolar disorder. *Curr Opin Psychiatry*, 22/1: 42–9.

Post RM, Altshuler L, Kupka R, McElroy SL, Frye MA, Rowe M, Grunze H, Suppes T, Keck PE, Leverich GS, and Nolen WA. (2015). Multigenerational positive family history of psychiatric disorders is associated with a poor prognosis in bipolar disorder. *J Neuropsychiatry Clin Neurosci*, 27/4: 304–10.

Selle V, Schalkwijk S, Vazquez GH, and Baldessarini RJ. (2014). Treatments for acute bipolar depression: meta-analyses of placebo-controlled, monotherapy trials of anticonvulsants, lithium and antipsychotics. *Pharmacopsychiatry*, 47/2: 43–52.

Szentagotai A and David D. (2010). The efficacy of cognitive-behavioral therapy in bipolar disorder: a quantitative meta-analysis. *J Clin Psychiatry*, 71/1: 66–72.

Taylor DM, Cornelius V, Smith L, and Young AH. (2014). Comparative efficacy and acceptability of drug treatments for bipolar depression: a multiple-treatments meta-analysis. *Acta psychiatrica Scandinavica*, 130/6: 452–69.

Treuer T and Tohen M. (2010). Predicting the course and outcome of bipolar disorder: a review. *Eur Psychiatry*, 25/6: 328–33.

Vázquez GH, Tondo L, Undurraga J, and Baldessarini RJ. (2013). Overview of antidepressant treatment of bipolar depression. *Int J Neuropsychopharmacol*, 16/7: 1673–85.

Vazquez GH, Holtzman JN, Lolich M, Ketter TA, and Baldessarini RJ. (2015). Recurrence rates in bipolar disorder: Systematic comparison of long-term prospective, naturalistic studies versus randomized controlled trials. *Eur Neuropsychopharmacol*, 25/10: 1501–12.

Vieta E, Torrent C, Garcia-Ribas G, Gilabert A, Garcia-Pares G, Rodriguez A, Cadevall J, García-Castrillón J, Lusilla P, and Arrufat F. (2002). Use of topiramate in treatment-resistant bipolar spectrum disorders. *J Clin Psychopharmacol*, 22/4: 431–5.

Vieta E, Langosch JM, Figueira ML, Souery D, Blasco-Colmenares E, Medina E, Moreno-Manzanaro M, Gonzalez MA, and Bellivier F. (2013). Clinical management and burden of bipolar disorder: results from a multinational longitudinal study (WAVE-bd). *Int J Neuropsychopharmacol*, 16/8: 1719–32.

van der Voort TYG, van Meijel B, Hoogendoorn AW, Goossens PJJ, Beekman ATF, and Kupka RW. (2015). Collaborative care for patients with bipolar disorder: Effects on functioning and quality of life. *J Affect Disord*, 179: 14–22.

Wang YT, Yeh TL, Lee IH, Chen KC, Chen PS, Yang YK, and Lu RB. (2009). Screening for bipolar disorder in medicated patients treated for unipolar depression in a psychiatric outpatient clinic using the Mood Disorder Questionnaire. *Int J Psychiatry Clin Pract*, 13/2:117–21.

Wilde A, Chan HN, Rahman B, Meiser B, Mitchell PB, Schofield PR, and Green MJ. (2014). A meta-analysis of the risk of major affective disorder in relatives of individuals affected by major depressive disorder or bipolar disorder. *J Affect Disord*, **158**: 37–47.

Woltmann E, Grogan-Kaylor A, Perron B, Georges H, Kilbourne AM, and Bauer MS. (2012). Comparative effectiveness of collaborative chronic care models for mental health conditions across primary, specialty, and behavioral health care settings: systematic review and meta-analysis. *Am J Psychiatry*, **169**/8: 790–804.

Yatham LN, Kennedy SH, O'Donovan C, Parikh S, MacQueen G, McIntyre R, Sharma V, Silverstone P, Alda M, Baruch P, Beaulieu S, Daigneault A, Milev R, Young LT, Ravindran A, Schaffer A, Connolly M, and Gorman CP; Canadian Network for Mood and Anxiety Treatments. (2005). Canadian Network for Mood and Anxiety Treatments (CANMAT) guidelines for the management of patients with bipolar disorder: consensus and controversies. *Bipolar Disord*, 7/Suppl 2: 5–69.

Yatham LN, Kennedy SH, Parikh SV, Schaffer A, Beaulieu S, Alda M, O'Donovan C, Macqueen G, McIntyre RS, Sharma V, Ravindran A, Young LT, Milev R, Bond DJ, Frey BN, Goldstein BI, Lafer B, Birmaher B, Ha K, Nolen WA, and Berk M. (2013). Canadian Network for Mood and Anxiety Treatments (CANMAT) and International Society for Bipolar Disorders (ISBD) collaborative update of CANMAT guidelines for the management of patients with bipolar disorder: update 2013. *Bipolar Disord*, **15**/1: 1–44.

Yildiz A, Vieta E, Leucht S, and Baldessarini RJ. (2011). Efficacy of antimanic treatments: meta-analysis of randomized, controlled trials. *Neuropsychopharmacology*, **36**/2: 375–89.

Chapter 12

Suicide and suicidal behaviour

Erkki Isometsä

Introduction

Completed suicide is a major cause of death. According to the World Health Organization (WHO) (2014), annually worldwide over 800000 people take their own lives. Suicide is a complex phenomenon, with multiple domains of risk factors, and valid perspectives for both scientific explanation and prevention. Suicide deaths form only the tip of an iceberg; for every suicide death there are more than ten-fold numbers of non-fatal suicide attempts; for any attempt, a manifold number of those who have suicidal ideas and plans.

For health care, however, a key fact is that according to numerous psychological autopsy studies (Cavanagh et al, 2003; Arsenault-Lapierre et al., 2004), almost all (~90%) subjects have suffered from some—usually multiple—mental disorders at time of death. Of all completed suicides, one-half to two-thirds are by people who have suffered from mood disorders, and up to one-half from substance use disorders (SUDs), most commonly of alcoholism or polysubstance abuse. Thus, preventing the suicide of subjects suffering from mood disorders or SUDs, or both, are key issues for suicide prevention overall (Mann et al., 2005), and therefore comprise the main foci of this review.

The vast majority of individuals suffering from mood or SUDs, if they are receiving treatment, are obtaining it within primary care services (Bruffaerts et al., 2011). Even though psychiatric settings usually are responsible for providing treatment for the most severe disorders and individuals with highest risk, from an epidemiological point of view, the role of primary health care is central for suicide prevention (Patel et al, 2015). Current epidemiological knowledge suggests that unfortunately, at present, the vast majority of suicidal individuals worldwide receives no treatment for their mental disorders or suicidal behaviour (Bruffaerts et al., 2011).

Epidemiology of suicide and suicidal behaviour

Suicide-related concepts

Suicidal behaviour is conceptually classified into suicide deaths (completed suicides), attempted suicide or self-harm, and suicidal ideation. However, not all self-harm involves intent to die and therefore a concept of non-suicidal self-injury (NSSI) has been developed. These concepts are debated, particularly around the question of whether or not deliberate self-harm with intent to die (attempted suicide) can be reliably differentiated from self-harm lacking this aim; i.e. whether a continuum can, in theory and practise, be categorized into separate phenomena or not.

This chapter refers to literature as classified in original research. If not otherwise stated, within this chapter the term 'suicide attempt' refers to intentional self-harm with at least some degree of intent to die. Due to limited space, NSSI is not covered (for a review see e.g. Whitlock & Selekman, 2014), except to the degree studies have included self-harm irrespective of intent to die.

Suicide process

Suicidal behaviour is usually conceptualized as a process, in which suicidal ideation progresses from thoughts of death to thinking of suicide, planning it, and eventually completing the act, which may then have a fatal or non-fatal outcome (Fig. 12.1). However, on some rare occasions suicide attempters describe their act as totally impulsive, and deny a phase of preceding suicidal ideation. Based on large-scale epidemiological studies, a common estimate is that of all individuals seriously considering suicide, about one-third will develop a plan for the act, and of those with a plan, about two-thirds eventually will attempt suicide (Kessler et al., 1999). In some cases, impulsive attempts occur in individuals with ideation but reportedly no planning. For every suicide death, there are more than tenfold number of non-fatal suicide attempts. The ratio of incidences of fatal to non-fatal acts is strongly related to age (Nock et al., 2008), with fatal acts being remarkably higher among the elderly than in adolescents and young adults, among whom incidence of non-fatal suicide attempts is highest.

What initiates the suicide process? Aetiology of suicidal behaviour is multifactorial. Mental disorders are important as risk factors for suicidal ideation and acts, and their presence is usually a precondition for a suicidal act to occur. However, not all individuals suffering from them are suicidal. Overall, most mental syndromes, and the associated hopelessness in particular, are found to predispose to suicidal ideation, whereas factors involving impaired self-control, such as impulsive-aggressive traits,

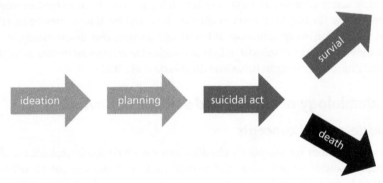

Fig. 12.1 Suicide process

use of substances, or neurocognitive deficits in decision-making, predispose to the transition to suicidal acts.

Current psychological theories of suicidal behaviour emphasize the role of psychological processes in the emergence of suicidal ideation, and deficits of decision-making for transition from ideation to acts (for a review, see O'Connor and Nock, 2014). Psychological vulnerability to suicidal behaviour has been conceptualized in multiple ways. In a cognitive model (Wenzel et al, 2009), activation of a suicide schema leads to hopelessness, selective attention towards suicide-relevant cues, and inability to disengage from them, all of which predispose to suicidal ideation. The frequency, duration, and severity of suicide-relevant cognitions will determine the probability that an individual will engage in a suicidal act. Furthermore, suicide schemas are postulated to strengthen with each suicidal act, so previous suicide attempts can be regarded as true risk factors for future suicidal acts, not merely indicators of vulnerability. Cognitive therapy has been shown in a randomized clinical trial among recent suicide attempters to reduce repetitions of suicide attempts.

Role of mental disorders as risk factors for suicide

It is ultimately impossible to know the mental state of an individual preceding the act of suicide. However, reasonable estimates can be constructed by using the methodology of a psychological autopsy. In brief, this method involves reconstruction of an individual's mental state and life situation based on information obtained from interviews of next of kin, attending health care personnel, medical and psychiatric records, plus police and forensic examination (Isometsä, 2001). Integration of information from multiple sources has been shown to result in reliable estimates of mental disorders, personality pathology and stressors. Since the late 1950s, numerous psychological autopsy studies have been conducted, and the view of mental disorder preceding suicide is consistent with few exceptions.

Suicides in the absence of a mental disorder are rare. Between one half and two thirds of suicides have suffered from mood disorders, about up to one half various types of substance use disorders, and between one third to one half from a personality disorder (Cavanagh et al, 2003; Arsenault-Lapierre et al., 2004) (Table 12.1). Approximately

Table 12.1 Typical prevalence of mental disorders among unselected suicides in psychological autopsy studies

Disorder	Prevalence
Depressive disorders	50–70%
Bipolar disorder	3–10%
Schizophrenia	5–10%
Substance use disorders	40–50%
Personality disorders	30–50%
Any mental disorder	*≈90%*

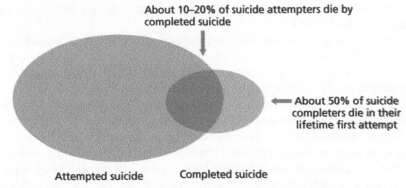

Fig. 12.2 The relationship between completed and attempted suicide
Reproduced from *The Canadian Journal of Psychiatry*, 59, Isometsä E., 'Suicidal Behaviour in Mood Disorders—Who, When, and Why?', pp. 120–130. Copyright (2014) with permission from Canadian Psychiatric Association.

up to one-quarter of suicides are estimated to have suffered from psychotic disorders at the time of death; this figure includes all types of mental disorders with psychotic symptoms (Henriksson et al., 1993). Overall, in about one in ten suicides, no diagnosis can be assigned, either due to no apparent psychopathology, conflicting or missing information, or difficulty of judging psychological health in the context of unusual circumstances (Henriksson et al.,1993). Large-scale prospective cohort studies of patients with mental disorders offer a complementary view of risk of suicide related to mental disorders (see e.g. Nordentoft et al., 2011), and find the same mental disorders to involve highest suicide risk.

By necessity, much of the literature focuses on suicide attempts as proxy for completed suicide. Studies on suicide attempts provide important information on suicidal acts, but it is important to remember differences in characteristics between populations of completed and attempted suicide. In general, completers are much more often males, have used more lethal methods than overdoses, are somewhat older, have in about 50% died in their lifetime first attempt, and suffered from more severe psychopathology than the attempters (Isometsä and Lönnqvist, 1998; Beautrais, 2001). Up to 20% of suicide attempters will eventually die by suicide (Fig. 12.2) (Suominen et al., 2004).

Elevated risk of suicide/death by suicide due to mood disorder

Early estimates of lifetime risk of patients with unipolar or bipolar mood disorders suggested that up to 19% will die by suicide. However, there were significant limitations both in the available data as well as the methodology, and the high estimates are incompatible with prevalence estimates of depression in the general population. Bostwick and Pankratz (2000) documented a gradient of lifetime suicide risk (case fatality prevalence) from general population to suicidal inpatients with mood disorders ranging from 0.5 to 8.6%. The most accurate current estimates of lifetime suicide risk are from a national study of suicide risk following all subjects treated in a psychiatric hospital or as outpatients in Denmark (Nordentoft et al., 2011). The study found life-time risk for men with depressive disorders at 6.7% and at 3.8% for females. However, these estimates do not generalize to primary care patients, or general population sub-jects not having treatment contacts for their disorder. In the longest follow-up study reported, Angst et al. (2005) found 11.1% of patients with mood disorders to have committed suicide in 40–44 years. All case fatality estimates unavoidably reflect treat-ments available during the past decades, not outcomes of patients in current settings.

Risk factors for suicide among subjects with depression

Information on risk factors for suicide death among patients with depression is rela-tively limited. The register-based Danish national study (Nordentoft et al., 2011) found male gender, history of a suicide attempt, and comorbid substance use disorder all asso-ciated with higher risk of completed suicide in unipolar mood disorders. Prospective clinical cohort studies of patients with mood disorders have found risk factors for completed suicide to include male gender, family history of suicide, previous suicide attempts, hopelessness, suicidal ideation, psychotic symptoms, comorbid personality disorders, alcohol dependence or misuse, and anxiety disorders. A systematic review by Hawton et al. (2013a) confirmed the role of these risk factors, except psychotic symptoms and suicidal ideation not reaching statistical significance.

Some psychological autopsy studies have specifically focused or reported on suicides with mood disorders, and present largely concordant findings (Isometsä, 2014). Almost all suicides with major depression have significant psychiatric or somatopsychiatric comorbidity, and substance use disorders and borderline per-sonality disorders are particularly prevalent. Impulsive-aggressive personality traits are important risk factors among suicides among young adults, particularly males, whereas the role of concurrent physical illness is more important among the middle-aged or elderly. Adverse life events, particularly losses, are the typical psychosocial context of suicide. Multiple stressors, some perhaps precipitating mood episodes, others more likely triggering the act, appear common among suicides by subjects with mood disorders.

Suicide among subjects with substance use disorders

Of all suicides, up to one half have suffered from substance use disorder, most com-monly alcohol use disorders or polysubstance abuse (Cavanagh et al., 2003; Arsenault-Lapierre et al., 2004). In addition, irrespective of preceding or concurrent disorders, about one-half of suicides have been under the influence of alcohol or other substances at the time of the act. The same is true for suicide attempters (Hawton et al., 2013b).

Ecological studies have documented a consistent correlation of consumption of alcohol and suicide mortality, particularly of middle-aged males. In epidemiologi-cal general population studies, alcohol use disorders have consistently been found to involve two-to-three-fold risk for suicidal ideation, attempts, and deaths (Borges and Loera, 2010; Darvishi et al., 2015). Use of illicit drugs is related to similar or higher risk (Borges and Loera, 2010).

In psychological autopsy studies, the vast majority of suicides with substance use disorders have been found to suffer from concurrent depressive syndromes and personality disorders, most commonly borderline personality disorder (Cavanagh et al, 2003). The life situation of these subjects has commonly been characterized by presence of interpersonal losses and conflicts during the final weeks (Heikkinen at al., 1994). However, in contrast to majority of suicides with depression, in a psychological autopsy study only a minority (30%) of those with alcoholism were found to have been in contact with health care services during their final month (Isometsä et al., 1995).

Suicide and suicidal behaviour in primary health care settings

Suicide deaths in primary care settings

Knowing risk factors for suicide is a precondition for rational preventive efforts. However, there are many limitations in the available literature, particularly pertaining to suicidal behaviour in primary care. Research on suicide specifically in primary health care settings is scarce, and much of what is known must be extrapolated from general population epidemiological studies, or clinical psychiatric studies. As findings related to central risk factors for suicidal behaviour are mostly robust (Nock et al., 2008), such extrapolations are usually valid. However, generalizability of findings related to incidence and prevalence of end-points, or predictive values of risk indicators from one primary care setting to another still remains uncertain. This is due to numerous factors, including major differences in organizations and funding of national health care systems, density of primary care doctors, availability of psychiatric consultations and psychiatric out- and in-patient or substance use disorder services, urban vs. rural settings, and most importantly, the characteristics of the populations served.

However, studies of unselected general population suicides allow some comparison of characteristics between suicides occurring in the context of primary care vs. psychiatric services. In general, suicides in primary care appear to involve relatively more often rural settings, older individuals, males, those with depression and with chronic somatic illnesses, and less communication of suicidal intent with health care professionals (Isometsä et al, 1994a; Conwell et all, 2000).

Risk of suicide among patients with physical diseases in primary care

Many somatic diseases (e.g. asthma, cancer, coronary heart disease, diabetes mellitus, epilepsy, and stroke) are associated with increased rates of suicide deaths. However, these diseases are also associated with increased prevalence of depression. A major issue is therefore whether the increased rate is due to illness per se or to co-occurring depression. A vast case-control study based on the General Practice Research Database in England (Webb et al., 2012) found suicide risks associated with 11 diseases were mostly explained by the presence of clinical depression. Nevertheless, in women with cancer or coronary heart disease, the physical disease appeared to involve elevated risk of suicide despite controlling for depression. This finding is consistent with the findings of psychological autopsy studies focusing on suicides in the elderly (Conwell et al., 2000) or on subjects with cancer (Henriksson et al., 1995).

Risk of suicide among patients with depression in primary care

Depressive patients with the highest risk of suicide are usually clustered into psychiatric settings, particularly among psychiatric in-patients. Consequently, incidence of suicide among primary care patient cohorts with depression is usually found to be lower than that of that of psychiatric out-patients, and markedly lower than that of psychiatric in-patients (Bostwick & Pankratz, 2000; Simon et al., 2007). However, characteristics of patients treated in these settings depend on availability and types of services, and are therefore likely to vary markedly.

Poor recognition of mild depression is a common problem in primary care. However, whether this is also true for depression eventually leading to attempted or completed suicide needs to be investigated; it is important to note that such depressions may be clinically more severe or complicated, and therefore more often recognized. Whether or not the risk for suicidal acts depends on severity, chronicity, or comorbidity, i.e. whether a meaningful risk is present in all depression, however mild, or clustered into a more ill subgroup, is decisive for creating optimal preventive strategies. Overall, suicide mortality among depressed patients is lower in primary care than in psychiatric settings (Simon et al., 2007). A psychological autopsy study focusing on depression in primary care (Isometsä et al, 1994, 1995) found the majority of suicides to be males with psychiatric comorbidity and untreated depression who rarely communicated their intent, particularly during the last appointment preceding suicide. Similarly, studies on suicide attempters in primary care report rare communication of suicidal ideation even if receiving treatment for depression (Houston et al., 2003; Vuorilehto et al., 2006; Riihimäki et al., 2014).

Suicidal behaviour among patients with depression in primary health care

Few studies have rigorously investigated suicidal ideation and attempts among primary care patients with depression. In a cohort study representative of a Finnish city, one-quarter of all patients with depressive disorder reported suicidal ideation during the current episode, and one-sixth had attempted suicide during their lifetime (Vuorilehto et al., 2006). The attempters were patients with moderate to severe major depressive disorder, psychiatric comorbidity with personality disorders, and a history of psychiatric care. Most were already receiving treatment for depression, but their suicidal ideation had usually remained unrecognized. A five-year follow-up of the cohort (Riihimäki et al., 2014) found that 10% of the patients attempted suicide, some multiple times. Riihimäki et al. also found suicide attempts to occur almost exclusively during major depressive episodes, often with concurrent substance abuse, but the attempts were hardly ever known by the attending primary care physician. Thus, the available studies accord that suicidal acts tend to cluster in major depressive episodes of complicated high-risk patients, but their suicidal intention or acts commonly remain unrecognized. Furthermore, primary care doctors were aware of the patient being depressed, but unaware of them having suicidal thoughts, and did not know about the suicide attempts during the follow-up. These findings are consistent with studies of suicide finding that suicidal intent was rarely communicated in the last appointments preceding suicide, and particularly so in primary care settings (Isometsä et al., 1995; Luoma et al, 2002). Thus, improving recognition of suicidal ideation and attempts appears important with regard to preventive measures.

Suicidal behaviour among subjects with substance use disorders in primary care

Clinical-epidemiological research on suicidal behaviour of patients with substance use disorders pertaining to primary health care is scarce. However, studies of depression in primary care highlight the potential importance of substance use disorders as a predictor for suicide attempts, as well as active substance use in precipitating the attempts (Riihimäki et al., 2014).

Assessment of suicide risk in primary care

Many of the general sociodemographic, psychosocial, and clinical risk factors for suicide are well known, as well as typical characteristics of suicides. However, most of the indicators of risk are prevalent, and suicide is a rare event. Therefore, the positive predictive value of these indicators of risk is low, while the proportion of false positive remarkably high, even when combining predictors.

A further problem is the conceptual and practical ambiguity of key concepts of suicidal ideation and suicide attempt or self-harm. Different operational definitions and temporal frameworks of assessment result in marked variations in who is considered to have suicidal ideation (Vuorilehto et al., 2014). Moreover, those with self-harm vs. suicide attempts are overlapping, but in partly dissimilar populations. Nevertheless, when robustly measured with a specified scale, presence of suicidal ideation may translate into risk of a suicide attempt of approximately 40% within the next six months (Vuorilehto et al., 2014). Use of structured measures of suicidal behaviour such as the Columbia-Suicide Severity Rating Scale (Posner et al., 2011) may markedly improve evaluation of risk, if sufficient training and time for evaluation are available.

Overall, primary care doctors need to be informed about the main risk factors for suicide, and feel capable of assessing suicidal ideation in order to target treatment efforts and referrals to those estimated to be at high risk. However, the difficulty of prediction must also be recognized.

Suicide prevention in primary health care settings

Potentials of treatment provision for mental disorders in preventing of suicide

The role of improved detection and management of depression in primary health care is one of the central cornerstones of national suicide prevention strategies. Earlier psychological autopsy studies uniformly indicated most suicides with depression to have occurred without the individual having received adequate, or any, treatment (Isometsä, 1994). Findings from representative forensic toxicological studies similarly have found that suicides were rarely positive for any antidepressant when the lethal method was not an antidepressant overdose (Isacsson et al., 2009). Despite remarkable increase in utilization of antidepressants, even recent studies have found the overwhelming majority of suicides to have been untreated. Information on psychotherapy, electroconvulsive therapy, or other treatments is quite limited, but the findings that do exist are similar (Isometsä et al., 1994).

Few studies have specifically examined suicides in primary care settings, generally finding evidence of adequate treatment in primary care even scarcer than among specialist settings. In most countries, because primary care doctors are responsible for treatment provision for the majority of patients with depression, it is clear that their role has been seen as central for suicide prevention. Overall, improving quality of care of primary care depression is in itself important, but whether education and training are the optimal strategy for preventing suicide remains open, and may depend on time and setting. As previously mentioned here, it is possible that the major problem in prevention may often be an unawareness of suicidal histories, ideas, and plans, rather than the fact that mere depression has remained unrecognized (Vuorilehto et al., 2006; Riihimäki et al., 2014). Nevertheless, benefits of screening for suicide risk are quite uncertain (O'Connor et al, AHRQ Task Force, 2013), and in the absence of clear benefit, some national guidelines advise against use of any risk evaluation scales (NICE, 2011).

Efficacy of specific treatments/interventions targeting mental disorders or suicidal behaviour

A central issue in the discussion of suicide prevention is whether or not providing pharmacological, psychotherapeutic, or other treatment for individuals suffering from mental disorders is effective as prevention. Given what is known about the role of mental disorders in suicide, the availability of treatments, and the public health impact of mental disorders overall, the expectation of improved services resulting in positive effects is rational (Cavanagh et al, 2003). With regard to depression, an ecological study of 28 European Union countries found consistent correlations between increasing antidepressant sales and reductions in suicide mortality in almost all of the countries (Guzmao et al., 2013). However, ecological studies are vulnerable to fallacies, are no proof of causality, and if a true effect of treatment exists, it is likely to reflect all facets of treatment provision (treatment-seeking, recognition, and benefits from both pharmacological and psychosocial treatment), rather than antidepressants alone. Unfortunately, randomized clinical trials (RCTs) of acute or maintenance phase antidepressant treatment cannot provide reliable evidence for efficacy in suicide prevention due to the lack of statistical power because of relative rarity of suicide, and exclusion of suicidal individuals from the RCTs.

Educating primary care doctors about the treatment of depression and suicide risk evaluation has been seen as one of the most plausible means of large-scale suicide prevention (Mann et al., 2005). However, the temporary success of the pioneering Gotland study in the 1980s (Rutz et al., 1992) has turned out to be difficult to replicate. Another major intervention study focusing on education and training of primary care doctors in Hungary in treatment of depression was to some extent successful in reducing suicide rate in the county of intervention (Szanto et al., 2007). A multimodal, population-level German intervention study involved also primary care doctors, and was successful in reducing non-fatal suicidal acts in the city of Nuremberg (Hegerl et al., 2006). The success of this work resulted in formation of the European Alliance Against Depression (EAAD) and consequently, various multi-country interventions studies. As effectiveness of educational interventions in changing doctors' behaviour is known to be limited overall (Gilbody et al., 2003), evaluation of the impact of stepped or collaborative care models in terms of suicide prevention is an important task. As numerous brief psychological interventions are currently being developed which target the high-risk group of suicide attempters in hospital and emergency room settings, integrating and coordinating such interventions into care provided in primary care settings will be an important future effort.

Conclusion

Primary health care is the first arena of suicide prevention in most countries. Given this central role, the knowledge in the context of primary care of suicidal behaviour and deaths remains inadequate. The majority of suicides attend primary care services the preceding year, and often also during the final weeks, before their suicidal act. However, these patients rarely communicate their intent, and are rarely correctly identified to be at risk. Most suicide deaths in primary care settings are by males suffering from depression, substance use disorders, or both, for which they have rarely received adequate treatment, or adhered to it. Co-occurrence of mental disorders and somatic illnesses is the rule, rather than an exception, among primary care suicides. Increasing provision of antidepressant treatment of depression may have reduced suicide rates in Europe, but this conclusion is tentative and based mainly on ecological findings. Some multimodal intervention studies have provided encouraging results for suicide prevention, but the generalizability of their findings remains open at present. For purposes of prevention, improving quality and continuity of care of depression and substance use disorders, as well as integrating targeted brief psychosocial interventions, are factors of central importance.

References

Angst J, Angst F, Gerber-Werder R, and Gamma A. (2005). Suicide in 406 mood-disorder patients with and without long-term medication: A 40 to 44 years' follow-up. *Archives of Suicide Research*, 9: 279–300.

Arsenault-Lapierre G, Kim C, and Turecki G. (2004). Psychiatric diagnoses in 3275 suicides: a meta-analysis. *BMC Psychiatry*, 4: 37.

Beautrais AL. (2003). Suicide and serious suicide attempts in youth: a multiple-group comparison study. *Am J Psychiatry*, 160: 1093–9.

Beautrais AL. (2001). Suicides and serious suicide attempts: two populations or one? *Psychol Med*, 31: 837–45

Borges G and Loera CR. (2010). Alcohol and drug use in suicidal behaviour. *Curr Opin Psychiatry*, 23/3: 195–204.

Bostwick JM and Pankratz VS. (2000). Affective disorders and suicide risk: a reexamination. *Am J Psychiatry*, 157:1925–32.

Bruffaerts R, Demyttenaere K, Hwang I, Chiu WT, Sampson N, Kessler RC, Alonso J, Borges G, de Girolamo G, de Graaf R, Florescu S, Gureje O, Hu C, Karam EG, Kawakami N, Kostyuchenko S, Kovess-Masfety V, Lee S, Levinson D, Matschinger H, Posada-Villa J, Sagar R, Scott KM, Stein DJ, Tomov T, Viana MC, and Nock MK. (2011). Treatment of suicidal people around the world. Br J Psychiatry, 199/1:64–70.

Cavanagh JT, Carson AJ, Sharpe M, and Lawrie SM. (2003). Psychological autopsy studies of suicide: a systematic review. *Psychol Med*, 33/3:395–405.

Conwell Y, Lyness JM, Duberstein P, Cox C, Seidlitz L, DiGiorgio A, and Caine ED. (2000). Completed suicide among older patients in primary care practices: a controlled study. *J Am Geriatr Soc*, 48/1: 23–9.

Darvishi N, Farhadi M, Haghtalab T, and Poorolajal J. (2015). Alcohol-related risk of suicidal ideation, suicide attempt, and completed suicide: a meta-analysis. *PLoS One*, 10/5: e0126870: doi: 10.1371/journal.pone.0126870. eCollection 2015.

Gilbody S, Whitty P, Grimshaw J, and Thomas R. (2003). Educational and organizational interventions to improve the management of depression in primary care: a systematic review. *JAMA*, 289: 3145–51.

Gusmão R, Quintão S, McDaid D, Arensman E, Van Audenhove C, Coffey C, Värnik A, Värnik P, Coyne J, and Hegerl U. (2013). Antidepressant Utilization and Suicide in Europe: An Ecological Multi-National Study. *PLoS One*, 8/6: e66455.

Hawton K, Casañas I Comabella C, Haw C, and Saunders K. (2013a). Risk factors for suicide in individuals with depression: a systematic review. *J Affect Disord*, 147: 17–28.

Hawton K, Saunders K, Topiwala A, Haw C. (2013b). Psychiatric disorders in patients presenting to hospital following self-harm: a systematic review. *J Affect Disord*, 151: 821–30.

Hegerl U, Althaus D, Schmidtke A, and Niklewski G. (2006). The alliance against depression: 2-year evaluation of a community-based intervention to reduce suicidality. *Psychol Med*, 36: 1225–33.

Heikkinen ME, Aro HM, Henriksson MM, Isometsä ET, Sarna SJ, Kuoppasalmi KI, Lönnqvist JK. (1994). Differences in recent life events between alcoholic and depressive nonalcoholic suicides. *Alcohol Clin Exp Res*, 18: 1143–9.

Henriksson MM, Isometsä ET, Hietanen PS, Aro HM, Lönnqvist JK. (1995). Mental disorders in cancer suicides. *J Affect Disord*, 36/1–2: 11–20.

Henriksson MM, Aro HM, Marttunen MJ, Heikkinen ME, Isometsä ET, Kuoppasalmi KI, and Lonnqvist JK. (1993). Mental Disorders and Comorbidity in Suicide. Am J Psychiatry, 150/6: 935–40.

Houston K, Haw C, Townsend E, and Hawton K. (2003). General practitioner contacts with patients before and after deliberate self-harm. *Br J Gen Practice*, 53: 365–70.

Isacsson G, Holmgren A, Osby U, and Ahlner J. (2009). Decrease in suicide among the individuals treated with antidepressants: a controlled study of antidepressants in suicide, Sweden 1995–2005. *Acta Psychiatr Scand*, 120: 37–44.

Isometsä ET, Aro HM, Henriksson MM, Heikkinen ME, Lönnqvist JK. (1994a). Suicide in major depression in different treatment settings. *J Clin Psychiatry*, 55: 523–7.

Isometsä ET, Henriksson MM, Heikkinen ME, Aro HM, Marttunen MJ, Kuoppasalmi KI, and Lönnqvist JK. (1994b). Suicide in major depression. *Am J Psychiatry*, 151: 530–36.

Isometsä ET. (2001). Psychological autopsy studies--a review. *Eur Psychiatry*, 16/7: 379–85.

Isometsä ET, Heikkinen, ME, Marttunen MJ, Henriksson MM, Aro HM, Lönnqvist JK. (1995). The last appointment before suicide: is suicide intent communicated? *Am J Psychiatry*, 152: 919–22.

Isometsä ET. Suicidal behaviour in mood disorders--who, when, and why? (2014). *Can J Psychiatry*, 59:120–30.

Isometsä ET and Lönnqvist JK. (1998). Suicide attempts preceding completed suicide. (1998). *Br J Psychiatry*, 173: 531–6.

Kessler RC, Borges G, and Walters EE. (1999). Prevalence of and risk factors for lifetime suicide attempts in the National Comorbidity Survey. *Arch Gen Psychiatry*, 56/7: 617–26.

Luoma JB, Martin CE, and Pearson JL. (2002). Contact with mental health and primary careproviders before suicide: a review of the evidence. *Am J Psychiatry*, 159/6: 909–16.

Mann JJ, Apter A, Bertolote J, Beautrais A, Currier D, Haas A, Hegerl U, Lonnqvist J, Malone K, Marusic A, Mehlum L, Patton G, Phillips M, Rutz W, Rihmer Z, Schmidtke A, Shaffer D, Silverman M, Takahashi Y, Varnik A, Wasserman D, Yip P, and Hendin H. (2005). Suicide prevention strategies: a systematic review. *JAMA*, 294: 2064–74.

National Institute for Health and Clinical Excellence (NICE). (2011). *Self-harm: longer-term management.* (Clinical guideline CG133.) Available at: http://guidance.nice.org.uk/CG133.

Nock MK, Borges G, Bromet EJ, Cha CB, Kessler RC, and Lee S. (2008). Suicide and suicidal behavior. *Epidemiol Rev*, 30: 133–54.

Nordentoft M, Mortensen PB, and Pedersen CB. (2011). Absolute risk of suicide after first hospital contact in mental disorder. *Arch Gen Psychiatry*, 68: 1058–64.

O'Connor R and Nock MK. (2014). The psychology of suicidal behavior. *Lancet Psychiatry*, 1: 73–85.

Patel V, Chisholm D, Parikh R, Charlson FJ, Degenhardt L, Dua T, Ferrari AJ, Hyman S, Laxminarayan R, Levin C, Lund C, Medina Mora ME, Petersen I, Scott J, Shidhaye R, Vijayakumar L, Thornicroft G, Whiteford H, and DCP MNS Author Group. (2015). Addressing the burden of mental, neurological, and substance use disorders: key messages from Disease Control Priorities, 3rd edition. *Lancet*, 387/10028: 1672–85.

Posner K, Brown GK, Stanley B, Brent DA, Yershova KV, Oquendo MA, Currier GW, Melvin GA, Greenhill L, Shen S, and Mann JJ. (2011). The Columbia-Suicide Severity Rating Scale: initial validity and internal consistency findings from three multisite studies with adolescents and adults. *Am J Psychiatry*, 168: 1266–77.

Riihimäki K, Vuorilehto M, Melartin T, Haukka J, and Isometsä E. (2014). Incidence and predictors of suicidal attempts among primary-care patients with depressive disorders: A five-year prospective study. *Psychol Med*, 44: 291–302.

Rutz W, von Knorring L, and Wålinder J. (1992). Long-term effects of an educational program for general practitioners given by the Swedish Committee for the Prevention and Treatment of Depression. *Acta Psychiatr Scand*, 85: 83–8.

Simon GE and Savarino J. (2007). Suicide attempts among patients starting depression treatment with medications or psychotherapy. *Am J Psychiatry*, 164/7: 1029–34.

Suominen K, Isometsä E, Suokas J, Haukka J, Achte K, and Lönnqvist J. (2004). Completed suicide after a suicide attempt: a 37-year follow-up study. *Am J Psychiatry*, 161: 562–3.

Szanto K, Kalmar S, Hendin H, Rihmer Z, and Mann JJ. (2007). A suicide prevention program in a region with a very high suicide rate. *Arch Gen Psychiatry*, 64: 914–20.

Vuorilehto M, Melartin T, and Isometsä E. (2006). Suicidal behaviour among primary care patients with depressive disorders. *Psychol Med*, 36: 203–210.

Vuorilehto M, Valtonen HM, Melartin T, Sokero P, Suominen K, and Isometsä ET. (2014). Method of assessment determines prevalence of suicidal ideation among patients with depression. *Eur Psychiatry*, 29/6: 338–44.

Webb RT, Kontopantelis E, Doran T, Qin P, Creed F, and Kapur N. (2012). Suicide risk in primary care patients with major physical diseases: a case-control study. *Arch Gen Psychiatry*, 69/3: 256–64.

Wenzel A, Brown GK, and Beck AT. (2009). *Cognitive therapy for suicidal patients. Scientific and clinical applications*. Washington, DC: American Psychological Association.

Whitlock J and Selekman MD. (2014). Nonsuicidal self-injury across the lifespan. In: *The Oxford Handbook of Suicide and Self-Injury*, Matthew K. Nock, ed. Oxford: Oxford University Press, 133–51.

World Health Organization. (2014). Preventing suicide: a global imperative. Geneva: World Health Organization.

Chapter 13

Somatic symptom and related disorders

Alexandra Murray, Anne Toussaint, and Bernd Löwe

Introduction

Primary Care Practitioners (PCPs) represent an integral part of mental health care (Jacob & Patel, 2014). As the patients' usual first point of contact with the health care system, PCPs not only connect patients to secondary and specialist services, but they also have the unique opportunity and obligation to comprehensively evaluate patients' health and psychosocial context (Starfield, 1994). For these reasons, a joint report from the World Health Organisation (WHO) and the World Organization of Family Doctors (WONCA) (2008) argues that integration of mental health and primary health care can improve outcomes, increase the provision of mental health services, be cost effective, and reduce stigma and discrimination by allowing patients to achieve functional recovery, while remaining in the community.

Arguably, the role of the PCP in the management of patients with somatoform symptoms is particularly important as there are a number of factors that necessitate the integrated management of mental and somatic aspects across different levels of the health care system. PCPs are positioned perfectly to gain a biopsychosocial understanding of patients and have the advantages of (1) often having an ongoing relationship with the patient which may facilitate care and knowledge of the patient's context (e.g. family), (2) being able to integrate examination and assessment of somatic and mental concerns in the first consultation, and (3) patients may be more comfortable in discussing psychological distress with their PCPs than in secondary or tertiary mental health care settings (Fritzsche, McDaniel, & Wirsching, 2014).

In addition to PCPs being well-positioned in the health care system to assist patients, somatoform and functional disorders comprise a large proportion of PCPs' consultations (Rief & Martin, 2014). It is estimated that up to two-thirds of symptoms presented in primary care are 'medically unexplained' (Steinbrecher, Koerber, Frieser, & Hiller, 2011) and 16–30% of patients have a diagnosable somatoform disorder depending on the criteria used (de Waal, Arnold, Eekhof, & van Hemert, 2004; Fink, Sorensen, Engberg, Holm, & Munk-Jorgensen, 1999; Steinbrecher et al., 2011). Apart from the sheer numbers of these patients, somatoform disorders are associated with high direct and indirect costs (Gustavsson et al., 2011), impairment (de Waal et al., 2004), health care utilization (Barsky, Orav, & Bates, 2005), and high rates of comorbidity and multi-morbidity (Hanel et al., 2009; Löwe et al., 2008; Steinbrecher et al., 2011).

Despite the costs, burden, and frequency of somatoform and related disorders, the diagnostic category was rarely used in the past (Levenson, 2011; Stein, 2013). Functional syndromes or the term medically unexplained symptoms (MUS) have been used as diagnostic labels, presumably because these options are more acceptable to patients (Kuruvilla & Jacob, 2012; Soler & Okkes, 2012). This, however, has led to confusion within the field and makes comparative research difficult. If we consider diagnosis as a gateway to targeted treatment, this confusion and underutilization of this nosologic category is particularly problematic (Stein, 2013). However, this argument may no longer be relevant given the recent changes to the diagnostic criteria (please see section Diagnostic process).

Unfortunately, previous reports have shown that PCPs find this patient group particularly difficult to manage (Rosendal et al., 2005), while some patients also report dissatisfaction or distrust with MUS management and treatment in primary care (Peters et al., 2009). It is important, therefore, to have clear diagnostic and management strategies within and beyond the primary care setting.

Foundations of optimal care

The biopsychosocial approach

The fundamental basis of psychosomatic medicine is the biopsychosocial approach which considers the biological, psychological, and social context of the patient, and his/her disease or suffering (Engel, 1977; Fritzsche et al., 2014). To do this, patient care should be essentially interdisciplinary and physicians should emphasise the importance of understanding patients' multifactorial context and psychosocial influences, regardless of the underlying pathology (Fritzsche et al., 2014). An awareness of psychosocial influences is especially important in somatoform disorders as patients may come to the consultation believing that their symptoms have a pure physical (i.e. somatic) aetiology (Aiarzaguenaet al., 2008), and thus could be unaware of psychosocial mechanisms or maintenance factors (Dwamena et al., 2009).

Patient-centred care

As part of the biopsychosocial approach, patient-centred care is also inherent to psychosomatic medicine (see also Hudonet al., 2011). Patient-centred care has been identified as one of the key elements of high quality health care and a central aim of the improvement of health care in general (Committee on Quality of Health Care in America, 2001; Epstein and Street, 2011). This approach has been linked to positive outcomes such as improvement in patients' emotional state and overall reduction in health care use (Bertakis and Azari, 2011; Hudon et al., 2011; Stewart et al., 2000). Although patient-centredness sounds upon first inspection self-explanatory, this concept is difficult to define, and there are several challenges to fully incorporate this model into routine care. The promotion of communication, the provision of information to patients, and the active involvement of patients in care are all parts of patient-centredness (Epstein and Street, 2011). If we consider patient-centred care as 'providing care that is respectful of and responsive to individual patient preferences, needs, and values and ensuring that patient values guide all clinical decisions' (Committee on Quality of Health Care in America, 2001: 6) then it is important to train both physicians to be mindful of patients, and patients to be more actively involved in consultations (Epstein and Street, 2011). This could include inviting patients to summarize treatment options with the idea of clarifying misunderstandings and making shared decisions (Epstein and Street, 2011). This is especially important for somatoform disorders because a satisfactory explanation of patients' symptoms is an important cornerstone of treatment but is often cited as an unmet patient need (Dowricket al., 2004). Ultimately, the aim is to develop a reliable patient-doctor collaborative relationship which is critical for the success of treatment (Fritzsche et al., 2014).

Doctor-patient communication

Open and effective doctor-patient communication is arguably the most important element of a good doctor-patient relationship. Good patient-doctor communication involves patient participation in both the diagnostic process and management of symptoms and co-operation throughout treatment (Fritzsche et al., 2014; Olde Hartman et al., 2013). The anamnesis interview can form the basis of 70% of all diagnoses (Fritzsche et al., 2014), and thus it is critical to include a discussion of patients' physical, social, and psychological history as well as the current situation. Communication techniques, such as active listening, asking open-ended questions, non-verbal encouragements, paraphrasing, and strategic use of pauses (Table 13.1) may enable the consultation to be focused on the patients' main concerns (for further information see Fritzsche et al., 2014).

Table 13.1 Some examples of useful communication techniques

Technique	Example
Active listening	Showing that doctors are actively engaged when the patient is talking can help the patient feel supported. E.g. use of encouraging words like 'yes', 'mmm hmm, I see' etc.
Open-ended questions	Asking open-ended questions encourages the patients to disclose more and focus on what is important for them. Doctor: e.g. 'What made you think these weren't normal stomach problems'?
Non-verbal communication	Nodding and keeping eye contact with the patient to show attentiveness and care.
Paraphrasing and summarizing	Summarizing and paraphrasing the patients' accounts shows that the doctor has been listening and gives the opportunity to clarify any misunderstandings. E.g. Doctor: 'So, just to re-cap, you have had these problems for three years but this is the first time they have affected your work'.
Strategic use of pauses	Giving patients some time and conversational space may encourage them to disclose more psychosocial information. E.g. Patient: 'I don't know, it has been tough ...' [*Pause*] '... tough because I don't know if I will get another job after my second child'

Diagnostic process

The changes to the latest version of the Diagnostic and Statistical Manual of Mental Disorders (American Psychiatric Association, 2013) have fundamentally shifted the way somatoform disorders are diagnosed and conceptualized. In the previous DSM edition (American Psychiatric Association, 2000), and according to the current ICD-10 system (World Health Organization, 1992), patients could only receive a diagnosis of a somatoform (somatization) disorder when physical symptoms were 'medically unexplained'. Not only did this dualism separate the somatic and psychological aspects of diagnosis and conceptualization, it also placed PCPs in a difficult professional and legal position. Under this model, PCPs were often hesitant to diagnose a somatoform disorder, possibly due to the fear of missing the diagnosis of a serious somatic illness (Ringsberg & Krantz, 2006). With the new conceptualization, however, patients with medical illnesses can also have the diagnosis of somatoform disorder (now referred to as Somatic Symptom and Related Disorders, or SSD) when they meet certain cognitive, affective or behavioural criteria (see Box 13.1). At least one of these psychological 'B' criteria must be present in addition to the presence of a distressing or disruptive

---

Box 13.1 Key Diagnostic Terms

Medically Unexplained Symptoms (MUS)—Symptoms which have no medical (organic) explanation. This term is sometimes used to avoid some of the problems with specific diagnostic criteria.

Functional Disorder—a disorder which is characterized by a dysfunction in the function of an organ or system rather than its structure.

Somatoform Disorder—general term for a mental disorder which is characterized by the presence of persistent physical symptoms. Most diagnostic criteria specify that the physical symptoms cannot be medically explained e.g. 'Somatization Disorder' in DSM-IV (American Psychiatric Association, 2000), or ICD-10 (World Health Organization, 1992).

Diagnostic and Statistical Manual of Mental Disorders, 5th Edition (DSM-5)—the current diagnostic criteria for mental disorders set out by the American Psychiatric Association.

Somatic Symptom Disorder (SSD)—the somatoform diagnostic category according to DSM-5. SSD differs from other conceptualizations of somatoform disorders because the medical 'explainability' of symptoms is not important and more emphasis is placed on the presence of positive psychological characteristics. The following three criteria must be fulfilled (American Psychiatric Association, 2013):

A. Presence of at least one disruptive physical symptom

B. Presence of excessive thoughts, behaviours, or feelings about the symptoms or health concerns

C. The patient should be persistently 'symptomatic' (usually more than six months)

Data from *Diagnostic and statistical manual of mental disorder*, 5th ed., 2013, American Psychiatric Association.

symptom, regardless of its aetiology (Criterion A). Finally, to fully meet DSM-5 diagnostic criteria patients must be symptomatic for six months or more (Criterion C).

Despite the shift away from a dualistic approach, changes to the diagnostic criteria have come under debate, with critics claiming that it will lead to large proportions of the population being diagnosed as 'mentally ill' (Frances, 2013) or the diagnostic category not being used at all (King, 2013). Certainly, the critical contrast to other somatoform diagnoses and the previous DSM-IV conceptualization brings about a new challenge in the diagnostic process. It is now important to assess patients' thoughts, behaviours, and affects associated with their symptoms, and to assess whether they are reasonable or 'proportionate' to their individual situation. This clinical judgement may be challenging and may require experience and training. It is still uncertain the impact these changes will have on the diagnostic process of SSD in primary care and other settings (Rief & Martin, 2014).

The DSM-5 criteria include the presence of 'disproportionate' thoughts, high levels of anxiety attached to symptoms, and excessive energy and time spent on symptoms (American Psychiatric Association, 2013), although the specific nature of these thoughts, feelings, or behaviours is unspecified. The utility and validity of certain features such as health anxiety, bodily weakness, and bodily scanning have been tested and data suggests they are helpful features to consider in this context (Voigt et al., 2012). Given that the diagnosis focuses on the impact of symptoms on the patient, and the psychological sequelae of this impact, psychological symptoms should also be targeted by treatment in addition to physical symptom management. Ideally, management should be undertaken in the primary care setting for patients with low levels of symptom severity, but more intensive care should be sought when certain warning signs are present (see the section Treatment in the primary care setting or other management strategies).

Even when placing more emphasis on the psychological component of symptoms, physical symptoms themselves should not be neglected. Neglecting them could indeed lead to missing a somatic illness or alienating the patient (Frances, 2013; Fritzsche et al., 2014). This is one of the central challenges to the diagnosis of somatoform disorders, i.e. knowing when to stop 'unnecessary' physical investigations or interventions, while also fully appreciating psychological aspects. Ideally, the possible somatoform nature of symptoms, or at least the psychosocial mechanisms leading to the formation of symptoms, should be discussed openly and early in the diagnostic process. Consistent with this approach, the introduction to the Dutch medical guidelines (Feltz-Cornelis et al., 2011) recently recommended that PCPs should concurrently pursue both somatic and psychological diagnostic procedures aiming to identify intertwined explanations for mental and physical symptoms. Firstly, it is important for PCPs to understand the patients' current concerns and symptoms, and to record any previous investigations and treatments they have already undergone.

There are a number of patient self-report questionnaires available to assist physicians assess the extent and severity of patients' symptoms (for example the 15 item Patient Health Questionnaire (PHQ-15; Kroenke et al., 2002) or the 25 item Bodily Distress Syndrome Checklist (Budtz-Lilly et al., 2015)). In addition, to aid the diagnosis of somatic symptom disorder in primary care and other settings, we have developed and validated a patient self-report questionnaire to measure the three 'B' sub-criteria

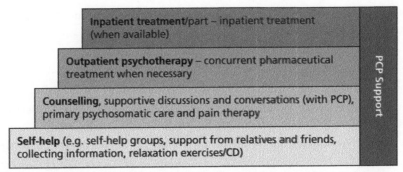

Fig. 13.1 Example of a stepped care model of treatment for somatoform disorders in primary care with links to other health care sectors. Patients' care is adapted to the appropriate level according to the severity of their symptoms and risk profile. As shown by the vertical side panel, although PCPs may not be the care provider for each step, they ideally should be a constant source of support throughout the treatment process (see also Schaefert et al., 2012)

(Toussaint et al., 2016). Other questionnaires such as the Whiteley Index-7 (Fink et al., 1999) or the Scale for the Assessment of Illness Behavior (SAIB; Riefet al., 2003) also cover aspects of these criteria. On their own, however, questionnaires are insufficient to form the basis of a diagnosis (Feltz-Cornelis et al., 2011) and should be used in conjunction with a comprehensive clinical evaluation. PCPs that have a long, ongoing relationship with patients may already be aware of some psychosocial stressors, which might play a role in the formation of symptoms, but clinicians should regularly ask patients about exposure to new stressors (e.g. life events).

Practical strategies

Table 13.2 presents some of the challenges to the diagnosis and care of patients with somatoform disorders, the effects they may have on treatment, and practical tips to overcome such barriers in routine practice (Murray et al., 2013; Murray et al., 2016). Ringsberg and Krantz (2006) also present some other practical strategies to overcome some of the challenges PCPs may face.

Treatment in the primary care setting or other management strategies

In some cases, it will become clear to the PCP that the patient needs more intensive or specialist care, which is beyond what they can directly provide in the primary care setting. When determining what type of care a patient needs, evidence-based medical guidelines (Feltz-Cornelis et al., 2011; Olde Hartman et al., 2013; Schaefert et al., 2012) suggest that a stepped care approach should be undertaken which varies in the intensity or 'dosage' of treatment according to patients' risk profiles (Fig. 13.1). Risk profiles refer to the extent that patients are at risk of chronic or sustained dysfunction. In their comprehensive guidelines, Schaefert et al. (2012; p. 808) identified a number of 'yellow flags' which may indicate a more moderate or severe course (i.e., a higher risk profile). These include:

◆ Several, frequent or persistent complaints

◆ Dysfunctional illness perception (e.g. marked health anxiety)

◆ Marked impairment (e.g. inability to work > 4 weeks, social withdrawal)

◆ Moderate to severe psychosocial stress (e.g. anxiety about the future, limited social support)

◆ Psychological comorbidity (e.g. depression, anxiety, post-traumatic stress disorder)

◆ Difficulties in the physician-patient relationship, which may include unfavourable PCP management strategies/behaviour (see Table 13.2)

Signs or characteristics indicative of more severe courses (i.e., 'red flags') include (Schaefert et al., 2012; 808):

◆ Very severe complaints or known warning signs of somatically defined diseases

◆ Self-harming behaviour or suicidality

◆ 'Physical sequelae'—the complaints lead to further physical health problems (e.g. limitation of movement due to 'sparing joints', marked weight gain)

◆ Severe psychological comorbidity (e.g. anxiety which prevents the patient from making social contacts)

◆ Frequent change of treating physicians or dropout of treatment

◆ Signs of severely poor management from PCP or health care system

As well as identifying factors that may indicate a more severe clinical course, it is also important to identify potential protective factors, which may support the patient and facilitate the management of patients' complaints, including but not limited to (i) active coping strategies (such as physical exercise, positive outlook and motivation for treatment; (ii) healthy lifestyle; (iii) social support (personal relationships and favourable work conditions); and (iv) openness to the biopsychosocial approach (Schaefert et al., 2012). PCPs should elicit patients' protective and worsening factors regularly to evaluate their current biopsychosocial context (Schaefert et al., 2012).

In consultation with the patient, the appropriate 'step' should be selected and then the intensity of the intervention can be 'stepped up' or 'stepped down' as needed. Patients with a low risk profile should be managed within the first two levels of the stepped care model. These approaches aim to motivate and educate the patient to take an active role in the management of his/her symptoms, with the support of the PCP (Feltz-Cornelis et al., 2011; Olde Hartman et al., 2013; Schaefert et al., 2012). On the other hand, patients with a moderate risk profile can also be managed in the primary care setting with proper support and consultation with specialist services. For high risk patients, specialist multidisciplinary/multimodal care including psychological inpatient/part-inpatient or psychiatric care is recommended (Schaefert et al., 2012).

Evidence suggests that somatoform disorders are treatable with the most studied approaches including psychotherapy (specifically cognitive-behavioural therapy), antidepressant medications, and the use of consultation letters (Kroenke, 2007). A Cochrane Review of the effects of pharmacological interventions in patients with

Table 13.2 Common mistakes, challenges, and potential strategies to overcome them

Mistake or challenge	Effect on patient and treatment	Potential management strategy
Problematic communication with patients such as not fully exploring, validating or explaining symptoms (Schaefert et al., 2012).	Patient may feel as though the PCP does not take their complaints seriously (Dirkzwager & Verhaak, 2007) and may search for alternative treatment options. This prevents a supportive on-going doctor-patient relationship.	◆ Acknowledge the bodily distress and attempt to reframe the symptom in terms of the patients' psychosocial context e.g. stress or lifestyle (Fritzsche et al., 2014).
Management of functional symptoms is inherently connected to the patients' socio-medico-legal context (e.g. the benefits of sick leave, PCP repercussions of missing a serious somatic diagnosis) (Mik-Meyer & Obling, 2012).	Some of the social advantages brought about by being in the 'sick role' may act as maintenance factors of the illness itself (Fritzsche et al., 2014).	◆ The influence of social factors should not be underestimated and taken into consideration during the consultation.
Giving patients their diagnosis in an unclear way, failing to give a diagnosis or dismissing the complaints as being 'all in the mind' (Schaefert et al., 2012).	Dismissing complaints may lead to patients developing strategies to convince PCPs that their suffering is real (Salmon, 2006). The effect can delay the start of appropriate treatment.	◆ It is important to validate and acknowledge the patients' suffering (Salmon, 2006). ◆ Attempt to give a clear diagnosis and explain how psychological and social influences can affect their symptoms.
Intolerance of uncertainty—in patients with diagnosed somatoform or functional disorders, PCPs may continue to perform diagnostic investigations to exclude somatic causes 'just to be sure' (Ringsberg & Krantz, 2006).	Unnecessary somatic investigations may send mixed signals to the patient. It is more difficult to understand the psychological contribution of symptoms if PCPS continue to focus on somatic results or investigations.	◆ Try to conduct somatic investigations only when necessary and be consistent when presenting explanations for symptoms. ◆ Try to avoid pressure from patients to perform somatic interventions (see also Salmon, Humphris, Ring, Davies, & Dowrick, 2006).
'Doctor shopping'—patients who constantly move from doctor to doctor to try to get the diagnosis, explanation, or treatment that they want.	Doctor shopping precludes integrated and coordinated care and an ongoing PCP-patient relationship.	◆ Attempt to improve the cooperation and communication with other health care professionals for successful referral (Schaefert et al., 2012). ◆ Schedule regular appointments with the patient to provide consistent and regular care which is determined by time rather than the severity of symptoms (Fritzsche et al., 2014; Olde Hartman et al., 2013).

(continued)

Table 13.2 Continued

Mistake or challenge	Effect on patient and treatment	Potential management strategy
Patients making unstructured 'complaint-led' appointments.	PCPs may feel pressured or unprepared to adequately explain the symptoms due to the ad-hoc nature of the appointments.	◆ Schedule regular appointments with the patient to provide consistent and regular care which is determined by time rather than the severity of symptoms (Fritzsche et al., 2014; Olde Hartman et al., 2013).
Maintaining a biomedical discussion and understanding of symptoms or presenting an 'either/or' biomedical or psychological model (Schaefert et al., 2012).	It is important to try to encourage a biopsychosocial understanding of patients' symptoms to help prevent patients constantly looking for non-existent 'medical' explanations.	◆ Recognize the contribution of psychosomatic factors on the illness. ◆ Undergo a parallel process of investigation of psychological and somatic aspects simultaneously (Feltz-Cornelis et al., 2011). ◆ Attempt to make the link between life stresses or personal context and physical symptoms clear. ◆ Encourage patients to keep a symptom diary to investigate the personal situations and context when patients experience symptoms (Fritzsche et al., 2014).

Data from *Journal of Psychosomatic Research*, 80, 2016, M.C. Shedden-Mora, et al, 'Collaborative stepped care for somatoform disorders: A pre–post-intervention study in primary care, , 80, pp. 23–30.

somatoform disorders found evidence that new-generation antidepressants and natural pharmacological products were more effective than placebo in treating somatoform symptoms (Kleinstauber et al., 2014). However, these findings were based on low-quality evidence (at best) and relatively high risks of adverse effects were found. In a meta-analysis of patients with chronic multiple MUS, Kleinstäuber et al. (2011) found an overall small but stable effect size of the efficacy of short-term psychotherapy (range: $d +=0.06$–$d +=0.40$; $n = 27$ studies). Although mental health professionals appeared to be more successful at performing psychotherapy, PCPs were more effective in addressing health care utilization. Another systematic review found small- to medium-effect sizes for psychotherapy compared to usual care (van Dessel et al., 2014), albeit with moderate heterogeneity and low quality of evidence. Psychotherapy has the advantage of actively involving patients in treatment while encouraging a biopsychosocial approach and reducing the risk of side effects, although the best treatment option should be tailored to the individual needs of each patient (Kleinstäuber et al., 2011).

When it is necessary for patients to be referred to secondary/tertiary services, it is important for PCPs to be well connected to specialist care clinics, psychotherapists, and other mental health care providers or support agencies in their local area (Schaefert et al., 2012). With the aim to improve the connection and communication between PCPs and mental health professionals, our group established a health network called Sofu-Net: Health network somatoform and functional disorders in Hamburg, Germany (please see Table 13.3 and Fig. 13.2). A basic premise of Sofu-Net was that if the communication between the stakeholders of care improved, then so would the flow of patients suffering from somatoform or functional symptoms through the health care system. Importantly, Sofu-Net was not only implemented on the level of the PCP and mental health care provider, but it also aimed to improve the understanding of the patient and general public of somatoform disorders. Specifically, a brief introduction to the disorder and possible treatment options were provided on the website and a psychoeducation group was established. Sofu-Net was implemented as part of a larger complex mental health intervention 'psychenet' (for more information, please see Härter et al., 2012).

We choose to present Sofu-Net here as an example of a complex intervention for patients suffering from somatic symptom and related disorders, because it draws in elements of many aspects of the management of patients suffering from somatic symptom and related disorders, which we discussed in this chapter:

1. Patients were screened and then treated according to a stepped care model (see Fig. 13.1).
2. The network aimed to improve the patient flow through the health care system Fig. 13.2 by minimizing the time between the first contact with the health system and the instigation of psychotherapy (when necessary). In this way, the PCP acts as the 'gatekeeper' of access to and co-ordinator of care.
3. Sofu-Net, as part of the larger project 'psychenet', attempted to address patients' needs within their local context. Public awareness campaigns (Härter et al., 2012) as well as psychoeducation groups were established (see Table 13.3).
4. The network emphasized the importance of the PCP communicating well with the patient and other health care providers. Communication between health professionals was facilitated by regular meetings, which were attended by Sofu-Net PCPs and psychotherapists as well as patient feedback forms (simplified consultation letters) and email distribution lists.
5. PCPs were continuously supported by specialists in the field.

Example intervention: A complex intervention to improve the management of patients with somatoform and functional complaints in primary care in Hamburg, Germany (Shedden Mora et al, 2015).

An alternative approach to referring patients outside of the primary care setting (such as in Sofu-Net) is integrated collaborative care. In such models, a team including PCPs, care management staff, and a psychiatric consultant are involved in the patients' care within a primary care setting (Unützer et al., 2013). Each patient is closely tracked using a validated scale (e.g. the PHQ-9 to measure depression; Kroenke et al., 2001) and treatment is adjusted according to their scores (Fig. 13.1).

Table 13.3 Sofu-Net network elements including diagnosis and stepped care.

Network element	Description
Stepped care approach	Management according to risk status for somatoform disorders including: ♦ Screening questionnaire to measure somatization (PHQ-15; Kroenke et al., 2002), depression (PHQ-9; Kroenke, Spitzer, & Williams, 2001), and anxiety (GAD-7; Spitzer, Kroenke, Williams, & Lowe, 2006) ♦ Use of a specialized outpatient clinic at the Department of Psychosomatic Medicine and Psychotherapy, University Medical Center Hamburg-Eppendorf
Improved communication and networking between stakeholders	One of major aims of the network is to promote communication and patient flow through the health care system. This involved the: ♦ Creation of a directory of all network partners including contact information as well as detailed information of individual specialties ♦ Creation of an email distribution list to enable PCPs to approach psychotherapists in search of free psychotherapy places ♦ Instigation of a short report form for psychotherapists to give back to PCPs to give feedback on patients' status.
Establishment of a co-ordinated network	The Sofu-Net was co-ordinated in the following fashion: ♦ The co-ordinating centre contacts all network partners every 4–6 weeks and is available in case of queries. ♦ Interdisciplinary quality circle meetings to discuss clinically relevant topics and case studies (three times per year) ♦ Network meetings and forum for evaluation of Sofu-Net operation, opportunities for improvement etc. (three times per year)
Improve communication with patients and the general public	In addition to co-ordinating care, the Sofu-net aimed to improve the provision of information to patients and the wider community by the: ♦ Creation and distribution of a patient information booklet which contains information on somatoform and functional disorders as well as key Sofu-Net details ♦ Instigation of a psychoeducation group to provide information about somatoform disorders, the bio-psycho-social illness model, different treatment options and steps into psychotherapy. ♦ Creation of a website with information on somatoform as well as other mental disorders, treatment options and steps into psychotherapy.

Data from *Journal of Psychosomatic Research*, 80, 2016, M.C. Shedden-Mora, et al, 'Collaborative stepped care for somatoform disorders: A pre–post-intervention study in primary care, 80, pp. 23–30.

Firstly, care is determined by the primary care team in consultation with a 'p-professional' (in this case a psychiatrist, but a psychologist or psychosomatic specialist could also fit well in this model). The care management staff member screens and regularly tracks the patient's progress and closely follows-up with the patient if they do not attend appointments, have problems with treatment effectiveness,

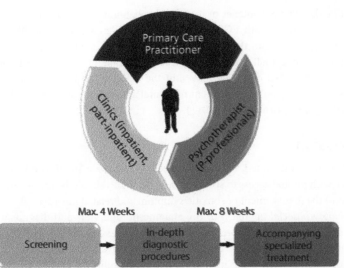

Fig. 13.2 Structure of 'Health network somatoform and functional disorders (Sofu-Net)'. Care and treatment of the patient in different settings is coordinated by the primary care practitioner (PCP; top panel). The sequence and timing of the steps in Sofu-Net to direct patients to appropriate treatment (bottom panel). It should take a maximum of four weeks between screening by the PCP and more in-depth diagnostic procedures (if the patient screened positive). If psychotherapy or in-patient treatment is indicated at the diagnostic stage, then a maximum of eight weeks should pass before treatment begins. *Note.* PCPs were linked with psychotherapists in Sofu-Net but this model could work for all p-professionals (including psychotherapists, psychiatrists, psychosomatic specialists)

or treatment side effects. This support can be conducted in person or via phone calls. In addition, care managers facilitate referrals and coordination by the PCP regarding psychiatric consultant and specialist referrals, while also being trained in evidence-based techniques such as motivational interviewing and problem-solving techniques. Consultant psychiatrists also regularly review the patient's progress and either report recommendations directly to the PCP or via the care manager. In rare cases, when the patient does not improve, they may be referred to specialist mental health care (Unützer et al., 2013).

There are good examples of trials of collaborative care for patients suffering from depression, and these trials have been shown to have positive effects on depressive and related symptoms, for example, the IMPACT trial (Unützer et al., 2002). Such collaborative care models have also been shown to be cost effective (Unützer et al., 2008) and well received by physicians (Levine et al., 2005). Similarly, another trial including patients with persistent somatic symptoms showed that patients in a collaborative care primary care practice with a consultant psychiatrist had reduced symptoms, improved social functioning, and decreased health care use post-intervention (van der Feltz-Cornelis, van Oppen, Ader, & van Dyck, 2006).

Despite the clear advantages of integrated collaborative care, its implementation is still not widespread. Both PCP support and systemic changes to health care provision are required to shift the delivery of mental health care to this integrated model. Changes in conceptualization and operationalization of the diagnosis of somatic symptom and related disorders may shift the emphasis to this integrated approach by focussing on a parallel assessment of mental and somatic symptoms (Aiarzaguena et al., 2008; Feltz-Cornelis et al., 2011).

Conclusion

Whether in an integrated, *collaborative care* setting, or a single rural primary care practice with limited access to specialist support, PCPs should be trained on the foundations of the management of somatic symptom and related disorders. By incorporating a *biopsychosocial approach* to the anamnestic interview and diagnostic process, PCPs should be aware of potential psychosocial stressors, which may contribute to the patients' distress. This is critically important given the changes to the *DSM-5 diagnostic criteria* where the medical 'non-explainability' of symptoms is no longer important, but rather where the presence of *positive psychological symptoms*, which lead to impairment in the patients' daily life, is the main focus of diagnostic evaluation. Psychotherapy, newer generation antidepressants, and natural pharmacological products may be effective treatment options. As the *first-contacts* and *co-ordinators of care*, PCPs are perfectly positioned in the health care system to manage patients who have lower levels of symptom severity, while referring patients to appropriate levels of care according to a *stepped care* approach. As such, PCPs should act as the central hub of a co-ordinated, *patient-centred* team.

References

Aiarzaguena JM, Grandes G, Salazar A, Gaminde I, and Sanchez A. (2008). The diagnostic challenges presented by patients with medically unexplained symptoms in general practice. *Scand J Prim Health Care*, 26/2: 99–105.

American Psychiatric Association. (2000). *Diagnostic and Statistical Manual of Mental Disorders, 4th edn, Text Revision (DSM-IV-TR)*. Washington, DC: American Psychiatric Association.

American Psychiatric Association. (2013). *Diagnostic and Statistical Manual of Mental Disorders, 5th end (DSM-5)*. Arlington, VA: American Psychiatric Publishing.

Barsky AJ, Orav EJ, and Bates DW. (2005). Somatization increases medical utilization and costs independent of psychiatric and medical comorbidity. *Arch Gen Psychiatry*, 62/8: 903–10.

Bertakis KD and Azari R. (2011). Patient-centered care is associated with decreased health care utilization. *J Am Board Fam Med*, 24/3: 229–39: doi: 10.3122/jabfm.2011.03.100170

Budtz-Lilly A, Fink P, Ornbol E, Vestergaard M, Moth G, Christensen KS, and Rosendal M. (2015). A new questionnaire to identify bodily distress in primary care: The 'BDS checklist'. *J Psychosom Res*, 78/6: 536–45: doi: 10.1016/j.jpsychores.2015.03.006

van Dessel N, den Boeft M, van der Wouden JC, Kleinstauber M, Leone SS, Terluin B, Numans ME, van der Horst HE, and van Marwijk H. (2014). Non-pharmacological interventions for somatoform disorders and medically unexplained physical symptoms (MUPS) in adults. *Cochrane Database Syst Rev*, 11/CD011142: doi: 10.1002/14651858. CD011142.pub2

Dirkzwager AJE and Verhaak PFM. (2007). Patients with persistent medically unexplained symptoms in general practice: Characteristics and quality of care. *BMC Family Practice*, 8/33): doi: 10.1186/1471-2296-8-33

Dowrick CF, Ring A, Humphris GM, and Salmon P. (2004). Normalisation of unexplained symptoms by general practitioners: A functional typology. *Br J Gen Pract*, 54/500: 165–70.

Dwamena FC, Lyles JS, Frankel RM, and Smith RC. (2009). In their own words: qualitative study of high-utilising primary care patients with medically unexplained symptoms. *BMC Fam Pract*, 10/67: doi: 10.1186/1471-2296-10-67

Engel GL. (1977). The need for a new medical model: a challenge for biomedicine. *Science*, 196/4286: 129–36.

Epstein RM and Street RL Jr. (2011). The values and value of patient-centered care. *Annals of Family Medicine*, 9/2: 100–3. doi: 10.1370/afm.1239

van der Feltz-Cornelis CM, van Oppen P, Ader HJ, and van Dyck R. (2006). Randomised controlled trial of a collaborative care model with psychiatric consultation for persistent medically unexplained symptoms in general practice. *Psychother Psychosom*, 75/5: 282–9.

van der Feltz-Cornelis, CM, Hoedeman R, Keuter EJW, and Swinkels JA. (2011). Presentation of the multidisciplinary guideline medically unexplained physical symptoms (MUPS) a somatoform disorder in the Netherlands: Disease management according to risk profiles. *J Psychosom Res*, 72: 168–9.

Fink P, Ewald H, Jensen J, Sørensen L, Engberg M, Holm M, and Munk-Jørgensen P. (1999). Screening for somatization and hypochondriasis in primary care and neurological in-patients: a seven-item scale for hypochondriasis and somatization. *J Psychosom Res*, 46/3: 261–73.

Fink P, Sorensen L, Engberg M, Holm M, and Munk-Jorgensen P. (1999). Somatization in primary care. Prevalence, health care utilization, and general practitioner recognition. *Psychosomatics*, 40/4: 330–8: doi: S0033-3182(99)71228-4 [pii] 10.1016/S0033-3182(99)71228-4

Frances A. (2013). The new somatic symptom disorder in DSM-5 risks mislabeling many people as mentally ill. *BMJ*, 346: f1580: doi: 10.1136/bmj.f1580

Fritzsche K, McDaniel SH and Wirsching M, eds. (2014). *Psychosomatic Medicine: An International Primer for the Primary Care Setting*. New York: Springer.

Gustavsson A, Svensson M, Jacobi F, Allgulander C, Alonso J, Beghi E, Dodel R, Ekman M, Faravelli C, Fratiglioni L, Gannon B, Jones DH, Jennum P, Jordanova A, Jönsson L, Karampampa K, Knapp M, Kobelt G, Kurth T, Lieb R, Linde M, Ljungcrantz C, Maercker A, Melin B, Moscarelli M, Musayev A, Norwood F, Preisig M, Pugliatti M, Rehm J, Salvador-Carulla L, Schlehofer B, Simon R, Steinhausen HC, Stovner LJ, Vallat JM, Van den Bergh P, van Os J, Vos P, Xu W, Wittchen HU, Jönsson B, and Olesen J; CDBE2010 Study Group. (2011). Cost of disorders of the brain in Europe 2010. *Eur Neuropsychopharmacol.*, 21/10: 718–79: doi: S0924-977X(11)00215-X [pii]; 10.1016/j.euroneuro.2011.08.008

Hanel G, Henningsen P, Herzog W, Sauer N, Schaefert R, Szecsenyi J, and Lowe B. (2009). Depression, anxiety, and somatoform disorders: Vague or distinct categories in primary care? Results from a large cross-sectional study. *J Psychosom Res*, 67/3: 189–97.

Härter M, Kentgens M, Brandes A, Bock T, Dirmaier J, Erzberger M, Fürstenberg W, Hillebrandt B, Karow A, von dem Knesebeck O, König HH, Löwe B, Meyer HJ, Romer G, Rouhiainen T, Scherer M, Thomasius R, Watzke B, Wegscheider K, and Lambert M. (2012). Rationale and content of psychenet: the Hamburg Network for Mental Health. *Eur Arch Psychiatry Clin Neurosci*, 262/Suppl 2: S57–63: doi: 10.1007/s00406-012-0359-y

Hudon C, Fortin M, Haggerty JL, Lambert M, and Poitras ME. (2011). Measuring patients' perceptions of patient-centered care: a systematic review of tools for family medicine. *Ann Fam Med*, 9/2: 155–64: doi: 10.1370/afm.1226

Institute of Medicine (US) Committee on Quality of Health Care in America. *Crossing the Quality Chasm: A New Health System for the 21st Century*. Washington, DC: National Academies Press.

Jacob KS and Patel V. (2014). Classification of mental disorders: a global mental health perspective. *Lancet*, 383/9926: 1433–5: doi: 10.1016/S0140-6736(13)62382-X

King SA. (2013). A step in the wrong direction. *BMJ*, 346/f2233: doi: 10.1136/bmj.f2233

Kleinstäuber M, Witthöft M, and Hiller W. (2011). Efficacy of short-term psychotherapy for multiple medically unexplained physical symptoms: A meta-analysis. *Clin Psychol Rev*, 31: 146–60.

Kleinstauber M, Witthoft M, Steffanowski A, van Marwijk H, Hiller W, and Lambert MJ. (2014). Pharmacological interventions for somatoform disorders in adults. *Cochrane Database Syst Rev*, 11/CD010628: doi: 10.1002/14651858.CD010628.pub2

Kroenke K. (2007). Efficacy of treatment for somatoform disorders: a review of randomized controlled trials. *Psychosom Med*, 69/9: 881–8: doi: 10.1097/PSY.0b013e31815b00c4

Kroenke K, Spitzer RL, and Williams JB. (2001). The PHQ-9: validity of a brief depression severity measure. *J Gen Intern Med*, 16/9: 606–13.

Kroenke K, Spitzer RL, and Williams JBW. (2002). The PHQ-15: Validity of a new measure for evaluating the severity of somatic symptoms. *Psychosom Med*, 64/2: 258–66.

Kuruvilla A and Jacob KS. (2012). Perceptions about anxiety, depression and somatization in general medical settings: a qualitative study. *Natl Med J India*, 25/6: 332–5.

Levenson JL. (2011). The somatoform disorders: 6 characters in search of an author. *Psychiatr Clin North Am*, 34/3: 515–24.

Levine S, Unützer J, Yip JY, Hoffing M, Leung M, Fan MY, Lin EHB, Grypma L, Katon W, Harpole LH, and Langston CA. (2005). Physicians' satisfaction with a collaborative disease management program for late-life depression in primary care. *Gen Hosp Psychiat*, 27/6: 383–91: doi: 10.1016/j.genhosppsych.2005.06.001

Löwe B, Spitzer RL, Williams JB, Mussell M, Schellberg D, and Kroenke K. (2008). Depression, anxiety and somatization in primary care: syndrome overlap and functional impairment. *Gen Hosp Psychiat*, 30/3: 191–9.

Mik-Meyer N and Obling AR. (2012). The negotiation of the sick role: General practitioners' classification of patients with medically unexplained symptoms. *Sociol Health Ill*, 34/7: 1025–38.

Murray AM, Toussaint A, Althaus A, and Löwe B. (2013). Barriers to the diagnosis of somatoform disorders in primary care: protocol for a systematic review of the current status. *Syst Rev*, 2/99: doi: 10.1186/2046-4053-2-99.

Murray AM, Toussaint A, Althaus A, and Löwe B. (2016). The Challenge of Diagnosing Somatoform Disorders: A Systematic Review of Barriers to Diagnosis in Primary Care. *J Psychosom Res*, 80: 1–10.

Olde Hartman T, Blankenstein N, Molenaar B, van den Berg DB, Horst, Van der Horst HE, Arnold, IA, Burgers JS, Wiersma TJ, and Woutersen-Koch H. (2013). NHG Guideline on Medically Unexplained Symptoms (MUS). *Huisarts Wet*, **56**/5: 222–30.

Peters S, Rogers A, Salmon P, Gask L, Dowrick C, Towey M, Clifford R, and Morriss R. (2009). What do patients choose to tell their doctors? Qualitative analysis of potential barriers to reattributing medically unexplained symptoms. *J Gen Intern Med*, **24**/4: 443–9.

Rief W, Ihle D, and Pilger F. (2003). A new approach to assess illness behavior. *J Psychosom Res*, **54**/5: 405–14.

Rief W and Martin A. (2014). How to use the new DSM-5 somatic symptom disorder diagnosis in research and practice: a critical evaluation and a proposal for modifications. *Annu Rev Clin Psychol*, **10**: 339–67: doi: 10.1146/annurev-clinpsy-032813-153745

Ringsberg KC, and Krantz G. (2006). Coping with patients with medically unexplained symptoms: Work-related strategies of physicians in primary health care. *J Health Psychol*, **11**/1: 107–16.

Rosendal M, Bro F, Sokolowski I, Fink P, Toft T, and Olesen F. (2005). A randomised controlled trial of brief training in assessment and treatment of somatisation: Effects on GPs' attitudes. *Fam Pract*, **22**/4: 419–27.

Salmon P. (2006). The potentially somatizing effect of clinical consultation. *CNS Spectrums*, **11**/3: 190–200.

Salmon P, Humphris GM, Ring A, Davies JC, and Dowrick CF. (2006). Why do primary care physicians propose medical care to patients with medically unexplained symptoms? A new method of sequence analysis to test theories of patient pressure. *Psychosom Med*, **68**/4: 570–7.

Schaefert R, Hausteiner-Wiehle C, Hauser W, Ronel J, Herrmann M, and Henningsen P. (2012). Clinical Practice Guideline: Non-specific, functional, and somatoform bodily complaints. *Dtsch Arztebl Int*, **109**/47: 803–13.

Shedden-Mora MC, Groß B, Lau K, Gumz A, Wegscheider K, and Löwe B. (2016). Collaborative stepped care for somatoform disorders: A pre–post-intervention study in primary care. *J Psychosom Res*, **80**: 23–30.

Shedden-Mora MC, Lau K, Kuby A, Groß B, Gladigau M, Fabisch A, and Löwe B. (2015). Verbesserte Versorgung von Patienten mit somatoformen und funktionellen Störungen: Ein koordiniertes gestuftes Netzwerk (Sofu-Net). *Psychiatrische Praxis*, **42**/Suppl 1: S60–64.

Soler JK and Okkes I. (2012). Reasons for encounter and symptom diagnoses: A superior description of patients' problems in contrast to medically unexplained symptoms (MUS). *Fam Pract*, **29**/3: 272–82.

Spitzer RL, Kroenke K, Williams JB, and Lowe B. (2006). A brief measure for assessing generalized anxiety disorder: the GAD-7. *Arch Intern Med*, **166**/10: 1092–7.

Starfield B. (1994). Is primary care essential? *Lancet*, **344**/8930: 1129–33.

Stein E. (2013). Somatic Symptom Disorders in DSM-5: A step forward or a fall back? [PowerPoint presentation]. Alberta Psychiatric Association.

Steinbrecher N, Koerber S, Frieser D, and Hiller W. (2011). The prevalence of medically unexplained symptoms in primary care. *Psychosomatics*, **52**/3: 263–71. doi: 10.1016/j.psym.2011.01.007

Stewart M, Brown JB, Donner A, McWhinney IR, Oates J, Weston WW, and Jordan J. (2000). The impact of patient-centered care on outcomes. *J Fam Pract*, **49**/9: 796–804.

Toussaint A, Murray AM, Voigt K, Herzog A, Gierk B, Kroenke K, Rief W, Henningsen P, and Löwe B. (2016). Development and Validation of the Somatic Symptom Disorder—B Criteria Scale (SSD-12). *Psychosom Med*, 78/1: 5–12.

Unützer J, Harbin H, Schoenbaum M, and Druss, B. (2013). *The Collaborative Care Model: An approach for integrating physical and mental health care in Medicaid health homes.* Princeton, NJ: Center for Health Care Strategies and Mathematica Policy Research.

Unützer J, Katon, W, Callahan CM, Williams JW Jr, Hunkeler E, Harpole, L, Hoffing M, Della Penna RD, Noël PH, Lin EH, Areán PA, Hegel MT, Tang L, Belin TR, Oishi S, Langston C, and IMPACT Investigators (Improving Mood-Promoting Access to Collaborative Treatment). (2002). Collaborative care management of late-life depression in the primary care setting: a randomized controlled trial. *JAMA*, **288**/22: 2836–45.

Unützer J, Katon WJ, Fan MY, Schoenbaum MC, Lin EH, Della Penna RD, and Powers D. (2008). Long-term cost effects of collaborative care for late-life depression. *Am J Manag Care*, 14/2: 95–100.

Voigt K, Wollburg E, Weinmann N, Herzog A, Meyer B, Langs G, and Löwe B. (2012). Predictive validity and clinical utility of DSM-5 Somatic Symptom Disorder--comparison with DSM-IV somatoform disorders and additional criteria for consideration. *J Psychosom Res*, 73/5: 345–50: doi: S0022-3999(12)00225-5 [pii] 10.1016/j.jpsychores.2012.08.020

de Waal, M. W. M., Arnold, I. A., Eekhof, J. A. H., & van Hemert, A. M. (2004). Somatoform disorders in general practice: Prevalence functional impairment and comorbidity with anxiety and depressive disorders. *British Journal of Psychiatry, 184*, 470–6.

World Health Organization. (1992). *The ICD-10 Classification of Mental and Behavioural Disorders: Clinical descriptions and diagnostic guidelines*, 10th edn. Geneva: World Health Organization.

World Health Organization and World Organization of Family Doctors (Wonca). (2008). *Integrating mental health into primary care: a global perspective.* Geneva: World Health Organization.

Chapter 14

Substance use disorders in primary care settings

Kathleen Broad and Tony P. George

Introduction

Substance use disorders (SUDs) are common clinical issues in primary care settings. According to the World Health Organization, the prevalence of any substance use disorder in the United States is 14.6% (Kessler et al., 2007). In 2013, an estimated 21.6 million persons aged 12 or older (8.2%) in the US were classified with substance dependence or abuse in the past year based on criteria specified in the Diagnostic and Statistical Manual of Mental Disorders, 4th edition (DSM IV-TR) (American Psychiatric Association, 2000) (Substance Abuse and Mental Health Services Administration (SAMSHA), 2014). More recently, there has been increased attention drawn to the rapidly growing incidence of prescription opioid use, now the second most common form of drug abuse after cannabis (SAMSHA, 2014).

The newest version of the diagnostic criteria for psychiatric and addictive disorders, the Diagnostic and Statistical Manual, 5th Edition (DSM-5), was published in 2013 by the American Psychiatric Association (APA). With this publication, the terms 'abuse' and 'dependence' were eliminated in preference of Substance Use Disorders. SUDs are defined as a cluster of symptoms suggesting that the affected individual continues using a substance despite significant substance-related problems. Box 14.1 shows eleven criteria for SUDs (APA, 2013). The individual must demonstrate at least two of these criteria of the past year for a diagnosis of an SUD.

It is notable that with DSM-5, most of the previous criteria from the DSM-IV regarding 'abuse' and 'dependence' were combined in 'substance use disorders', with the exception that *'legal' issues were excluded*, and ***craving was added*** as a new feature. A list of substance use disorders and their descriptions are listed in Table 14.1.

Given the high prevalence of SUDs in the primary care setting, it is essential that primary care providers (PCPs) develop a practical and evidence-based approach to the screening, assessment, and treatment of SUDs. With that in mind, this chapter provides a framework for the screening, assessment, and treatment of substance use disorders in the primary care setting.

Box 14.1 Criteria indicating a substance use disorder

1. Substance taken in larger amounts or over a longer period than intended.
2. Unsuccessful efforts to cut down or control substance use.
3. Significant time spent in activities necessary to obtain the substance, or to use and recover from its effects.
4. Craving for the substance.
5. Substance use resulting in failure to fulfil major obligations at work, school, or home.
6. Continued substance use despite recurrent social or interpersonal problems.
7. Important social, occupational, or recreational activities are altered due to substance use.
8. Substance use in situations in which it is physically hazardous.
9. Presence of a psychological or physical problem likely caused or exacerbated by the substance.
10. Tolerance; a) need for markedly increased amounts to achieve substance intoxication or desired effect; or b) markedly diminished effect with continued use of the same amount of the substance.
11. Withdrawal; a) withdrawal syndrome for the substance upon discontinuation or reduction of use; or b) the substance is taken to relieve or avoid withdrawal symptoms.

Remission Criteria: a) Early Remission—Does not meet criteria in past three–12 months; b) Sustained Remission—Does not meet criteria for 12 months or longer.

    Severity: Mild—Presence of 2–3 symptoms; Moderate—Presence of 4–5 symptoms; Severe—Presence of 6 or more symptoms.

Data from Diagnostic and Statistical Manual of Mental Disorder, 5th edn. (2013): American Psychiatric Association.

Screening for substance use disorders in primary care

Screening, Brief Intervention, Referral, and Treatment (SBIRT) is a comprehensive, integrated, public health approach to the delivery of early intervention and treatment services for persons with SUDs, or those who are at risk (McCance-Katz, 2012). Screening quickly assesses the severity of substance use and identifies the appropriate level of treatment; brief intervention focuses on increasing insight and awareness regarding substance use and motivation toward behavioural change (McCance-Katz, 2012).

Screening and brief intervention for unhealthy alcohol use is among the most efficacious and cost-effective of preventive services. The United States Preventative Services Task Force provides a Grade B recommendation to screen adults aged 18 or older for alcohol misuse, and to provide brief counselling interventions for those engaged

Table 14.1 Description of substances of abuse

Substance	Epidemiology	Acute intoxication effects	Potential harms with chronic use	Withdrawal effects
Alcohol	**Low risk drinking guidelines (NIAAA, 2015):** **Women:** no more than 3 drinks per day, no more than 7 drinks per week. **Men:** no more than 4 drinks per day, no more than 14 drinks per week. **Alcohol misuse:** 21.3% of primary care patients report risky drinking (Vinson et al., 2010). 16.6 million adults age 18 and older had an alcohol use disorder in 2013 (NIAAA, 2015). Responsible for 85,000 deaths per year in US (Moyer et al., 2013).	Signs and symptoms of vary according to the blood alcohol level. **Mild:** mild speech, memory, attention, and balance impairments. **Severe:** loss of consciousness, vomiting, blackouts, death.	Cardiomyopathy, hypertension, gastric bleeding and gastritis, liver cirrhosis, osteoporosis, pancreatitis, anaemia, cognitive impairment, depression, anxiety, insomnia, suicidal tendencies, injury, and violence.	**Signs and symptoms include:** tremulousness, anxiety, seizures, and hallucinations **Onset:** 6–48 hours from the last drink. **Delirium tremens:** a serious syndrome characterized by marked mental status changes, confusion, hallucinations, and severe autonomic instability; requires inpatient medical management.
Opioids	Over 100 Americans/day died from opioid overdose in 2010; ~50% overdose deaths in 2010 due to opioid pain relievers and 8% overdose deaths in 2010 related to heroin (CDC, 2013).	Analgesia, drowsiness, nausea, constipation, euphoria, confusion, slowed breathing, and death.	Chronic use of opioids can lead to physiological dependence. **Injection use:** risk of hepatitis and HIV from sharing needles. **Older adults:** accidental misuse and drug-drug interactions. **Use during pregnancy:** miscarriage, low birth weight, and neonatal abstinence syndrome.	**Signs and Symptoms:** Restlessness, muscle and bone pain, insomnia, diarrhoea, vomiting, cold flashes with goosebumps, and leg movements.

(continued)

Table 14.1 Continued

Substance	Epidemiology	Acute intoxication effects	Potential harms with chronic use	Withdrawal effects
Stimulants	34 million people in the United States have reported using cocaine in their lifetime. **Promote consistency:** 2 million Americans report current use of cocaine. Men are more likely to use than women. Adults aged 18–25 have higher rates of use than any other age group (SAMSHA, 2015).	**Immediate psychological effects:** euphoria, energy, alertness, confidence, feelings of sexual desire. **Immediate physical effects:** constricted blood vessels, increased pupil size, heart rate, temperature, and blood pressure; and decreased appetite and need for sleep. Cocaine can cause vasospasm of the coronary arteries resulting in sudden death. When alcohol and cocaine are mixed, the risk of sudden death increases.	**Chronic psychological effects:** irritability, depression, increased restlessness, paranoia, auditory hallucinations, and decreased ability to feel pleasure. **Chronic physical effects:** arrhythmias, heart attacks, pneumonia, respiratory failure, strokes, weight loss and malnutrition, headaches, and seizures. **Injection use:** risk of blood-borne illnesses such as Hepatitis C and HIV, and abscesses at injection sites. **Use during pregnancy:** can result in premature birth, low birth weight, and deleterious neurodevelopment effects on the child. In general, the higher the dose of cocaine, the increased risk of toxic effects.	**Signs and Symptoms:** Strong craving for more cocaine, fatigue, lack of pleasure, anxiety, irritability, sleepiness, and sometimes agitation or extreme suspicion or paranoia.

Cannabis	Delta-9-tetrahydracannabinol (THC) is the main psychoactive ingredient. ~9% of those who try cannabis develop an addiction (Anthony et al., 1994). Risk is increased to 17% if use began in adolescence and to 35% of those who use cannabis daily (Wagner and Anthony, 2002).	**Most users:** mild euphoric state, reduction of anxiety, stimulates appetite. **Immediate cognitive effects:** impaired judgment, problem-solving, and learning, which can last up to 5–12 hours. **High doses:** can cause anxiety and dysphoria.	Cognitive decline, increased risk of lung-cancer in those who smoke cannabis, and increased risk of psychosis. Negative effects mediated by total dose of cannabis used and early initiation of use (e.g. adolescence). Some individuals may have a genetic vulnerability to developing psychosis, as mediated through allelic variations in catechol-O-methyltransferase (COMT) genotype (Caspi et al., 2005).	**Onset:** 24–48 hours after last use. **Signs and Symptoms:** irritability, restlessness, sweating, sleep disturbance, fatigue, anxiety, depression, and cravings. Withdrawal symptoms likely contribute to the maintenance of chronic use.
Nicotine and Tobacco	**Route:** typically, cigarette smoking; other forms of tobacco use include pipe tobacco, cigars, smokeless tobacco, and e-cigarettes. Nicotine is the reinforcing component of tobacco. The prevalence of tobacco use in the United States is decreasing (~19%), due to widespread public health efforts CDC, 2015. Most smokers are daily users and have some degree of physiological dependence.	Induces a feeling of a 'rush' in most users, and results in feelings of relaxation, satisfaction, and reduction of anxiety. These effects produced by non-nicotine ingredients in tobacco such as tar. Airway stimulation and conditioned cues mediate the maintenance of smoking and smoking relapse.	Causes COPD, lung cancer, cardiovascular diseases, and stroke. Approximately 470,000 Americans die from tobacco-related disease annually (Giovino, 2007). Abstinence from smoking decreases health risks in smokers.	**Signs and Symptoms:** Insomnia, irritability, difficulty concentrating, anxiety, depressed mood, increased hunger and caloric intake

in risky or hazardous drinking (Moyer, 2013). There are several potential screening instruments to detect alcohol misuse in adults. A single-question screen (covering the past 12 months) using the Alcohol Use Disorders Identification Test (AUDIT) appears to be the best overall instrument to screen adults for the full spectrum of alcohol misuse in primary care, considering sensitivity, specificity, and time burden (Jonas et al., 2012a). The CAGE (Cut Down, Annoyed, Guilty and Eye Opener) has very low sensitivity for detecting risky/hazardous drinking and is therefore not a good screening test for identifying risky/hazardous drinking (Jonas et al., 2012b).

In contrast to alcohol misuse, there is no conclusive evidence to support the screening for illicit drug use in the primary care setting (Polen et al., 2008). There is some evidence that standardized questionnaires (CAGE) have acceptable accuracy and reliability in screening for drug use/misuse; however, the evidence is not sufficient to establish the positive predictive value of these tests when used in the primary care setting (Lanier et al., 2008).

Assessment of substance use disorders in primary care

Assessment of readiness to change: transtheoretical model and motivational interviewing

When a patient presents with substance use in the primary care setting, the primary care clinician should first complete an assessment, which will direct treatment setting and modality.

The Transtheoretical Model, which conceptualizes behaviour change as a process that unfolds overtime and involves progression through a series of five stages: precontemplation, contemplation, preparation, action, and maintenance (Norcross et al., 2011). It is useful to assess the stage of a client's readiness for change and to tailor treatment according to their stage.

Motivational interviewing (MI) is a person-centred approach for strengthening a person's own motivation and commitment to change (Miller and Rollnick, 2002). This approach has been used successfully to reduce use of alcohol, tobacco, and cannabis use in various populations. MI involves helping patients to say why and how they might change, and is based on the use of a guiding style (Rollnick et al., 2010). Strategies for the primary clinician include agenda-setting with the patient, eliciting pros and cons of making a change, and assessing the importance and confidence a patient has in making change (Rollnick et al., 2010). The essential parts of MI include: (1) Express empathy, (2) Develop discrepancies, (3) Roll with resistance, and (4) Believe in the patient's self-efficacy and ability to be masterful in making a change. The PCP can intentionally utilize certain techniques to achieve the MI tasks, represented by the acronym 'OARS': Open questions, Affirmations, Reflective listening, and Summarizing.

Assessment of medical and psychiatric comorbidities

It is estimated that approximately 4.6 million American adults have both SUDs and psychiatric disorders (SAMSHA, 2005a). In persons presenting with substance misuse, PCPs should screen for co-occurring mental disorders or medical illnesses and, in particular, for the presence of HIV, Hepatitis B and C, and injection drug use (SAMSHA, 2006a).

Injection drug use is often associated with increased risk of HIV (HCV) and Hepatitis B (HBV) and C infection. The primary care clinician should distinguish 'track marks' from other dermatological lesions in order to facilitate accurate diagnosis, promote the delivery of effective treatments, and to reduce patient risk. SAMSHA has recommended a six-level classification system that categorizes lesion characteristics according to their consistency with injection drug use (Cagle et al., 2002).

Because substance use is associated with the risk of HIV infection, it is recommended that clients receiving SUD treatment be screened for HIV/AIDS (SAMSHA, 2008). The primary care clinician should screen for risky behaviours, including:

(1) Unprotected vaginal, oral, or anal intercourse, or unprotected sex with a man who has had sex with another man, persons using injection drugs, or someone who has HIV or AIDS;

(2) Used injection drugs, steroids, or vitamins, has shared potentially contaminated paraphernalia (cooker, cotton rinse water);

(3) Blood transfusion between 1978–1985;

(4) Multiple sexual partners, has a sexually transmitted infection, has received money or substances in exchange for sex, or has had sexual partners who did any of the above

(Data from *Substance Abuse Treatment for Persons with HIV/AIDS.* (2008). Treatment Improvement Protocol (TIP) Series, 37. Rockville, MD: Substance Abuse and Mental Health Services Administration.)

After screening, the PCP should provide HIV education and counsel the patient about risk reduction. Substance abuse can lower inhibitions and increase impulsiveness, thereby contributing to risky behaviours. PCPs should refer the patient for HIV antibody testing and know how to provide appropriate pre- and post-test counselling (SAMSHA, 2008). SUDs may interfere with effective HIV care because of many factors, including poor adherence to antiretroviral therapy. In addition, the presence of HIV infection may result in more severe co-occurring symptoms (SAMSHA, 2008).

The signs and symptoms of viral hepatitis often become evident only after the disease has caused severe liver damage; thus, many infected people are unaware that they have the disease and do not seek treatment (SAMSHA, 2011). According to SAMSHA, all people who use or have used illicit substances are at risk of contracting viral hepititis (2011). Commonly, people can contract or spread some types of viral hepatitis by sharing needles and other drug paraphernalia, though injection drug use is the principle means of contracting HCV (SAMSHA, 2011).

The PCP should promote the prevention, screening, and treatment of viral hepatitis. They should utilize screening as an opportunity to speak with patients about hepatitis, its health effects, and prevention strategies, and clearly explain that the hepatitis screening test is optional and follow-up with the patient should be offered regardless of the results. Patients who are diagnosed with chronic hepatitis require a full medical evaluation and should be referred to a specialist.

Some medications used to treat HCV may initiate or exacerbate psychiatric symptoms such as depression, anxiety, and irritability, and have the potential to interact with medications used for other psychiatric conditions (SAMSHA, 2011). However, according to SAMSHA, the rates of adherence to hepatitis treatment and successful outcome for those with psychiatric disorders are comparable to those who do not have psychiatric disorders (2011).

Determination of treatment setting: ASAM criteria

The American Society of Addiction Medicine Patient Placement Criteria (ASAM PPC) are the most widely used and comprehensive set of guidelines for assessment and service planning of patients with addiction and co-occurring conditions (Mee-Lee, 2013). The ASAM PPC recommend six dimensions to guide service planning and treatment, including acute intoxication and relapse.

Primary care clinicians can use the PPC to determine where to focus treatment and services and to determine the intensity and frequency of service needed using the PPC's detailed guides to levels of care (Mee-Lee, 2013).

Clinical effects of substances of abuse

The epidemiology, acute and chronic effects, and withdrawal syndromes associated with the use of alcohol, opioid, stimulant, cannabis, and nicotine are summarized in Table 14.1.

Behavioural interventions for substance use disorders: relapse-prevention

Brief counselling by PCPs is an easy-to-deliver intervention for alcohol use disorder that focuses on relapse-prevention. This intervention focuses on identification and avoidance of high-risk situations as well as training patients in coping skills, which can be activated in high-risk situations and when they are tempted to lapse (Brandon et al., 2007). This approach also prepares a patient for possible lapse in order to prevent the 'abstinence violation effect' and improve a patient's sense of self-efficacy when a relapse occurs (Brandon et al., 2007).

Evidence supports brief (ten to 15-minute) multi-contact interventions, which reduces total alcohol consumptions and fewer heavy drinking episodes in both treatment seeking and non-treatment seeking individuals (Jonas et al., 2012a; Moyer et al., 2002). In contrast, brief intervention does not demonstrate efficacy for decreasing unhealthy drug use in patients identified by screening in the primary care setting (Saitz et al., 2014). When a treatment-seeking individual with illicit drug use presents to the primary care setting, the principles of motivational interviewing should be applied in order to enhance and strengthen that individual's motivation for change and to set goals regarding future treatment.

Pharmacotherapy for substance use disorders

Medical withdrawal

In the primary care setting, the clinician should assess the need for medical withdrawal. This should determine whether the patient is currently intoxicated and the degree of intoxication, type and severity of the withdrawal syndrome, previous withdrawal episodes, and the presence of co-occurring psychiatric, medical, and surgical conditions that might require specialized care (SAMSHA, 2006b). The goal of medical withdrawal is to palliate otherwise intolerable withdrawal symptoms and reduce the risk of serious medical consequences (Lee et al., 2015).

For example, in alcohol use disorder, a long half-life benzodiazepine, such as diazepam, may be given every one to two hours until significant clinical improvement occurs (such as reducing the Clinical Institute Withdrawal Assessment for Alcohol (CIWA-Ar) score to eight or under for three consecutive measurements). The CIWA-Ar is a valid and reliable method of determining alcohol withdrawal syndrome (AWS) (Lee et al., 2015). If a patient has mild symptoms (CIWA-Ar score < 8), AWS can be managed as an outpatient using a fixed dose schedule of long-acting benzodiazepine (e.g. oral diazepam 10mg every six hours for four doses, followed by 5mg every six hours for eight doses). Any history of severe withdrawal, delirium tremens (a potentially fatal syndrome associated with alcohol withdrawal), seizures, or patients with a CIWA-Ar score >15 would necessitate medical management of AWS (SAMSHA, 2006b; Lee et al., 2015)

Detoxification from opioids is not typically medically dangerous; however, opioids are highly addicting, and chronic use leads to withdrawal symptoms that can produce intense discomfort. Additionally, opioids are often combined with alcohol and benzodiazepines. Opioid withdrawal can be managed using medications such as methadone (μ-opioid agonist) or buprenorphine (μ-opioid partial agonist) in order to relieve most opioid withdrawal symptoms without producing opioid intoxication or drug reward. Alternatively, clonidine (an alpha-adrenergic agonist) can be used to relieve autonomic withdrawal symptoms (but not opioid craving).

Pharmacotherapy for alcohol use disorder

There are three US Food and Drug Administration (FDA) approved approved medications for the treatment of alcohol dependence: disulfiram, naltrexone, and acamprosate.

Disulfiram inhibits aldehyde dehydrogenase, an enzyme involved in alcohol metabolism. The inhibition of this enzyme results in the build-up of acetaldehyde, which leads to a disulfiram-ethanol reaction and results in aversive symptoms such as nausea, headaches, flushing, warmness, vomiting, shortness of breath, and blurred vision (Garbutt, 2009). Disulfiram is one of the few demonstrably effective interventions for alcohol dependence, both alone and as an adjunct to psychosocial methods. However, its success is highly correlated with compliance (Brewer, 2000), and it is ineffective if taken intermittently.

Naltrexone is an opioid receptor antagonist and is thought to reduce both cravings and euphoria related to alcohol consumption (O'Brien et al., 1996; O'Malley et al.,

1992). Studies have demonstrated its effectiveness in decreasing alcohol consumption and increasing the time to relapse (Anton and Swift, 2003). Naltrexone has also been shown to be effective in treating opioid dependence (Roozen et al., 2006). It is FDA-approved in both oral (ReVia) and depot injection (Vivitrol) formulations.

Acamprosate has a novel mechanism of action that supports abstinence by restoring homeostasis in N-methyl-D-aspartate (NMDA)–mediated glutamatergic neurotransmission, which is dysregulated in alcohol use disorder (Mason et al., 2010). Acamprosate has been found to have a significant effect compared to placebo in improving abstinence rates in both men and women with alcohol dependence (Mason et al., 2012); patients with more severe alcohol dependence and who were abstinent at treatment initiation may experience the greatest benefit from acamprosate (Maisel et al., 2013). In addition, acamprosate is not metabolized in the liver and has been shown to be safe in patients with hepatic impairment. Interestingly, in the COMBINE study of light drinking community samples, patients receiving medical management with naltrexone, combined behavioural intervention, or both, fared better on drinking outcomes, whereas acamprosate showed no evidence of efficacy, with or without combined behavioural intervention (Anton et al., 2006). This may relate to the fact that acamprosate appears to be more effective in heavy drinkers (Maisel et al., 2013).

Pharmacotherapy for opioid use disorder

Methadone is an agonist used to treat opioid dependence (Bao et al., 2009). The opioid-withdrawing brain cannot distinguish between methadone and the abused opioid (e.g. heroin, oxycodone, morphine), as both relieve withdrawal symptoms such as body aches, nausea, diarrhoea, anxiety, and elevated pulse. Methadone is readily absorbed and is long-lasting, with a half-life ~12–100 hours (Reisine and Pasternak, 1996). Methadone is effective in blocking craving and withdrawal for 24 to 36 hours (Scimeca et al., 2000). It improves treatment retention, reduces their use of injection drugs (and of thus acquiring or transmitting diseases), and reduces overdose risk. Methadone decreases opioid abuse more successfully than treatments that do not incorporate this therapy. The best outcomes are observed with extended treatment of six months or longer (Kleber, 2007).

Buprenorphine is a newer treatment option for opioid-dependence, with a higher safety profile and easier accessibility. Methadone patients generally require once-daily dosing, but many people on buprenorphine can be treated once every two or three days. Buprenorphine is a μ-opioid receptor partial agonist. It has very high affinity and low intrinsic activity at the mu-receptor and thus will displace opioid full agonists, such as abused opioids, from the receptor, contributing to its long duration of action. At increasing doses, buprenorphine has a ceiling effect—it reaches a maximum euphoric effect and subsequently does not continue to increase linearly with increasing doses of the drug; in fact, at higher doses, the antagonist effects of this drug become more prominent. Accordingly, these properties explain why overdose of buprenorphine is rare and why it is unlikely to cause respiratory depression, a major concern with full opioid agonists such as heroin and methadone. Furthermore, buprenorphine may be less sedating than full μ-opioid agonists while still decreasing cravings for other opioids and preventing opioid withdrawal. Having opioid-dependent patients comply with buprenorphine therapy remains a clinical issue (Boothby and Doering, 2007). The Suboxone formulation provides a potential advantage, in that buprenorphine is combined with naloxone, a μ-opioid antagonist, which reduces the possibility of diversion and illicit use if crushed and injected. Buprenorphine is also available in individually wrapped sublingual and film strip formulations, which may reduce the risk of tampering or diversion.

Pharmacotherapy for tobacco use disorder

Three pharmacotherapies are approved by the US Food and Drug Administration (FDA) for the treatment of tobacco use disorders: varenicline (Chantix), nicotine replacement therapies (NRTs), and sustained-release bupropion (Zyban).

Varenicline acts as a partial agonist at the nicotinic acetylcholine receptor (nAChR), the same receptor on which nicotine itself acts. The target dose is 2mg/day in BID dosing and the typically duration is 12 weeks, with up to 24 weeks' total treatment recommended in the package insert if abstinence is not achieved at 12 weeks. The main adverse effect of varenicline is nausea, but mostly at mild to moderate levels, and which subsides over time. Association of varenicline with serious psychiatric or cardiovascular events has also been described, and frequent monitoring is suggested.

NRT comprises several formulations, including transdermal patch, gum, lozenge, inhaler, and sublingual tablet; and each form varies in its duration of action (George, 2011). While the more slowly absorbed vehicles (gum and patch) reduce withdrawal symptoms, the more rapidly absorbed agents (inhaler and spray) treat both nicotine withdrawal and craving, and achieve higher smoking cessation rates. NRTs deliver nicotine without the additional exposure to carcinogens and other aromatic hydrocarbons in cigarettes.

Sustained-release bupropion is an antidepressant which increases brain dopamine and norepinephrine levels and acts as an antagonist at the nAChR. It has efficacy comparable with NRT monotherapy (Hughes et al., 2014). Bupropion is started at least one week prior to smoking cessation and taken for a 9-week course, with a target dose of 300mg/day in BID dosing. The side effects of bupropion include insomnia, dry mouth, and nausea, and rarely, (1:1000) seizures (Hughes et al., 2014). It is contraindicated in patients with a history of seizures, eating disorders, head trauma, and alcohol dependence.

Pharmacotherapy for benzodiazepine use disorder

There is no approved pharmacotherapy for the treatment of benzodiazepine dependence, although medications such as carbamazepine and antidepressants have been studied (Denis et al., 2006). Benzodiazepines should be tapered as abrupt cessation can cause severe withdrawal symptoms and seizures. There is no clear evidence to support the optimum rate of tapering; aiming for withdrawal in <6 months is a reasonable goal with reduction of benzodiazepine by no more than 25% per week (Lader et al., 2009).

Pharmacotherapy for stimulant and cannabis use disorder

There is no clear evidence to support the use of pharmacotherapy for the management of cannabis or stimulant use disorders. As such, psychological interventions form the basis of their treatment. Cognitive behavioural therapy (CBT) and contingency management are well tolerated and moderately effective in achieving drug abstinence.

Conclusion

Substance use is common in primary care settings. PCPs should develop a practical and evidence-based approach to the screening, assessment, and treatment of these disorders in the primary care setting.

Screening and brief interventions are important first steps in addressing SUDs. All patients presenting with concerns regarding substance misuse should be screened for **medical** and psychiatric comorbidities, including HIV and Hepatitis B/C. The ASAM PPC can guide primary care clinicians in matching patients to the appropriate level of care. Motivational interviewing utilizes a guiding style of interacting with the patient that can enhance and strengthen an individual's motivation for change, and to set goals regarding future treatment. There are approved medications for tobacco, alcohol, and opioids, which should be used as adjuncts to behavioural interventions, including relapse-prevention therapies for maintenance treatment.

References

American Psychiatric Association. (2013). *Diagnostic and statistical manual of mental disorders: DSM-5 (5th ed.)*. Arlington, VA: American Psychiatric Publishing, Inc.

Anthony J, Warner L, and Kessler R (1994). Comparative epidemiology of dependence on tobacco, alcohol, controlled substance and inhalants: Basic findings from the National Comorbidity Survey. *Exp Clin Psychopharmacol*, 2/3: 244–68.

Anton RF and Swift RM. (2003). Current pharmacotherapies of alcoholism: A U.S. perspective. *Am J Addict*, 12/Suppl 1: s53–s68.

Bao Y, Liu Z, Epstein DH, Du C, Shi J, and Lu L. (2009). A meta-analysis of retention in methadone maintenance by dose and dosing strategy. *Am J Drug Alcohol Ab*, 35: 28–33.

Boothby LA and Doering PL. (2007). Buprenorphine for the treatment of opioid dependence'. *Am J Health-Syst Pharm*, 64: 266–72.

Brandon TH, Vidrine JI, and Litvin EB. (2007). Relapse and Relapse Prevention. *Annu Rev Clin Psychol*, 3: 257–84.

Brewer C, Meyers RJ, and Johnsen J. (2000). Does disulfiram help to prevent relapse in alcohol abuse? *CNS Drugs*, 14: 329–41.

Budney AJ, Roffman R, Stephens RS, and Walker D. (2007). Marijuana dependence and its treatment. *Addict Sci Clin Pract*, 4/1: 4–16.

Cagle HH, Fisher DG, Senter TP, Thurmond RD, and Kastar AJ. (2002). *Classifying Skin Lesions of Injection Drug Users: A Method for Corroborating Disease Risk*. DHHS Pub. No. (SMA) 02-XXX. Rockville, MD: Center for Substance Abuse Treatment, Substance Abuse and Mental Health Services Administration.

Caspi A, Moffitt TE, Cannon M, McClay J, Murray R, Harrington H, Taylor A, Arseneault L, Williams B, Braithwaite A, Poulton R, and Craig IW. (2005). Moderation of the effect of adolescent-onset cannabis use on adult psychosis by a functional polymorphism in the catechol-O-methyltransferase gene: longitudinal evidence of a gene X environment interaction. *Biol Psychiatry*, 57/10: 1117–27.

Centers for Disease Control and Prevention, National Center for Health Statistics. Underlying Cause of Death 2000–2010, on CDC WONDER Online Database. Accessed June 24 2015. Available from: http://wonder.cdc.gov/wonder/help/ucd.html

Centers for Disease Control and Prevention. (2015). Current cigarette smoking among adults—United States, 2005–2014. *Morb Mortal Wkly Rep* 64/44: 1233–40. Accessed October 24, 2016. Available from: http://www.cdc.gov/mmwr/preview/mmwrhtml/mm6444a2.htm?s_cid=mm6444a2_w

Denis C, Fatseas M, Lavie E, and Auriacombe M. (2006). Pharmacological interventions for benzodiazepine mono-dependence in outpatient settings. *Cochrane Database Syst Rev*, 3: CD005194.

Garbutt JC. (2009). The state of pharmacotherapy for the treatment of alcohol dependence. *J Subst Abuse Treat*, 36/1: S15–23; quiz S24–5.

George TP. (2003). Biological basis of drug addiction. In: JC Soares and S Gershon eds. *Handbook of Medical Psychiatry*. New York: Marcel Dekker, 581–94.

George TP. (2011). Nicotine and tobacco. In: L Goldman and A Schafer eds. *Cecil Textbook of Medicine*, 24th edn. New York: Elsevier, 142–6.

Giovino GA. (2007). The Tobacco epidemic in the United States. *Am J Prev Med*, 33: S318–26.

Hughes JR, Stead LF, Hartmann-Boyce J, Cahill K, and Lancaster T. (2014). Antidepressants for smoking cessation. *Cochrane Database Syst Rev*, 1: CD000031.

Jonas DE, Garbutt JC, Amick HR, Brown JM, Brownley KA, Council CL, Viera AJ, Wilkins TM, Schwartz CJ, Richmond EM, Yeatts J, Evans TS, Wood SD, and Harris RP. (2012a). Behavioral counseling after screening for alcohol misuse in primary care: a systematic review and meta-analysis for the U.S. Preventive Services Task Force. *Ann Intern Med*, 157/9: 645–54.

Jonas DE, Garbutt JC, Brown JM, Amick HR, Brownley KA, Council CL, et al. (2012b). Screening, behavioral counseling, and referral in primary care to reduce alcohol misuse. *Comparative Effectiveness Review No. 64*. Rockville, MD: Agency for Healthcare Research and Quality. Accessed October 24, 2016. Available from: http://www.ncbi.nlm.nih.gov/books/NBK99199

Jorenby DE, Hays JT, Rigotti NA, Azoulay S, Watsky EJ, Williams KE, Billing CB, Gong J, and Reeves KR; Varenicline Phase 3 Study Group. (2006). Efficacy of varenicline, an alpha4beta2 nicotinic acetylcholine receptor partial agonist, vs placebo or sustained-release bupropion for smoking cessation: A randomized controlled trial. *JAMA*, 296: 56–63.

Kessler RC, Angermeyer M, Anthony JC, De Graaf R, Demyttenaere K, Gasquet I, DE Girolamo G, Gluzman S, Gureje O, Haro JM, Kawakami N, Karam A, Levinson D, Medina Mora ME, Oakley Browne MA, Posada-Villa J, Stein DJ, Adley Tsang CH, Aguilar-Gaxiola S, Alonso J, Lee S, Heeringa S, Pennell BE, Berglund P, Gruber MJ, Petukhova M, Chatterji S, and Ustün TB; The WHO World Mental Health Survey Consortium. (2007). Lifetime prevalence and age-of-onset distributions of mental disorders in the World Health Organization's World Mental Health Survey Initiative. *World Psychiatry*, 6/3: 168–76.

AUDIT PCF

Kleber HD. (2007). Pharmacologic treatments for opioid dependence: Detoxification and maintenance options. *Dialogues Clin Neurosci*, **9**: 455–70.

Lader M, Tylee A, and Donoghue J. (2009). Withdrawing benzodiazepines in primary care. *CNS Drugs*, **23**/1: 19–34.

Lanier D and Ko S. (2008). Screening in primary care settings for illicit drug use: assessment of screening instruments—a supplemental evidence update for the US Preventive Services Task Force. *Evidence Synthesis*, No. 58/2. AHRQ Publication No. 08-05108-EF-2. Rockville, MD: Agency for Healthcare Research and Quality.

Lee J, Kresina TF, Campopiano M, Lubran R, and Clark HW. (2015). Use of pharmacotherapies in the treatment of alcohol use disorders and opioid dependence in primary care. *BioMed Res Int*, **2015**: ID137020. doi: 10.1155/2015/137020. Epub 2015 Jan 5.

Maisel NC, Blodgett JC, Wilbourne PL, Humphreys K, and Finney JW. (2013). Meta-analysis of naltrexone and acamprosate for treating alcohol use disorders: when are these medications most helpful? *Addiction*, **108**/2: 275–93.

Mason BJ and Heyser CJ. (2010). Acamprosate: a prototypic neuromodulator in the treatment of alcohol dependence. *CNS Neurol Disord Drug Targets*, **9**/1: 23–32

Mason BJ and Lehert P. (2012). Acamprosate for alcohol dependence: a sex-specific meta-analysis based on individual patient data. *Alcohol Clin Exp Res*, **36**/3: 497–508.

McCambridge J and Strang J. (2004). The efficacy of single-session motivational interviewing in reducing drug consumption and perceptions of drug related risk and harm among young people: results from a multi-site cluster randomized trial. *Addiction*, **99**: 39–52.

McCance-Katz EF and Satterfield J. (2012). SBIRT: A key to integrate prevention and treatment of substance abuse in primary care. *Am J Addict*, **21**/2: 176–7.

Mee-Lee D., Ed. (2013). *The ASAM Criteria: Treatment Criteria for Addictive, Substance-Related, and Co-Occurring Conditions*. Chevy Chase, MD: American Society of Addiction Medicine.

Miller WR and Rollnick S. (2002). *Motivational interviewing*. New York: Guilford.

Moyer VA; Preventative Services Task Force. (2013). Screening and behavioral counseling interventions in primary care to reduce alcohol misuse: US Preventive Services Task Force Recommendation Statement. *Ann Intern Med*, **159**/3: 210–8. doi: 10.7326/0003-4819-159-3-201308060-00652.

Moyer A, Finney JW, Swearingen CE, and Vergun P. (2002). Brief interventions for alcohol problems: a meta-analytic review of controlled investigations in treatment-seeking and non-treatment-seeking populations. *Addiction*, **97**/3: 279–92.

National Institute on Alcohol Abuse and Alcoholism (NIAAA). (2015). Alcohol & your health. Accessed June 25 2015. Available from: http://www.niaaa.nih.gov/alcohol-health

Norcross JC, Krebs PM, and Prochaska JO. (2011). Stages of change. *J Clin Psychol*, **67**/2: 143–54.

O'Malley SS, Jaffe AJ, Chang G, Schottenfeld RS, Meyer RE, and Rounsaville B. (1992). Naltrexone and coping skills therapy for alcohol dependence. *Arch Gen Psychiat*, **49**: 881–7.

Polen MR, Whitlock EP, Wisdom JP, Nygren P, and Bougatsos C. (2008). Screening in primary care settings for illicit drug use: staged systematic review for the US Preventive Services Task Force. *Evidence Synthesis*, No 58/1. Rockville, MD: Agency for Healthcare Research and Quality.

Reisine T and Pasternak G. (1996). Opioid analgesics and antagonists. In: AG Gilman, TW Rall, AS Nies, and P Taylor eds. *Goodman and Gilman's The Pharmacological Basis of Therapeutics*, 9th edn. New York: McGraw Hill, 521–55.

Roozen HG, de Waart R, van der Windt DA, van den Brink W, de Jong CA, and Kerkhof AJ. (2006). A systematic review of the effectiveness of naltrexone in the maintenance treatment of opioid and alcohol dependence. *Euro Neuropsychopharmacol*, **16**: 311–23.

Saitz R, Palfai TPA, Cheng DM, Alford DP, Bernstein JA, Lloyd-Travaglini CA, Meli SM, Chaisson CE, and Samet JH. (2014). Screening and Brief Intervention for Drug Use in Primary Care: The ASPIRE Randomized Clinical Trial. *JAMA*, **312**/5: 502–13.

Scimeca MM, Savage SR, Portenoy R, and Lowinson J. (2000). Treatment of pain in methadone-maintained patients. *Mt Sinai J Med*, **67**: 412–22.

Shapiro B, Coffa D, and McCance-Katz EF. (2013). A primary care approach to substance misuse. *Am Fam Physician*, **88**/2: 113–21.

Substance Abuse and Mental Health Services Administration. (2006b). *Detoxification and substance abuse treatment*. Treatment Improvement Protocol (TIP) Series, No. 45. HHS Publication No. (SMA) 134131. Rockville, MD: Substance Abuse and Mental Health Services Administration.

Substance Abuse and Mental Health Services Administration. (2008). *Substance abuse treatment for persons with HIV/AIDS*. Treatment Improvement Protocol (TIP) Series 37. HHS. Publication No. (SMA) 08-4137 Rockville, MD: Substance Abuse and Mental Health Services Administration.

Substance Abuse and Mental Health Services Administration. (2011). *Addressing viral hepatitis in people with substance use disorders*. Treatment Improvement Protocol (TIP) Series 53. HHS. Publication No. (SMA) 11-4656. Rockville, MD: Substance Abuse and Mental Health Services Administration.

Substance Abuse and Mental Health Services Administration. 2015. *Session 4: Methamphetamine and cocaine*. Accessed June 24 2015. Available at: https://store.samhsa.gov/shin/content/SMA12-4153/methamphetamine_and_cocaine.ppt

Vinson DC, Manning BK, Galliher JM, Dickinson LM, Pace WD, and Turner BJ. (2010). Alcohol and sleep problems in primary care patients: a report from the AAFP National Research Network. *Ann Fam Med*, **8**: 484–92.

Chapter 15

Motivational interviewing: Its role for the management of mental disorders in primary care

Jeffrey P. Haibach, Elizabeth A. DiNapoli,
Deborah S. Finnell, John W. Kasckow,
and Adam J. Gordon

Introduction

Motivational Interviewing (MI) is a counselling approach practitioners can use to facilitate behaviour change, including for the management of mental disorders. MI emerged in addiction and mental health treatment in the 1980s and has since been adapted to overall health behaviour change and mental health management applications across various settings. It has a strong evidence base with over 200 randomized clinical trials in print and 25,000 research article citations (Miller and Rollnick, 2013).

Miller and Rollnick's (2013) practitioner definition of MI is, '... *a person-centered counseling style for addressing the common problem of ambivalence about change'*. Although patients generally want to lead a healthier lifestyle, they often struggle in doing so. Practitioners can also help or hinder the change process through the way they interact with their patients. When practitioners use a person-centred approach in addressing their patients, patients are more likely to participate in maintaining or enhancing their own health status. However, when practitioners overly dictate what patients should do and why they should do it, patients tend to become more ambivalent, frustrated, and reluctant to integrate healthy changes into their lives. This is not to say that practitioners should never provide information, but rather that information is generally better received when shared in a manner that respects the patient's values, treatment goals, and autonomy. As a primer for the MI method, Miller and Rollnick set the stage with a quote from Blaise Pascal, '*People are generally better persuaded by the reasons which they have themselves discovered than by those which have come into the mind of others*' (Miller and Rollnick, 2013).

Mental Disorders, Health, Behaviour, and MI

Compared to individuals without mental disorders, individuals with mental health disorders are more likely to have physical health problems, health-risk behaviours, and to die prematurely (Felker et al., 1996; Newcome and Hennekens, 2007). Worldwide, mental disorders account for the largest burden of non-fatal disabling conditions, with the top two categories being depressive disorders and alcohol use disorders (Lopez et al., 2006). The health-risk behaviours of cigarette smoking, physical inactivity, poor diet, and at-risk alcohol use are among the top behavioural causes of death worldwide (Lopez et al., 2006; WHO, 2014). Many health-risk behaviours (e.g., cigarette smoking, heavy alcohol use, and illicit drug use) can contribute to mental disorders (Balfour and Ridley, 2000; Lopresti et al., 2013; McKenna and Eyler, 2012; Sarris et al., 2014; Sullivan et al., 2005) and can also lead to diagnostic substance use disorders from their influence on neurobiology and associated pathological behaviour patterns with prolonged use (APA, 2003). There is a growing evidence base for the treatment of mental disorders with positive health behaviours such as physical activity or exercise and dietary improvement (Merrill et al., 2008; Sarris et al., 2014, 2015; Scheewe et al., 2013; United States Department of Health and Human Services; 2008; Walsh, 2011). MI is one of the leading evidence-based methods for positive health behaviour change counselling and the management of mental disorders across settings (Appiah-Brempong et al., 2014; Heckman et al., 2010; Macdonald et al., 2012; Naar-King et al., 2012; O'Halloran et al., 2014; Romano and Peters, 2015; Shingleton and Palfai, 2015; Wells et al., 2012), including in primary health care (Barnes and Ivezaj, 2015; Haibach et al., 2014; Purath et al., 2014; VanBuskirk and Wetherell, 2014).

MI in Primary Care

MI is a patient-centred counselling method that seeks to empower patients as they make decisions about how to manage their health. For persons with mental disorders, the management of their health may be compounded by their emotional, cognitive, and motivational symptoms associated with their acute or chronic mental disorders and co-occurring health conditions. In more recent years, mental health treatment has increasingly become integrated into primary care environments, largely as a result of 1) the increased awareness of the interrelated nature of mental health, physical health, and health-related behaviour; 2) patients often presenting in primary care with multimorbidity among mental and physical health conditions; and 3) the reachable opportunity in primary care to address health behaviour and mental health. MI can be used as a method to interact with patients in brief encounters (e.g. five to 15 minutes), psychotherapy appointments, in a group setting, or collectively by an interdisciplinary team who share responsibility for their patients. MI is also used to promote initial treatment engagement (e.g. to promote utilization of specialty care services such as addiction treatment, a nutritionist, or a psychiatrist), to maintain treatment engagement (e.g. medication adherence), as well as through integration with psychotherapeutic treatments such as cognitive behavioural therapy.

This chapter provides an overview of MI for primary care practitioners (PCPs) who care for patients with mental disorders. It covers the central processes, skills, and other considerations for MI and includes a case example demonstration. We also present and discuss tools for evaluating practitioner competence in MI and provide a narrative review of MI research.

MI practice

Method and flow of MI

There are four central processes within the method and flow of MI: *engaging, focusing, evoking*, and *planning* (Miller and Rollnick, 2013). When a practitioner first meets the patient, there is a period of *engaging* the patient, which is the process by which the patient and practitioner begin to establish a trusting, respectful, and collaborative relationship. Establishing rapport and mutual understanding through the process of engaging is helpful to begin patient-practitioner collaboration for the patient's health. Engaging then flows into a period of *focusing*, where both parties move toward a particular agenda for the appointment and the patient's health. Focusing is generally a balance of the patient's purpose in scheduling the visit (e.g. depression and anxiety symptoms) and the practitioner's insight into the patient's health (e.g. neurochemical imbalance, inadequate sleep, physical inactivity, need for preventive health services).

Once the patient and practitioner have one or more change goals as a focus (e.g. within categories of medication management, improving sleep, increasing physical activity), the practitioner then begins the *evoking* process, where the practitioner elicits the patient's own motivations and ideas for change. Evoking empowers the patient to use their own ideas and feelings as to why they would like to change their health-related behaviour and how they might accomplish it. One of the primary concepts in the evoking process is to promote change talk and reduce sustain talk. Change talk is primarily the patient discussing reasons why and how to change, whereas as sustain talk is the patient discussing reasons to not change. Methods to evoke and support change talk are discussed in the next section on core skills; these skills include asking open questions, affirming, and reflective listening.

Once a patient has moved through the process of why and how they would like to change their behaviour for their health, the culminating process in the MI method is *planning*. In the planning process, the practitioner assists the patient in making a commitment to change and in developing a specific plan of action. An example plan for a patient with depression or anxiety could be meeting with a sleep specialist, starting a physical activity program, or better medication management. The plan should also include specific goals such as taking 15-minute brisk walks in the morning and afternoon five days per week to increase physical activity, calling and starting a smoking cessation group, or calling and taking the next available stress management class.

The four MI processes are not linear; they are fluid and circular, and therefore engaging can occur during the evoking process, and focusing during planning, etc., to some degree. The method of moving through the processes may restart on each appointment and, in any particular appointment, may not cover all of the processes. Health behaviour change is also an ongoing course of action where goals may change over time through continuous development across the continuum of health-risk to health-positive behaviour. In addition to the skills and other considerations presented in the next three subsections, this chapter also includes a case example that moves through the MI processes and outlines the MI skills with a patient as they move through an integrated primary care system.

Core Skills

Across the four MI processes, there are core communication skills to promote a collaborative, supportive, and productive patient-provider relationship (Miller and Rollnick, 2013). The core skills include asking open questions, affirming, reflective listening, and summarizing; these can be remembered with the acronym OARS (Open questions, Affirming, Reflective listening, Summarizing).

Open questions

Open questions are designed to prompt a more thoughtful and reflective response from the patient, whereas closed questions generally result in shorter, yes or no style, responses. Both open and closed questions are important for gathering information; however, open questions tend to better provide a common feeling of understanding between practitioner and patient, and are beneficial in first developing a collaborative relationship through the engaging process. Open questions can also help the patient-practitioner team to narrow the discussion to a specific area of focus that is most warranted (*focusing*), help patients think and discuss the why and how of their potential health behaviour change (*evoking*), and assist with the development and initiation of a plan for health behaviour change (*planning*). See Table 15.1 for examples of open-ended questions, other core skills, and questions for self-evaluation throughout the MI processes.

Affirming

Affirming has two uses in MI. First, it is a general MI action where the practitioner respects and honours the patient as someone of value and independence with their own freedom to choose growth and change for health. Second, it is a specific counselling action where the practitioner supports client strengths and successes through positive encouragement.

Reflective listening

A reflective listening statement is a practitioner's attempt at stating back to the patient a brief paraphrase (simple reflections) or an intuitive extension of what the patient has said (complex reflections). Reflections not only allow the provider to both gain and express understanding of the patient, but they also help the patient to have greater self-awareness of what they are saying, thinking, and doing. While simple and complex reflections are both useful in MI, complex reflections tend to motivate the patient to think seriously about their willingness to change, and to move the conversation forward.

Table 15.1 Core practitioner skills and self-evaluation across the 4 MI processes

Skills	MI Process	Examples
Open Questions	Engaging	Can you please describe your symptoms? (Closed question: How many nights per week do you have sleep trouble?)
	Focusing	What would you like to work on most to improve your health and why? (Closed: Do you think you should eat healthier?)
	Evoking	What are some of the reasons you would like to exercise more? (Closed: Would you like to exercise more?)
	Planning	What are some things that might get in the way of your plan and how might you overcome them? (Closed: If you feel you have to do more, will you still go to bed at 10?)
Affirming	Engaging	It sounds like you have made great progress since our last appointment!
	Focusing	That sounds like a good area to work on.
	Evoking	You are quite creative.
	Planning	Sounds like a good plan!
Reflective Listening	Engaging	Things have been difficult for you lately. [complex reflection]
	Focusing	You would like to focus on your feelings of anxiety today. [simple reflection]
	Evoking	You think something else would probably be better. [complex reflection]
	Planning	That goal would be more manageable with all you have going on. [complex reflection]

Summarizing	You have a lot going on in raising three children with two jobs as a single parent and are having a tough time getting enough sleep.
Focusing	You have been in a lot of pain and you would like to try a different medication because your current prescription makes you feel tired.
Evoking	You would like to stop drinking because it is causing problems in your life, and you are thinking about a few different options as a next step.
Planning	Your plan to lose weight and start feeling better is to take a 15-minute brisk walk in the morning and afternoon, five days per week, replace your unhealthy snacks with fruits and vegetables, and your confidence level for successfully completing these goals is an eight.
Self-Evaluation Questions	
Engaging	Have I connected with the patient? Do I understand the patient's situation and perspective? Am I moving the conversation forward with reflective listening and open questions?
Focusing	Are the patient and I moving in a similar direction in the appointment agenda? Am I moving the conversation forward with complex reflections?
Evoking	What are the patient's concerns, goals, or values that could encourage healthful change? Am I bringing out and supporting change talk? Am I affirming the patient's positive reasons for change, past successes, and future goals?
Planning	Is the patient ready to begin planning? Am I asking permission before providing information or advice? Did I help the patient collect the specifics of their plan for change through summarizing?

Summarizing

Summarizing is a type of reflection the practitioner conveys to the patient to pull together a collection of what the patient has been saying. It can be used to sum up one section or task of an appointment and transition to the next (e.g. at the end to collect an appointment) or to go over a collection of information across time. Across the different processes, especially engaging and focusing, summarizing can help the patient feel understood and valued by the practitioner while also providing an opportunity for the practitioner to confirm they have documented key points and details mentioned by the patient. During the evoking process, summarizing can also help the practitioner collect change talk and move forward along the change continuum. It can also assist the practitioner to help the patient establish a specific and finite plan.

Other skills

Among and beyond the four MI processes and OARS, there are a number of other skills or actions for use within the MI method including: *asking permission, informing, advising, positivity*, and providing *hope*. Asking *permission* before giving advice or information generally results in the least level of defensiveness and greatest level of engagement, acceptance, or adherence. *Informing* and *advising* are important aspects of the practitioner's service to the patient; however, in the MI method this is generally done in small amounts and through asking permission (e.g. 'Would you like to hear about options for help to quit smoking?'). It is also best to maintain an overall *positive* atmosphere within the appointment with the patient so that the patient leaves feeling good about their successes and *hopeful* for positive change.

Actions to avoid

There are many actions or traps to avoid or divert in MI, as patients can become quickly disengaged or unmotivated. Some common traps or actions to avoid include the *assessment trap, expert trap, labelling*, and *chatting*. An *assessment trap* can occur when learning about the patient and their health is structured as an intake interview that the patient feels is a requirement for assistance rather than an engaging conversation. An assessment-intensive practitioner asks a lot of questions and subsequently the patient takes a more passive role and may respond with only short answers. The client has little opportunity to talk themselves through and participate in the change process before the provider has assessed the situation and provided a directive prescription or solution. A closely related situation to avoid is the *expert trap*. Through the questioning process and in utilizing a directive style, the practitioner maintains the control and power as the 'expert' in the relationship, while the patient again assumes a more passive role. Utilizing an assessment-intensive, expert, and directive style can work or even may be warranted for more clear and acute health concerns such as severe flu-like symptoms; however, for longer-term health behaviour change, a directive expert style will tend to prevent the necessary motivation for patient success.

Another action to avoid is *labelling*. When a practitioner is quick to label a patient with a diagnosis (e.g. 'you have diabetes') or a patient adopts a label ('addict', 'alcoholic'), this can provoke defensiveness or despair. Labelling is generally unhelpful and may be counterproductive to moving forward with positive change. Additionally, using terms like 'addict' or 'alcoholic' can be pejorative and perpetuate the negative stigma often experienced by people struggling with addiction (Broyles et al., 2014). In contrast, by using respectful and dignified language, i.e. people-first language, a practitioner can address the person's harmful substance use as a behaviour rather than an identity. With people-first language, patients are represented as people with heavy alcohol use, or people with blood sugar in a diabetic range, and thus patients may better understand the behaviours they can change to stop an addiction or to prevent full onset of a disease.

A final action to avoid is *chatting*. As a relatively conversational and collaborative style of counselling, an MI session can easily turn over to periods of chatting or small talk, resulting in lack of substantial focus or meaningful relevance to the health agenda. While a bit of small talk may be okay or warranted for engagement, it must be kept to a minimum so that the practitioner ensures the appointment sticks to the agenda of the patient's health and the main reason for the visit.

Moving forward

Ultimately, a patient is more likely to take beneficial steps and change for their health when they sense understanding, respect, and empathy from the practitioner while he or she provides information and advice. The patient's visit will likely be even more effective when the patient feels involved in the process, positive about the experience, and hopeful about the necessary actions to improve their health. In essence, through effective use of MI in practice, practitioners can help to empower patients in behaviour change to restore and maintain their health.

To become skilled in MI, it is recommended that practitioners engage in formal MI training and review the publications referred to in this chapter. There are in-person and online courses that can assist practitioners to learn both beginning and advanced MI skills (e.g. www.motivationalinterviewing.org or through your employer or university). MI is a learned method of patient-centred counselling that must also be practised and evaluated through continuous improvement over time for proficiency.

MI case example

The following case example highlights the MI method and flow in action. Zora is a 58-year-old married female who presented to her PCP with complaints of anxiety and difficulty controlling her diabetes. Zora reported that she frequently forgets to take her insulin, struggles to maintain a healthy diet with portion control and low carbohydrates, and her BMI is 39. Zora's PCP is concerned that Zora may begin to experience other health complications secondary to diabetes and obesity. In an integrated care model, Zora's PCP places a consult for her to be seen by a psychologist embedded within the primary care clinic. Box 15.1 exhibits example dialogue from the PCP appointment where MI is used.

Psychologist in primary care consult

In her later appointment with the health psychologist in primary care, the psychologist conducted an initial evaluation with Zora to determine her treatment needs.

Box 15.1 PCP appointment dialogue to exhibit the MI method and flow in action

Practitioner: Good morning Zora.

Patient: Good morning.

Practitioner: What brings you in today? [*open question*]

Patient: I am not sure if you can help, but I am having a difficult time with taking care of myself. I worry a lot about my health because I can't get my diabetes under control.

Practitioner: Your health is very important to you. [*complex reflection*]

Patient: It is. I try to do the right things to take care of myself but I just have so much going on in my life right now. I sometimes forget to take my insulin with dinner and eat too much. I also have a hard time keeping my carbs low. It causes me to feel down and I am nervous that something bad may happen to me.

Practitioner: You are feeling overwhelmed. [*complex reflection*]

Patient: I am. I would love to get some additional support to help me. What do you think I should do?

Practitioner: Would you like to hear about some different options? [*asking permission* before *informing* and *advising*]

Patient: Yes.

Practitioner: [*Zora's PCP offered her a few options for assistance in managing her mood and diabetes from pharmacotherapy, to a support group, to a primary care-based health psychologist*]. What do you think you'd like to do next?

Patient: I think the health psychologist might help. Can I do that?

From here the PCP answered additional questions and had a brief concluding dialogue with Zora. The PCP also supported Zora in putting in the referral to meet with the health psychologist in primary care.

Because of Zora's complaints of anxiety, and since depression commonly co-occurs with both anxiety and diabetes, the psychologist administered the Patient Health Questionnaire-9 (PHQ-9) (Kroenke et al., 2001) and Generalized Anxiety Disorder 7-item survey (GAD-7) (Spitzer et al., 2006). Her PHQ-9 score of 13/27 was suggestive of moderate depression. Specifically, Zora's score indicated that she has little interest or pleasure in doing things, feels down/depressed, has little energy, has low self-esteem, overeats, and experiences trouble concentrating. Her total GAD-7 score of 10/21 was indicative of a probable anxiety disorder. Zora reported that she feels nervous, has trouble relaxing/sitting still, and is afraid that something awful might happen to her. She has had these feelings for several months. Both her symptoms of depression and anxiety make it difficult for her to take care of her work and household responsibilities. Zora denies suicidal or homicidal thoughts.

When in discussion with her health psychologist, Zora attributed her anxiety and depression to being in an unhappy marriage, financial strain, and having trouble managing her diabetes. Lastly, Zora divulged feeling 'overwhelmed' by having to constantly monitor her diet, take insulin, and check her sugar levels (See Box 15.2 for

Box 15.2 Psychologist first appointment dialogue example

Practitioner: [*After initial engagement, the practitioner then moves on to the more formal agenda of the appointment*] Since this is our first visit together, we will start with a brief written assessment and I would also like to hear more about your concerns. We can start with either—do you have a preference? [*closed question*]

Patient: Could we do the written assessment first?

Practitioner: Sure! [with additional dialogue, Zora was administered the PHQ-9 and GAD-7 to complete, thanked on their completion, and transitioned to hear more about the concerns that brought her in]. Your PCP referred you to me because of concerns about your health. What's been going on? [*open question*]

Patient: I have tried really hard to manage my diabetes but have not been successful. I feel like a failure. So I am hoping that you might be able to help me do this better.

Practitioner: It has been difficult for you lately. [*complex reflection*]

Patient: Very difficult. My husband and I have been arguing a lot lately about finances. Then to add to the stress I am struggling with having to monitor my diabetes. It seems like every time I check my blood sugar, it is way too high.

Practitioner: You have a lot going on with your marriage, financial strain, and health concerns. Where would you like to start? [*simple reflection* followed by a *closed question* for *focusing*]

Patient: I would like to start with my health. I need to get better … be healthier.

Practitioner: How do you think you might go about being healthier? [*open question* for both *focusing* and *evoking*]

Patient: I'm not sure, I have to do something. I feel just … horrible all the time (shakes head in despair).

Practitioner: It sounds like you are ready to do whatever it takes to feel better and get healthy. [*complex reflection* and *affirming*]

Patient: I am. I need to get better; I'm tired of living this way. [change talk]

Practitioner: I could tell you a bit about managing your mood and health with individual therapy. Would that be okay? [*asking permission* before *informing* and *advising*]

Patient: Yes.

Practitioner: Individual therapy using motivational interviewing has been found to help patients manage their mood and with healthy lifestyle behaviours, such as managing your diabetes, increasing physical activity, or improving diet. This would involve us meeting each week for an appointment so we could talk about how you might change your health behaviours. How does that sound? [*informing* and *advising* followed by a *closed question*, providing a rapid transition from *focusing* and *evoking* to *planning*]

Patient: That would be great! I'm excited to start.

After additional and minor discussion, in concluding the appointment, the practitioner scheduled Zora for the next session to occur in a week.

a psychologist dialogue example). After completing her initial consultation with the primary care psychologist, Zora is invited and scheduled for additional motivational interviewing appointments to help with mood management and healthy living.

In the next appointment, the health psychologist engaged Zora by actively listening, using the core MI interviewing skills (OARS), and exploring Zora's values and goals. Zora quickly decided that she would like to focus on making adjustments to her diet. Box 15.3 shows an example dialogue from the second session that goes more into the *evoking* and *planning MI processes* than the prior examples. In the next section we discuss MI evaluation from self-evaluation by the practitioner, to independent observation by an evaluator, and to the research that has evaluated and informs evidence-based MI practice.

Box 15.3 Psychologist follow-up appointment dialogue example

This *excerpt begins after an initial engagement period and with the patient focusing on wanting to improve diet.*

Patient: I need to eat better.

Practitioner: What are some reasons why you would like to eat better? [*open question* for *evoking*]

Patient: It would help me control my diabetes and feel better. I think I would have more energy and be able do things I enjoy more, like gardening. That would make me happier.

Practitioner: On a scale from zero to 10, how confident are you about being able to eat healthier? With zero being 'not at all confident' and 10 being 'very confident'? [*closed question*]

Patient: I would say seven.

Practitioner: And why are you at a seven rather than, say, a two or nine? [*open question*]

Patient: Because I need to get my diabetes under control. I know that if I don't start controlling my bloods sugar I'm going to have other health complications. A healthy diet can improve my blood sugar. I have been able to eat healthy in the past and know that I can do it again. But it is also hard sometimes.

Practitioner: What are some more specific things you think you can do to eat healthier? [*open question* for *focusing, evoking,* and to move into *planning*]

Patient: I need to lower my carbohydrate intake. I plan to start tracking my food intake again.

Practitioner: You definitely want to improve your eating habits, and to do that you know you need to control your carbohydrate intake. What you're thinking of doing is to track your food intake. Is that right? [*summarizing* and using a *closed question*]

Patient: Yes. That is my plan.

Practitioner: When could you do that?

Patient: Every time after I eat, I will update my food log, and I will keep my log in my wallet.

Practitioner: If it's all right, I'd like to suggest one thing about your plan. Would that be ok? [*asking permission* before *informing and advising*]

Patient: Sure.

Practitioner: Changing your eating, especially controlling your carbohydrate intake is a great step. It is generally recommended that women eating a below-average 2,000 calories a day would consume 250–325 grams of carbohydrates a day. Does that sound like a reasonable amount? [*informing, advising*, and asking a *closed question* for clarification]

Patient: Yes, I would like to have less than 325 grams of carbohydrates a day.

Practitioner: Great plan! [*affirming*] Just to summarize: you have decided to improve your eating by logging your food intake every time after you eat, and your goal is to reduce your carbohydrates to less than 325 grams a day. [*summarizing*]

Patient. That's right! [*ending in a collaborative and positive way*]

After additional and minor discussion, in concluding the appointment, the practitioner scheduled Zora for the next session to occur in a week.

MI evaluation

Self-evaluation (am I doing MI?)

Self-evaluation for MI competency ranges from self-reflection during or after the appointment with the patient to reviewing an audio or video recording of the interaction. Overarching example questions for MI self-evaluation may include: 'Am I directing the patient to do what I feel they should for the reasons I value (using a directing style instead of MI)?; Am I seeking to understand and support the patient's own situation, motivation, and action steps for healthful change?; Who is talking more, me or the patient?'. Self-evaluation questions will also vary as a practitioner moves through the four MI processes, as conveyed in Table 15.1. The assessment tools in the next section may also be useful for self-evaluation.

Evaluation of practitioner competence of MI

There are many evaluation instruments to assess practitioner competence in MI and MI-based counselling by an independent evaluator or supervisor. Two instruments that have particular relevance to MI for treatment of mental disorders and health behaviour change in primary care are the Motivational Interviewing Treatment Integrity (MITI) Code (Jelsma et al., 2015; Moyers et al., 2015) and the MD3 Screening, Brief Intervention, and Referral to Treatment (MD3 SBIRT) Coding Scale (DiClemente et al., 2015). Evaluation of MI competence during initial training and over time is crucial for development and maintenance of MI proficiency (Hall et al., 2015; Miller and Rollnick, 2013).

Motivational Interviewing Treatment Integrity (MITI) Code

The MITI was developed for use in both research and clinical practice to evaluate practitioner competence in MI (Moyers et al., 2015), and it is the most frequently used instrument to evaluate MI treatment fidelity in research (Jelsma et al., 2015). The MITI evaluates the four MI processes and has two overarching components: Global Scores and Behaviour Counts. The Global Score component consists of the following: (1) Cultivating Change Talk, (2) Softening Sustain Talk, (3) Partnership, and (4) Empathy. The Behavior Count component of the MITI is measured as a running tally of specific provider MI behaviours (giving information, persuading, questions, reflections, affirming, seeking collaboration, emphasizing autonomy, confronting) and assesses the percentage or ratio of MI aligned practitioner behaviours. MI competency is exhibited when a practitioner scores an average 3.5/5.0 or higher for the relational global scores (Partnership, Empathy) and 3.0/5.0 for technical global scores (Change Talk, Sustain Talk), ≥ 40% of reflections are 'complex reflections', there is a ≥ 1:1 ratio of reflections to questions, and ≥ 90% of the practitioner's responses are 'MI consistent' (e.g. asking permission before giving advice, affirming and supporting the patient with positive statements about the person or expressing compassion). For MI proficiency, the global scores will average ≥ 4.0/ 5.0, ≥ 50% of reflections are 'complex', ≥ 2:1 ratio of reflections to questions, and ≥ 98% of practitioner responses are 'MI consistent'. These targets were established through expert opinion and warrant further validity and reliability testing (Moyers et al., 2015).

MD3 Screening, Brief Intervention, and Referral to Treatment (MD3 SBIRT) Coding Scale

The MD3 SBIRT Coding Scale was developed to assess provider skills and fidelity to Screening, Brief Intervention and Referral to Treatment (SBIRT)—a set of clinical strategies used to promote behaviour change among persons with health-risk behaviours and substance use disorders (DiClemente et al., 2015). Since skilful delivery of motivationally based brief interventions is emphasized in SBIRT, the MD3 SBIRT Coding Scale was developed with MI core competencies in mind.

Three subscales of the MD3 SBIRT Coding Scale parallel those of the MITI: adherent behaviours, non-adherent behaviours, and global ratings. The 14 SBIRT-adherent behaviours address MI-related principles such as respect, expressing genuine concern, and the MI-directed core skills of OARS. The 7 SBIRT-nonadherent behaviours (e.g. being paralyzed/unable to respond to patient concerns) are coded as behaviour counts with a value of −1 assigned to each. Thus, the total points range from 0 to −7. The global ratings are rated on a 5-point scale to capture the extent to which the provider works synergistically with the patient (collaboration) and the extent to which the provider makes an effort to grasp the patient's perspectives, feelings, and goals (empathy). Higher scores reflect the provider's general interactions as being more collaborative and empathic (DiClemente et al., 2015).

The MD3 SBIRT scale has demonstrated excellent inter-rater reliability (DiClemente et al., 2015). Experienced coder pairs had higher reliability scores than those with limited experience. However, even the limited experience coder pairs scored excellent for both adherent and non-adherent behaviours and fair for global ratings. Evaluation of the validity of the MD3 SBIRT Coding Scale is still needed, yet this scale has promise for a reliable evaluation of SBIRT competence, fidelity, and training outcomes and applicable to MI evaluation.

Research evaluation of MI

Overall, there is solid support for the efficacy of MI across settings, across health behaviours, and among a variety of health conditions (Appiah-Brempong et al., 2014; Barnes and Ivezaj, 2015; Haibach et al., 2014; Heckman et al., 2010; Macdonald et al., 2012; Naar-King et al., 2012; O'Halloran et al., 2014; Purath et al., 2014; Romano and Peters, 2015; Shingleton and Palfai, 2015; Wells et al., 2012; VanBuskirk and Wetherell, 2014). A *MEDLINE* search for recent peer-reviewed articles with 'motivational interviewing' in the title or abstract and published between years 2005–2015 revealed over 1,900 articles and over 50 reviews, largely systematic reviews and meta-analyses of randomized controlled trials (RCTs). The majority of reviews evaluated research in medical settings and some in community or other settings. The reviews evaluated MI among the general patient population, among those with chronic conditions, across age groups, and were conducted for many health-related behaviours or substance use disorders, primarily in areas of alcohol use, smoking cessation, physical activity, diet, weight management, and medication adherence. In this section, we highlight key points from the reviews that are most relevant to the treatment of mental disorders and health behaviour change in primary care.

In a systematic review and meta-analysis of MI RCTs among primary care populations, VanBuskirk and Wetherell (2014) found MI interventions to be more effective than comparison conditions for favourable outcomes overall (Effect Size [ES] = 0.18; $p < .05$; average of 12 studies). Outcomes were related to weight management, physical activity, blood pressure, substance use, and medication adherence. However, in assessing individual subcategory outcomes, results were only significant for medication adherence (ES = 0.19; $p < .05$). They attributed the lack of significance as likely due to the small number of studies for each subcategory. The authors found professional credentials of the practitioner to moderate the association between MI and outcomes overall as well as for the substance use subcategory. As few as one MI session was also found to be useful in enhancing readiness to change and promoting action toward health behaviour change goals. Purath and colleagues (2014) reviewed MI RCTs in primary care among older adults aged 60 years or older, and concluded that the use of MI with older adults can be effective in promoting positive health behaviour change across a diversity of practitioners and settings. However, they cautioned that this was based on a limited number of eight studies and that MI competence can vary considerably by clinician and context.

In a review and meta-analysis evaluating the mechanisms of change for MI treatment of persons with mental disorders, Romano and Peters (2014) found that MI was effective at promoting patient treatment attendance (ES = 0.38, $p < .05$) and in-session engagement (ES = 0.42, $p < .01$) across 20 studies meeting inclusion criteria. However, MI treatment did not appear to increase patient motivation above comparison conditions (ES = 0.18; $p > .05$). In another meta-analysis of 12 studies comprising 1,721 patients, Riper and colleagues (2014) found combined MI-CBT for the treatment of comorbid alcohol use disorder and depression to be effective compared to control conditions (e.g. treatment as usual) at decreasing alcohol consumption (ES = 0.17, $p < .001$) and reducing depressive symptoms (ES = 0.27, $p < .001$). In a review to inform integrated behavioural intervention in primary care for chronic pain, depression, and substance use disorders, an MI-CBT approach that addressed multiple health behaviour change emerged as a promising treatment method (Haibach et al., 2014).

Across studies, MI interventions have been found to promote positive health behaviour change and improve health outcomes. When evaluated through meta-analysis, the effect sizes for MI-alone interventions tend to be small. However, the authors generally point out that study quality and MI fidelity is often unclear or poor, there is a large heterogeneity of studies, and there are a number of limitations of existing reviews and meta-analyses for search strategies, article screening, data abstraction, and effect size estimation. As a result, the reviews almost universally call for future studies and practise to ensure practitioner competence in MI through training and continued evaluation. In a review of studies assessing sustained MI practice change after practitioner training in MI, less than one-third of MI trained practitioners reached beginner proficiency initially (Hall et al., 2015). The authors of the review concluded in agreement with Miller and Rollnick (2013) that it may take years and the support of supervisor evaluation and feedback over time to achieve and maintain MI proficiency. To assess and report MI fidelity in RCTs, it is recommended to 1) audio record all sessions and select a random representative sample of them for evaluation; 2) train and evaluate coders prior to starting the study; 3) double code a percentage of sessions; and 4) report raw and summary assessment scale results as well as inter-rater (coder) reliability scores (Jelsma et al., 2015). It is also generally recommended to use formal systematic review and meta-analysis procedures such as the PRISMA method (Moher et al., 2009).

Conclusion

Motivational interviewing is one of the leading counselling methods for the management of mental disorders, for health behaviour change, and it can be particularly useful in the primary care setting. We have provided a background, overview, and primer for motivational interviewing with an outline of the MI processes and skills. Through a case study, we provided an example of how the processes and skills of MI can be applied in primary care. Finally, we summarized methods for evaluation and maintenance of MI proficiency and provided a brief review of the research on MI. There is much more to MI than can be covered in one chapter and it takes formal training and evaluation for basic competency. To gain and maintain MI proficiency it requires periodic evaluation with feedback to the practitioner and years of practise. With MI competency or proficiency, practitioners can better motivate patients to utilize health services and to improve their health-related behaviour for the management of mental disorders through primary care.

Acknowledgements

The contents of this chapter do not necessarily represent the views of the US Department of Veterans Affairs or the United States Government.

References

American Psychiatric Association. (2013). *Diagnostic and Statistical Manual of Mental Disorders, Fifth Edition.* Arlington, VA: American Psychiatric Association.

Appiah-Brempong E, Okyere P, Owusu-Addo E, and Cross R. (2014). Motivational interviewing interventions and alcohol abuse among college students: a systematic review. *Am J*

Wells SA, Smyth T, and Brown TG. Patient attitudes towards change in adapted motivational interviewing for substance abuse: a systematic review. *Subst Abus Rehab*, 3: 61–72.

Balfour DJK and Ridley DL. (2000). The effects of nicotine on neural pathways implicated in depression: a factor in nicotine addiction? *Pharmacol Biochem Behav*, 66/1: 79–85.

Barnes RD and Ivezaj V. (2015). A systematic review of motivational interviewing for weight loss among adults in primary care. *Obes Rev*, 16/4: 304–18.

Broyles LM, Binswanger IA, and Jenkins JA, Finnell DS, Faseru B, Cavaiola A, Pugatch M, and Gordon AJ. (2014). Confronting inadvertent stigma and pejorative language in addiction scholarship: a recognition and response. *Subst Abus*, 35/3: 217–21.

DiClemente CC, Crouch TB, Norwood AE, Delahanty J, and Welsh C. (2015). Evaluating training of screening, brief intervention, and referral to treatment (SBIRT) for substance use: reliability of the MD3 SBIRT Coding Scale. *Psychol Addictive Behav*, 29/1: 218.

Felker B, Yazel J Joe, and Short D. (1996). Mortality and medical comorbidity among psychiatric patients: a review', *Psychiatric Serv*, 47/12: 1356–63.

Haibach JP, Beehler GP, Dollar KM, and Finnell DS. (2014). Moving toward integrated behavioral intervention for treating multimorbidity among chronic pain, depression, and substance-use disorders in primary care. *Med Care*, 52/4: 322–7.

Hall K, Staiger PK, Simpson A, Best D, and Lubman DI. (2015). After 30 years of dissemination, have we achieved sustained practice change in motivational interviewing? *Addiction*, 111/7: 1144–50.

Heckman CJ, Egleston BL, and Hofmann MT. Efficacy of motivational interviewing for smoking cessation: a systematic review and meta-analysis. *Tob Control*, 19/5: 410–6.

Jelsma JG, Mertens V-C, Forsberg L, and Forsberg L. (2015). How to measure motivational interviewing fidelity in randomized controlled trials: practical recommendations. *Contemp Clin Trials*, 43: 93–9.

Kroenke K, Spitzer RL, and Williams JBW. (2001). The PHQ-9: validity of a brief depression severity measure. *J Gen Intern Med*, 16/9: 606–13.

Lopez AD, Mathers CD, Ezzati M, Jamison DT, and Murray CJ. (2006). Global and regional burden of disease and risk factors, 2001: systematic analysis of population health data. *Lancet*, 367/9524: 1747–57.

Lopresti AL, Hood SD, and Drummond PD. (2013). A review of lifestyle factors that contribute to important pathways associated with major depression: diet, sleep and exercise. *J Affect Disord*, 148/1 (2013: 12–27.

Macdonald P, Hibbs R, Corfield F, and Treasure J. (2012). The use of motivational interviewing in eating disorders: a systematic review. *Psychiatry Res* 200/1: 1–11.

McKenna BS and Eyler LT. (2012). Overlapping prefrontal systems involved in cognitive and emotional processing in euthymic bipolar disorder and following sleep deprivation: a review of functional neuroimaging studies. *Clin Psychol Rev*, 32/7: 650–63.

Merrill RM, Taylor P, and Aldana SG. (2008). Coronary Health Improvement Project (CHIP) is associated with improved nutrient intake and decreased depression. *Nutr*, 24/4: 314–21.

Miller W and Rollnick S. (2013). *Motivational Interviewing: Helping People Change*, 3rd edn. New York: The Guilford Press.

Moher D, Liberati A, Tetzlaff J, and Altman DG. (2009). Preferred reporting items for systematic reviews and meta-analyses: the PRISMA statement. *Ann Intern Med*, 151/4: 264–9.

Moyers TB, Manuel JK, and Ernst D. (2015). Motivational Interviewing Treatment Integrity Coding Manual 4.2.1. Revised June 2015: Unpublished Manual: http://casaa.unm.edu/download/MITI4_2.pdf. Accessed August 15, 2015.

Naar-King S, Parsons JT, and Johnson AM. (2012). Motivational interviewing targeting risk reduction for people with HIV: a systematic review. *Curr HIV/AIDS Rep* 9/4: 335–43.

Newcomer JW and Hennekens CH. (2007). Severe mental illness and risk of cardiovascular disease. *JAMA*, 298/15: 1794–6.

O'Halloran PD, Blackstock F, Shields N, Holland A, Iles R, Kingsley M, Bernhardt J, Lannin N, Morris ME, and Taylor NF. (2014). Motivational interviewing to increase physical activity in people with chronic health conditions: a systematic review and meta-analysis. *Clin Rehabil*, 28/12: 1159–71.

Purath J, Keck A, and Fitzgerald CE. (2014). Motivational interviewing for older adults in primary care: a systematic review. *Geriatr Nurs*, 35/3: 219–24.

Riper H, Andersson G, Hunter SB, de Wit J, Berking M, and Cuijpers P. (2014). Treatment of comorbid alcohol use disorders and depression with cognitive-behavioural therapy and motivational interviewing: a meta-analysis. *Addiction* 109/3: 394–406.

Romano M and Peters L. (2015). Evaluating the mechanisms of change in motivational interviewing in the treatment of mental health problems: a review and meta-analysis', *Clin Psychol Rev*, 38: 1–12.

Romano M and Peters L. (2014). Understanding the process of motivational interviewing: a review of the relational and technical hypotheses. *Psychother Res*, 26/2: 220–40.

Sarris J, O'Neil A, Coulson CE, Schweitzer I, and Berk M. (2014). Lifestyle medicine for depression. *BMC Psychiatry*, 14: 107.

Sarris J, Logan AC, Akbaraly TN, Amminger GP, Balanzá-Martínez V, Freeman MP, Hibbeln J, Matsuoka Y, Mischoulon D, Mizoue T, Nanri A, Nishi D, Ramsey D, Rucklidge JJ, Sanchez-Villegas A, Scholey A, Su KP, and Jacka FN; International Society for Nutritional Psychiatry Research. (2015). Nutritional medicine as mainstream in psychiatry. *Lancet Psychiatry* 2/3: 271–74.

Scheewe T, Backx F, Takken T, Jörg F, van Strater AC, Kroes AG, Kahn RS, and Cahn W. (2013). Exercise therapy improves mental and physical health in schizophrenia: a randomised controlled trial. *Acta Psychiatri Scand*, 127/6: 464–73.

Shingleton RM and Palfai TP. Technology-delivered adaptations of motivational interviewing for health-related behaviors: a systematic review of the current research. *Patient Educ Couns*, 99/1: 17–35.

Spitzer RL, Kroenke K, Williams JB, and Löwe B. (2006). A brief measure for assessing generalized anxiety disorder: the GAD-7. *Arch Intern Med*, 166/10: 1092–7.

Sullivan LE, Fiellin DA, and **O'Connor PG.** The prevalence and impact of alcohol problems in major depression: a systematic review. *Am J Med* **118**/4: 330–41.

United States Department of Health and Human Services. (2008). *2008 Physical Activity Guidelines Advisory Comittee Report.* Washington, DC: United States Department of Health and Human Services.

VanBuskirk KA and **Wetherell JL,** 'Motivational interviewing with primary care populations: a systematic review and meta-analysis', *J Behav Med,* **37**/4 (2014), 768–80.

Walsh R. Lifestyle and mental health. *Am Psychol,* **66**/7: 579.

World Health Organization. (2014). The top 10 causes of death. Geneva: World Health Organization.

Chapter 16

Psychosis

Jayashri Kulkarni, Emorfia Gavrilidis,
Shainal Nathoo, and Jasmin Grigg

Introduction

Psychosis is a broad term for a set of symptoms impairing a person's perception of reality. The key clinical features of psychotic disorders are delusions, hallucinations, disorganized thinking, bizarre behaviour, and/or negative symptoms (Austin, 2005). Psychotic disorders affect functioning and personality, and are among the most severe of the psychiatric disorders (American Psychiatric Association, 2013). Onset tends to occur during young adulthood, which interferes with this critical period of educational, occupational, and social development. Psychosis can result in lifelong disability, increased physical morbidity, and shortened life expectancy, and exerts significant emotional and economic burden for the individual as well as their families. Psychosis represents a heavy economic burden due to costs of care and treatment, and loss of productivity.

As the first point of contact for many patients experiencing psychotic symptoms, primary care practitioners (PCPs) play a critical role in early diagnosis and treatment initiation (Gavin et al., 2006). Early identification, referral, and intervention have a direct, positive impact on prognosis (Yung et al., 2004). Further, approximately 10% of patients will be in contact *only* with their PCP (Conway et al., 1994). The sound diagnostic and management skills of the PCP are essential to optimizing care and outcomes for patients experiencing psychotic illness.

Epidemiology

Although lifetime prevalence of schizophrenia has been estimated at 1%, and more than 3% for *any* psychotic disorder (Perälä et al., 2007), it is now recognized that there are significant differences among populations. While both sexes are at risk of developing psychosis, younger male and older female age groups have a slightly higher prevalence. Oestrogen is hypothesized to raise the vulnerability threshold in women during adolescence, until menopause (Kulkarni et al., 2008). The aetiology and pathogenesis of psychotic disorders are still largely unknown (Perälä, 2013). Genetic influence, life events, and other risk factors play a role in their development. A consistent finding in the epidemiology of psychosis is its high incidence among migrant and ethnic minority groups (Cantor-Graae and Selten, 2014).

Disease classification

Psychotic disorders are classified using symptom-based diagnostic criteria established by the Diagnostic and Statistical Manual of Mental Disorders 5th Edition (DSM-5) (American Psychiatric Association, 2013) or the International Classification of Diseases 10th Edition (ICD-10) (World Health Organization, 1992), which are periodically revised based on research findings and expert consensus. Psychosis is not a diagnosis per se, but rather a class of illness characterized by the following key features:

* Hallucinations—perception-like experiences that can occur in any sensory modality, and which occur in the absence of external stimuli.

* Delusions—fixed beliefs that are not amenable to change in light of conflicting evidence, which can be persecutory, referential, somatic, religious, or grandiose.

* Disorganized thinking –thoughts that appear illogical, lacking in sequence, and may be delusional or bizarre in content.

* Disorganized behaviour—problems with goal-directed behaviour can manifest in a number of ways and impair daily functioning. Behaviours may include agitation, purposeless or excessive motor activity, odd expressions (staring, grimacing), and catatonia (which includes decreased responsiveness and odd posturing).

* Negative symptoms—these can manifest in diminished emotional expression (reduced facial expression, eye contact, gestures), decreased self-initiated purposeful activities (avolition), diminished speech output (alogia), decreased enjoyment from activities (anhedonia), and loss of interest in social interactions.

(Data from *Diagnostic and statistical manual of mental disorder*, 5th ed., 2013, American Psychiatric Association)

Engaging with a psychotic patient

An effective therapeutic relationship is the foundation for clinical care, and can be pivotal in promoting and maintaining patient engagement in treatment. Box 16.1 outlines several techniques that can be helpful in engaging a patient who is experiencing psychosis.

Emergency management of presenting psychosis

It is critical for the PCP to evaluate risk, assess the ability of the patient to accept treatment, and determine the need for immediate hospitalization if required (Simon et al., 2014). Mental health laws tend to be primarily concerned with protecting individuals from harming themselves and others, and allow the involuntary treatment of individuals at high risk of self-harm or violence. Involuntary hospitalization may be warranted if the patient is in a crisis and poses a risk to themselves or others, or is seriously impaired in their capacity for self-care. In these extreme cases, police intervention and rapid sedation may be required. If sedation is required while awaiting admission, oral medication lorazepam 1–2mg or chlorpromazine 50–100mg can be used if the patient is compliant. If the patient is resistive, they should be allowed to leave and the police called.

Box 16.1 Techniques to engage a patient experiencing psychosis

1. Be conscious that your patient may be wary/anxious.
2. Be aware that psychosis may impair your patient's ability to interact or process information.
3. Avoid confrontational behaviour (e.g. sit to you patient's side rather than front on; consider their personal space and access to the exit; use a degree of eye contact that does not distress your patient).
4. Listen carefully, and acknowledge your patient's viewpoint
5. Spend time building trust.
6. Gather information at your patient's pace.
7. Be respectful and empathic.

Preliminary assessment

Whilst the presence of psychotic symptoms usually results in referral to a specialist psychiatric service, the PCP plays an important role in initial management, and evaluation of any underlying organic causes. (Saunders et al., 2011). In the early phase of assessment, the goal is to stabilize the crisis rather than to establish a final diagnosis.

Diagnostic evaluation should involve a thorough evaluation of current psychotic symptoms, a complete psychiatric history including a timeline of symptoms, a complete medical history (including family history and history of substance use), and a physical examination.

The PCP should make careful note of the patient's overall behaviour, appearance, hygiene, speech, and gait. Of particular interest are any acute changes in these behaviours, as well as the presence of disorganized or bizarre thinking and behaviour.

If carried out by the PCP, a final diagnosis is often best determined via a longitudinal assessment process that includes: direct patient questioning (e.g. query on hearing/seeing things, feeling suspicious, having special powers such as reading minds, receiving messages via TV or radio) (Marder and Davis, 2014), clinical observation, collateral information from family/friends, and a review of the patient's available documented history (Saunders et al., 2011).

Organic causes must be excluded prior to attributing psychosis to a primary psychiatric disorder. Some organic causes of psychosis to be considered during initial assessment are outlined in Box 16.2.

Box 16.3 outlines important factors to be considered in the patient's medical history.

During the physical examination, carefully evaluate vital signs, thyroid, nutritional status, any dysmorphic features, and conscious state. Tachycardia, hypertension, and pupillary responses possibly indicate drug intoxication or drug withdrawal, or fever/infection (also inspect for rashes) (Freudenreich et al., 2009). Box 16.4 outlines screening tests for organic causes of psychosis.

Box 16.2 Organic causes of psychosis

- Toxicity due to prescription medication, recreational drugs, over the counter medication, or other substance exposure.

- Neurological conditions—neoplasms, cerebrovascular disease, Huntington's disease, multiple sclerosis, epilepsy, auditory or visual nerve injury, deafness, migraine, central nervous system infections.

- Metabolic abnormalities—hypoxia, hypercarbia, hypoglycaemia.

- Endocrine condition—hyper- and hypothyroidism, hyper- and hypoparathyroidism, hyper- and hypoadrenocorticism, thyrotoxicosis.

- Fluid/electrolyte imbalances

- Hepatic or renal disease

- Autoimmune disorders with central nervous system involvement (e.g. systemic lupus erythematosus)

Data from *Diagnostic and statistical manual of mental disorder*, 5th ed., 2013, American Psychiatric Association.

Box 16.3 Medical history to assist in diagnosis of psychosis

- History of recent or past head injury, which could result in a seizure disorder that increases the risk of schizophrenia.

- Recent seizures—it is important to establish the timing of the patient's presentation (post-ictal, ictal, or intra-ictal)

- Neurological symptoms often indicate organic CNS pathology. Symptoms to screen for include headaches, focal neurological signs, visual changes, speech impediments, memory disturbances, and alterations of consciousness (delirium).

- Drug history, including prescription medication, over-the-counter medication, recreational drugs, and herbal medications.

- Recent history of surgery—which could be a cause for hypoxia.

- Recent history of travel—consider infectious diseases that may lead to encephalitis and psychosis

- HIV positive patients—AIDS can mimic psychosis symptoms

- Family history—psychiatric history, auto immune disorders, and genetic disorders.

Box 16.4 Tests for organic causes of psychosis

- Full blood count and ESR
- Urea, creatinine, and electrolytes
- Fasting glucose, cholesterol, triglycerides
- Liver function
- Thyroid function
- Urine drug screen
- Vitamin B12 and folate
- Hepatitis and other blood-borne diseases (HIV if indicated)
- Anti-NMDAR, Anti-VGKC, Anti-GAD antibodies

Computerized tomography or magnetic resonance imaging is indicated when the patient presents with a history of head trauma, focal neurological signs, headache or change in pattern of headache, late age onset (30+ years), or pronounced cognitive deficits.

Differential diagnoses

The major psychoses are illustrated in Fig. 16.1. Psychotic symptoms can be brief, episodic, or enduring in their occurrence, may involve an affective component, and can be induced by various psychiatric or organic conditions. Substance abuse can

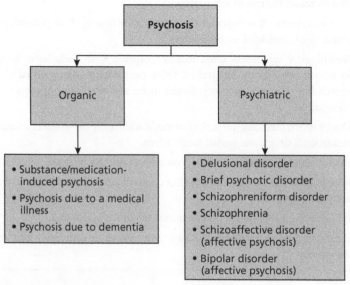

Fig. 16.1 The major psychoses

trigger a psychiatric disorder, and can also cause a transient organic psychotic illness (Saunders et al., 2011). Symptom severity (e.g. degree of disorganized thinking or mood symptoms) and duration (e.g. remitting within a month, or lasting more than six months) carry prognostic value and can guide treatment.

Organic psychosis

Substance/medication-induced psychosis

This diagnosis is indicated when prominent delusions and/or hallucinations occur as a physiological effect of the substance/medication. Symptoms occur soon after exposure, intoxication, or withdrawal; they can also persist for weeks. This diagnosis is distinguished from a psychiatric disorder *triggered* by substance use (American Psychiatric Association, 2013).

Psychosis due to a medical condition

This diagnosis can be made when the presence of a medical condition can be identified, and is considered to be the aetiology of the psychosis through a *physiological* mechanism (i.e. not a psychologically mediated response to the condition). The presence of a temporal association between the medical condition and psychotic symptoms regarding onset, exacerbation, and remission can indicate aetiology and assist with diagnosis (American Psychiatric Association, 2013).

Psychosis due to dementia or depression

Psychotic symptoms, such as delusions and hallucinations, are frequently observed in dementing neurodegenerative diseases (e.g. Alzheimer's disease and dementia with Lewy bodies) (Shinagawa et al., 2013). Psychotic symptoms in older persons are also commonly caused by depression, which has been estimated to account for 20% of presenting psychotic symptoms in this cohort (Saunders et al., 2011). PCPs can encounter therapeutic difficulties in managing psychotic symptoms in older patients; antipsychotics or antidepressants may have limited efficacy or may not be well tolerated by this cohort (Shinagawa et al., 2013). Diligent treatment is necessary, as psychosis in older persons is associated with additional disability, poorer quality of life, and caregiver burden.

Psychiatric psychoses

Schizophrenia

Schizophrenia is a complex, severely disabling disorder characterized by psychosis, negative symptoms, and cognitive dysfunction. The diagnosis of schizophrenia can be made when two or more psychotic symptoms are clearly prominent for at least one month (active-phase symptoms), with continuous signs of disturbance persisting for at least six months. During prodromal or residual periods, level of disturbance may be limited to negative symptoms or psychotic symptoms in an attenuated form (e.g. odd beliefs). Schizophrenia causes significant impairment in social, interpersonal, or occupational functioning. Schizophrenia is a heterogeneous diagnosis, and individual presentations will vary considerably (American Psychiatric Association, 2013).

Schizoaffective disorder

Prominent mood symptoms, in addition to the occurrence of the core symptoms of schizophrenia, feature in schizoaffective disorder. A diagnosis of schizoaffective disorder is made when there is a major mood episode (depressive or manic) concurrent with the presence of two or more psychotic symptoms for a significant proportion of time over at least one month. Differing from depressive or bipolar disorder with psychotic features, delusions or hallucinations must be present for at least two weeks in the absence of a major mood episode at some point during the illness (American Psychiatric Association, 2013).

Bipolar disorder

Bipolar disorder is recognized to be related to both the schizophrenia spectrum and depressive disorder classifications (American Psychiatric Association, 2013). A diagnosis of bipolar I disorder can be considered when there has been a distinct manic episode—abnormal, persistently elevated, and persistently increased activity/energy for at least one week—which is preceded by, and may be followed by, major depressive episodes. Rapid shifts in mood can occur, and irritability can predominate (hypomanic episodes). During a manic episode, inflated self-esteem, grandiosity reaching delusional proportions, poor judgement, and reckless behaviour is common. The need for sleep can be greatly reduced, speech and thoughts can be rapid, and increased goal-directed activity, psychomotor agitation, and distractibility occurs (American Psychiatric Association, 2013).

People at risk of psychotic disorders

The ability to identify individuals at high risk of developing a psychotic disorder is an important goal of PCPs; early treatment in this group can improve prognosis considerably, with the potential to reduce illness progression and chronicity (Yung et al., 2004) (Yung and McGorry, 2007). Some evidence suggests early intervention may be able to delay or even prevent onset of psychosis patients who are high-risk, or *prodromal* (Morrison et al., 2004, McGorry et al., 2002). Poor prognosis is associated with a longer duration of symptoms prior to treatment, family history of psychotic disorders, pronounced negative symptoms, non-compliance, and substance abuse comorbidity.

Several clinical and psychopathological variables, shown in Table 16.1, are known to predict the imminent onset of psychosis.

Management of first episode psychosis

Box 16.5 (adapted from EPPIC, 2002; Buckley, 2009) comprises a step-by-step guide for the initiation of treatment for first-episode psychosis. Please note that for patients presenting with a first episode, commencement of antipsychotic medication is best

Table 16.1 Predictors of psychosis onset

Predictor	Example
Schizotypal features	Odd beliefs/behaviour, social withdrawal or isolation, social anxiety
Sub-threshold positive symptoms	Perceptual disturbances, unusual thoughts and ideas, suspiciousness, conceptual disorganization
Negative symptoms	Impaired concentration/attention, subjectively abnormal emotional experiences, impaired energy, anhedonia, blunted affect, social withdrawal
Basic symptoms	Subjectively defined thought, language, perception, and motor disturbances
Affective disturbance	Depression, anxiety and/or distress in relation to psychotic experiences
Poor functioning	Decline in school/work performance
Substance use	Use of cannabis or other illicit drugs
Stressful life events	The subjective experience of stressful/distressing major and minor life events, lifetime experience of major stressors
Neurocognitive Symptoms	Cognitive deficits (e.g. working memory, 'concentration difficulties'), olfactory identification deficits
Neurobiological features	Increased cortisol levels, abnormal circadian cortisol rhythms, increased volume of pituitary gland corticotrophs, progressive hippocampal volume loss

Data from *The British Journal of Psychiatry*, 191, 2007, Yung, A. R. & MCGorry, P. D., 'Prediction of psychosis: setting the stage', pp. s1–s8.

done in consultation with a specialist psychiatric service (Saunders et al., 2011). Older persons presenting with first-episode psychosis require special treatment considera-tion (e.g. optimize social care, consider treatment with acetylcholinesterase inhibi-tors, consider low-dose trazodone, discuss and minimize cardiovascular risk factors) (National Collaborating Centre for Mental Health, 2011).

Benzodiazepines can be used initially to treat distress, insomnia, and agitation. Other symptoms such as mania and severe depression require treatment with mood stabilizers and antidepressants. If the patient is recognized to be experiencing first-episode psychosis of an affective nature (e.g. schizoaffective disorder, bipolar disor-der), follow the steps in Box 16.5; however, consider prescribing a mood stabilizer in conjunction with atypical antipsychotic.

◆ Day 1—start 500mg lithium or 500mg sodium valproate oral daily
◆ Day 2—500mg lithium or 500mg sodium valproate oral twice daily
◆ After 5 days—Increase dose according to clinical response if required (serum levels of lithium should be performed, with a target level of 0.9–1.2mmol/l)
◆ If not sufficient clinical response, switch to alternate mood stabilizer

Box 16.5 Management of first episode psychosis

1. Initial medical and psychiatric assessment
2. Period of observation of 24 hours
   - if psychiatric emergency, manage as above
   - consider prescribing diazepam if patient is aggressive/agitated
   - consider prescribing lorazepam if patient is anxious
3. If symptoms persist, prescribe an atypical antipsychotic with a low starting dose, for example:
   - olanzapine, start 2.5–5mg oral daily
   - risperidone, start 0.5–1mg oral daily
   - quetiapine, start 25mg oral twice daily
4. Gradually titrate atypical antipsychotic up to an effective level, according to clinical response and tolerability
5. Monitor adherence and side effects continuously from early on, and intervene as appropriate.
6. If not sufficient clinical response after six–seven weeks, or if not well-tolerated, switch to a different atypical antipsychotic using slow cross-over titration.

Regular investigation of renal function, lithium levels, full blood examination, and thyroid function are integral to the management of a patient taking lithium (National Collaborating Centre for Mental Health, 2014). Sodium valproate should not be prescribed to women of child-bearing age.

Medicines concordance and adherence

Choice of antipsychotic, including the expected benefits, side effects, and potential long-term adverse effects, should be discussed with the patient. The patient's questions and concerns should be addressed, and tolerability of and response to previously trialled medications should be considered. Patients who are able to participate in decisions about their own treatment are more likely to adhere to medication regimes (de Almeida Neto and Aslani, 2008). Concordance and adherence can be challenged depending on the psychotic symptoms present (e.g. thought disorder, lack of insight), although generally the patient will still be capable of meaningful communication and will usually appreciate the opportunity to participate in clinical decision-making (Galletly and Crichton, 2011). See Box 16.6 for actions aimed at enhancing treatment adherence.

Treatment-resistant psychosis

Treatment resistance is usually defined as unremitting positive symptoms despite treatment with at least two different antipsychotic medications. In refractory schizophrenia,

Box 16.6 Actions to increase treatment adherence

- Educate the patient about their illness and treatment—discuss treatment options, regimens, and adverse effects, and involve them in clinical decision-making.
- Prescribe drug regimens that are simple to follow.
- Monitor medication use and screen for adverse effects—prompt resolution of adverse effects improves adherence.
- Devise a treatment and ongoing support plan, discuss realistic expectations, and goals of treatment.
- With patient permission, involve family members in ensuring adherence
- If considering the use of long-acting injectable antipsychotics, discuss this with the patient.

negative symptoms are usually also prominent. The antipsychotic clozapine can be very effective for patients who do not respond to other antipsychotics, and is most effective when treatment resistance is identified early (within 6–12 months) and is commenced without delay. It can take up to twelve months for clozapine to take full effect. Clozapine treatment requires strict monitoring; it can cause serious adverse effects, including cardiomyopathy, agranulocytosis, and other blood dyscrasias, as well as weight gain and diabetes mellitus.

Other interventions for treatment-resistant psychosis include the use of transcranial magnetic stimulation (TMS), applied to the temporoparietal cortex to treat auditory hallucinations (Fitzgerald et al., 2013). There is limited evidence for the efficacy of TMS applied to the left dorsolateral prefrontal cortex to treat negative symptoms of schizophrenia (Freitas et al., 2009). TMS is generally well tolerated.

Many emerging adjunctive treatments for persistent psychosis are currently being investigated and include repurposed drugs such as aspirin, celecoxib, estrogen, selective estrogen receptor modulators (SERMs), folate, minocycline, mirtazapine, omega-3 fatty acids, pramipexole, and pregnenolone (Torrey and Davis, 2011; Kulkarni et al., 2015, 2016).

Psychosis relapse

Relapses of active-phase symptoms may occur, and can result from non-adherence, substance use/abuse, psychological stress (e.g. death of a loved one), physical ill health, poor sleep, or for a non-discernible reason. Relapse can have a detrimental impact on the long-term course of psychotic disorders (Emsley et al., 2013). Relapse management involves early detection of psychotic symptoms, intervention, and consulting with others the patient knows whenever possible. It is important to try to identify the 'relapse signature', which is the recognizable pattern of symptoms that can emerge with each new episode. This pattern of symptoms should be discussed with the patient and known others (when possible), so that there is awareness of what the early signs of relapse look like. Practitioner-patient rapport increases reporting of symptom relapse, and of factors that can precipitate relapse (e.g. medication issues that lead to non-adherence).

When relapse does occur, ensure the patient is taking antipsychotic medication as prescribed. Re-starting the same medication in the correct dose may be an important first step to treating a relapse (however careful, gradual titration must be used if re-starting clozapine to prevent arrhythmias (Merrill et al., 2005)). Additional sedation may be needed to treat agitation or anxiety. There are many choices available for sedation, including low-dose, short-term (7 days or fewer) use of benzodiazepines, or using an increased dose of the primary antipsychotic medication if it is sedating (e.g. olanzapine, quetiapine). Rarely, two or more antipsychotics may be required to manage an acute relapse. In this situation, the pharmacological profile of medications including side effects need to be carefully considered. Additional psychiatric conditions such as depression or mania, drug-induced psychosis, or other comorbid disorders will need special management. Negative symptoms of schizophrenia can be difficult to distinguish from depression. A careful history for symptoms of depression and a trial of antidepressant medication, in addition to the primary antipsychotic, may be useful. Adding a mood stabilizer such as lithium to antipsychotic treatment can be useful in treating a relapse of bipolar disorder with psychosis.

Harm minimization from substance abuse

The use of substances such as alcohol, cannabis, and crystal methamphetamine is widespread, and poses significant challenges for treatment providers. Substance use can trigger first-episode and also relapse of psychotic symptoms, often presenting in crisis (Grant et al., 2012).

A comprehensive assessment, including physical examination and mental health review, is essential for determining the most appropriate approach to minimizing substance use. Early engagement and intervention should be incorporated into a comprehensive and tailored treatment plan, which the patient can assist in developing. Treatment should focus on controlling medical and psychiatric symptoms while eliminating the offending substance, or reducing its impact when cessation is not possible.

Maintenance of good physical health

Patients with psychosis tend to experience poor physical health (Kulkarni et al., 2013). It is critical to address physical health early in the course of psychosis. Obesity and tobacco smoking are significant factors in this cohort's high mortality (Thornicroft, 2011). Weight gain due to medication side effects requires patient education, and ongoing monitoring with the goals of prevention and early intervention. The modification of lifestyle factors such as diet, exercise, alcohol consumption, and smoking is important, and PCPs are ideally placed to have an impact on outcomes related to these factors (Kulkarni et al., 2013). Smoking alters the concentration-to-dose ratio of some antipsychotics (e.g. olanzapine, clozapine, haloperidol), therefore smoking reduction or cessation warrants the appropriate adjustment of antipsychotic dose (Tsuda, 2014).

Many of the psychotropic medications prescribed to patients with psychosis increase risk of serious adverse events. An important role of the PCP is to regularly monitor adverse events, paying particular attention to cardiovascular and metabolic side effects, as well as extrapyramidal effects, with prompt intervention and/or referral as required. A range of other side effects (e.g. sexual, endocrine, sedative) should be routinely assessed and managed accordingly.

Psychosocial treatment

While medical management is often unavoidable, current pharmacotherapy treatments are far from ideal (Kulkarni et al., 2012). It is now accepted that for optimal outcomes, the treatment of psychotic disorders requires a multidimensional approach that combines biological, psychological, and social strategies (Kulkarni et al., 2013).

Psychosocial interventions have a positive effect on recovery, functioning, readmission rates, and quality of life (McGorry et al., 2005). Additionally, providing education and support to the family leads to improved care of the unwell individual (McGorry et al., 2005). Several psychosocial interventions have shown promising results in targeting symptoms of psychosis, as well as addressing the wider psychosocial consequences of this group of disorders. These include:

◆ Cognitive-Behavioural Therapy for Psychosis (CBTp)—CBTp aims to increase awareness of the connections between thoughts, behaviours, and feelings to promote changes in symptoms and functioning (Turner et al., 2014).

◆ Social Skills Training—A behavioural intervention addressing social function (e.g. responding to social cues, non-verbal communication) (Turner et al., 2014).

◆ Family-Based Intervention—focuses on key elements of illness education, crisis intervention, emotional support, and training to cope with illness symptoms. It should be offered whenever there is ongoing contact between the individual and their relatives and/or significant others. Family-based intervention has been found to significantly reduce rates of relapse and hospitalization, improve medication adherence, and increase satisfaction with family relationships (Dixon et al., 2010).

◆ Cognitive Remediation—targets basic cognitive processes (i.e. working memory, attention, executive functioning) implicated in the development and course of psychosis, with the aim of improving these aspects of functioning (Turner et al., 2014).

◆ Psycho-education—relevant information is provided to patients about their diagnosis with the aim of improving understanding, coping, and medication adherence (Turner et al., 2014).

◆ Vocational Interventions—for individuals with psychosis, unemployment is a significant area of disability. Individual placement and support (IPS) is a particularly promising form of supported employment that has been shown to engage a significant proportion of patients in school/work for a sustained period of time (i.e. at least two years) (Rinaldi et al., 2010).

Special issues for women with psychosis

Pregnancy and postpartum

The desire to reproduce is both a powerful urge and a basic human right for women, regardless of mental health status. Deinstitutionalized treatment for mental illness, better pharmacotherapies, and generally higher expectations for a normal quality of life all have the potential to raise the incidence of pregnancy in women with psychosis (Miller et al., 1992). It has been estimated that more than 50% of women with psychotic illness are mothers (Howard et al., 2001, McGrath et al., 1999). Many of these women will therefore require ongoing antipsychotic treatment during pregnancy and the postpartum period to avoid severe psychosis relapse, and optimize their wellbeing and capacity to care for their newborn.

The right of women with mental illness to become a parent places responsibility upon health care professionals to ensure sound antenatal and ongoing care is available. Antipsychotic medications are being prescribed to a growing number of women with mental illness. However, there is currently insufficient evidence regarding their safety in pregnancy, which complicates decision-making for clinicians and patients. This clinical dilemma is the driving force behind the establishment of The National Register of Antipsychotic Medication in Pregnancy (NRAMP) (Kulkarni et al., 2014), an ongoing Australia-wide observational study that follows mothers who take antipsychotic medications during pregnancy and tracks progress of both woman and infant.

The preliminary results of the NRAMP study highlight the need to be particularly vigilant for metabolic complications during pregnancy (e.g. excess weight gain, gestational diabetes) and worsening of psychotic symptoms, particularly during postpartum (Kulkarni et al., 2014). Women should be screened regularly for diabetes and hypercholesterolemia. Attention to lifestyle factors such as diet, exercise, smoking, and alcohol cessation are important, and the PCP is ideally placed to have a positive impact on these health behaviours.

Fertility and pre-pregnancy care

Fertility and pre-pregnancy planning seems to be rarely discussed between women with psychosis and their PCP, with the focus of psychosis symptoms dominating the clinical interaction. Women with psychotic disorders have a lower fertility rate when matched with women without a mental illness (Howard et al., 2002), and early referral to a fertility specialist should be considered when appropriate.

Pre-pregnancy care is vital, and the key goals should be to optimize the woman's mental and physical health. Education regarding nutrition, cessation of smoking and illicit drugs, taking folate, and minimizing alcohol intake before and during pregnancy is important in ensuring better outcomes for both mother and infant.

Early referral to a psychiatrist who specializes in women's mental health or perinatal psychiatry, to optimize psychotropic use and mental health outcomes, is imperative. It is also important that, in planning the birth, the woman is booked into a hospital that has access to relevant psychiatric facilities (e.g. a mother-baby unit). This ensures an immediate response if her mental state deteriorates after she gives birth.

The identification of a history of serious mental illness, and a holistic management strategy that addresses well-being and safety while aiming to keep mother and infant together after the birth, are essential aspects of care for this cohort.

Menopause

Perimenopause refers to the reproductive stage immediately prior to menopause—usually around the age of 47—when due to endocrine, biological, and clinical changes in women may lead to the onset of depression or psychosis for the first time, or may experience a relapse of symptoms.

Both hormone therapies and antidepressants can effectively treat the mood symptoms associated with menopause, and a combination of the two can at times be indicated. For psychosis, the augmentation of a primary antipsychotic with a SERM (e.g. raloxifene hydrochloride) might be beneficial for women during peri- and postmenopause (Kulkarni et al., 2010; Kulkarni et al., 2016). A detailed history should be taken prior to prescribing, especially in regard to stroke, thromboembolic disease, and family history of breast or ovarian cancer. Regular mammograms and pap smears are particularly important in ensuring the safe use of hormone therapy. Many women with psychosis will have experienced sexual abuse and may therefore find mammograms and pap smears very traumatic. A sensitive approach is required and a referral to a female doctor should be considered.

Other health issues associated with menopause including weight gain, hypercholesterolemia, diabetes, and osteoporosis—which may be exacerbated by the use of antipsychotic medication—also require ongoing monitoring. Psychosocial issues such as fears of ageing, loss of fertility, change in domestic life, and changes in career (e.g. retirement) can also be assessed by the PCP, so that a holistic approach to treatment can be achieved.

Conclusion

Psychosis can severely disrupt the afflicted individual's life. Early intervention has the potential to change illness progression and chronicity, and primary health care plays a critical role in the pathway to optimal care. PCPs are well-placed to recognize early symptoms, stabilize the crisis, provide initial management, identify any underlying organic pathogenesis, use a sound working knowledge of local specialist services for referral, consider special management issues relating to different patient cohorts, and use good clinical judgment to hospitalize if required. In the longer term, PCPs facilitate ongoing medication adherence and optimize physical health through follow-up care. High quality primary care continues even after referral to specialist services, wherein ongoing physical health and chronic disease care, health promotion, and shared care arrangements can ultimately improve patient prognosis.

References

American Psychiatric Association. (2013). *Diagnostic and Statistical Manual of Mental Disorders, Fifth Edition (DSM-5)*. London: American Psychiatric Publishing.

Austin J. (2005). Schizophrenia: an update and review. *Journal of genetic counseling*, 14: 329–40.

Buckley P, Foster AE, Patel NC, and Wermert A. (2009). *Adherence to mental health treatment.* Oxford: Oxford University Press.

Cantor-Graae E and Selten JP. (2014). Schizophrenia and migration: a meta-analysis and review. *Am J Psychiatry*, 162/1: 12–24.

Conway AS, Melzer D, and Hale AS. (1994). The outcome of targeting community mental health services: evidence from the West Lambeth schizophrenia cohort. *BMJ*, 308: 627–30.

De Almeida Neto AC and Aslani P. (2008). Medicines concordance in clinical practice. *British journal of Clinical Pharmacology*, 66: 453–4.

Dixon LB, Dickerson F, Bellack AS, Bennett M, Dickinson D, Goldberg RW, Lehman A, Tenhula WN, Calmes C, and Pasillas RM. (2010). The 2009 schizophrenia PORT psychosocial treatment recommendations and summary statements. *Schizophrenia Bulletin*, 36: 48–70.

Emsley R, Chiliza B, Asmal L, and Harvey BH. (2013). The nature of relapse in schizophrenia. *BMC Psychiatry*, 13: 50.

Early Psychosis Prevention and Intervention Centre (EPPIC). (2002). *EPPIC Pharmacotherapy Guide: Prolonged recovery in early psychosis: A treatment manual and video*. Melbourne: Early Psychosis Prevention and Intervention Centre.

Fitzgerald PB and Hoy KE. (2013). Neuromodulation techniques to treat hallucinations. In: R Jardri, A Cachia, P Thomas, and D Pins, eds. *The Neuroscience of Hallucinations* New York: Springer, 493–511.

Freitas C, Fregni F, and Pascual-Leone A. (2009). Meta-analysis of the effects of repetitive transcranial magnetic stimulation (rTMS) on negative and positive symptoms in schizophrenia. *Schizophrenia Research*, 108: 11–24.

Freudenreich O, Charles Schulz S, and Goff DC. (2009). Initial medical work-up of first-episode psychosis: a conceptual review. *Early Intervention in Psychiatry*, 3: 10–18.

Galletly C and Crichton J. (2011). Accomplishments of the thought disordered person: A case study in psychiatrist–patient interaction. *Medical Hypotheses*, 77: 900–4.

Gavin B, Cullen W, O'Donoghue B, Ascencio-Lane JC, Bury G, and O'Callaghan E. (2006). First episode schizophrenia in general practice: a national survey. *Irish journal of Psychological Medicine*, 23: 6–9.

Grant KM, Levan TD, Wells SM, Li M, Stoltenberg SF, Gendelman HE, Carlo G, and Bevins RA. (2012). Methamphetamine-associated psychosis. *Journal of Neuroimmune Pharmacology*, 7: 113–39.

Howard LM, Kumar C, Leese M, and Thornicroft G. (2002). The general fertility rate in women with psychotic disorders. *American Journal of Psychiatry*, 159: 991–7.

Howard LM, Kumar R, and Thornicroft G. (2001). Psychosocial characteristics and needs of mothers with psychotic disorders. *British Journal of Psychiatry*, 178: 427–32.

Kulkarni J, De Castella A, Fitzgerald PB, Gurvich CT, Bailey M, Bartholomeusz C, and Burger H. (2008). Estrogen in severe mental illness: a potential new treatment approach. *Archives of General Psychiatry*, 65: 955–60.

Kulkarni, J, Gavrilidis E, Hayes E, Heaton V, and Worsley R. (2012). Special biological issues in the management of women with schizophrenia. *Expert Reviews of Neurotherapeutics*, 12: 823–33.

Kulkarni J, Gavrilidis E, and Worsley R. (2013). Biological aspects of treating women with severe mental illness. *Medicine Today*, 14: 44–48.

Kulkarni J, Gurvich C, Lee SJ, Gilbert H, Gavrilidis E, De Castella A, Berk M, Dodd S, Fitzgerald PB, and Davis SR. (2010). Piloting the effective therapeutic dose of adjunctive selective estrogen receptor modulator treatment in postmenopausal women with schizophrenia. *Psychoneuroendocrinology*, 35: 1142–7.

Kulkarni J, Worsley R, Gilbert H, Gavrilidis E, Van Rheenen TE, Wang W, Mccauley K, and Fitzgerald P. (2014). A prospective cohort study of antipsychotic medications in pregnancy: the first 147 pregnancies and 100 one-year-old babies. *PLoS One*, 9: e94788.

Kulkarni J, Gavrilidis E, Wang W, Worsley R, Fitzgerald B, Gurvich C, Van Rheenen T, Berk M, and Burger H. (2015). Estradiol for treatment-resistant schizophrenia: a large-scale randomized-controlled trial in women of child-bearing age. *Mol Psychiatry*, 20/6:695–702.

Kulkarni J, Gavrilidis E, Gwini SM, Worsley R, Grigg J, Warren A, Gurvich C, Gilbert H, Berk M, and Davis SR. (2016). Effect of adjunctive raloxifene therapy on severity of refractory schizophrenia in women: a randomized clinical trial. JAMA Psychiatry, 73: 947–54.

Marder SR and Davis M. (2014). Clinical manifestations, differential diagnosis, and initial management of psychosis in adults. Available at: http://www.uptodate.com/contents/clinical-manifestations-differential-diagnosis-and-initial-management-of-psychosis-in-adults Accessed 14 May, 2015.

McGorry P, Killackey, E, Lambert T, Lambert M, Jackson H, and Codyre D. (2005). Royal Australian and New Zealand College of Psychiatrists clinical practice guidelines for the treatment of schizophrenia and related disorders. *Australian and New Zealand Journal of Psychiatry*, 39: 1–30.

McGorry PD, Yung AR, Phillips LJ, Yuen HP, Francey S, Cosgrave EM, Germano D, Bravin J, McDonald T, and Blair A. (2002). Randomized controlled trial of interventions designed to reduce the risk of progression to first-episode psychosis in a clinical sample with subthreshold symptoms. *Archives of General Psychiatry*, 59: 921–8.

McGrath JJ, Hearle J, Jenner L, Plant K, Drummond A, and Barkla JM. (1999). The fertility and fecundity of patients with psychoses. *Acta Psychiatrica Scandinavica*, 99: 441–6.

Merrill DB, Dec GW, and Goff DC. (2005). Adverse cardiac effects associated with clozapine. *Journal of Clinical Psychopharmacology*, 25: 32–41.

Miller WH Jr, Bloom JD, and Resnick MP. (1992). Chronic mental illness and perinatal outcome. *General Hospital Psychiatry*, 14: 171–6.

Morrison AP, French P, Walford L, Lewis SW, Kilcommons A, Green J, Parker S, and Bentall RP. (2004). Cognitive therapy for the prevention of psychosis in people at ultra-high risk- A randomised controlled trial. *The British Journal of Psychiatry*, 185: 291–7.

National Collaborating Centre for Mental Health. (2011). CG42. *Dementia: supporting people with dementia and their carers in health and social care*. London: NICE.

National Collaborating Centre for Mental Health. (2014). *Psychosis and Schizophrenia in Adults: Treatment and Management*. London: National Institute for Health and Care Excellence.

Perälä J. (2013). *Epidemiology of Psychotic Disorders*. Tampere: National Institute for Health and Welfare.

Perälä J, Suvisaari J, Saarni SI, Kuoppasalmi K, Isometsä E, Pirkola S, Partonen T, Tuulio-Henriksson A, Hintikka J, and Kieseppä T. (2007). Lifetime prevalence of psychotic and bipolar I disorders in a general population. *Archives of General Psychiatry*, 64: 19–28.

Rinaldi M, Killackey E, Smith J, Shepherd G, Singh SP, and Craig T. (2010). First episode psychosis and employment: a review. *International Review of Psychiatry*, 22: 148–62.

Saunders K, Brain S, and Ebmeier K. (2011). Diagnosing and managing psychosis in primary care. *The Practitioner*, 255: 17–20, 2–3.

Shinagawa S, Nakajima S, Plitman E, Graff-Guerrero A, Mimura M, Nakayama K, and Miller BL. (2013). Psychosis in frontotemporal dementia. *Journal of Alzheimer's Disease*, 42: 485–99.

Simon C, Everitt H, Van Dorp F, and Burkes M. (2014). *Oxford Handbook of General Practice*, 4th edn. Oxford: Oxford University Press.

Thornicroft G. (2011). Physical health disparities and mental illness: the scandal of premature mortality. *The British Journal of Psychiatry*, 199: 441–2.

Torrey E and Davis J. (2011). Adjunct treatments for schizophrenia and bipolar disorder: what to try when you are out of ideas. *Clinical Schizophrenia & Related Psychoses*, 5: 208–16C.

Tsuda Y, Saruwatari J, and Yasui-Furukori N. (2014). Meta-analysis: the effects of smoking on the disposition of two commonly used antipsychotic agents, olanzapine and clozapine. BMJ open, 4/3: e004216.

Turner DT, Van Der Gaag M, Karyotaki E, and Cuijpers P. (2014). Psychological interventions for psychosis: a meta-analysis of comparative outcome studies. *The American Journal of Psychiatry*, 171: 523–38.

World Health Organization. (1992). *The ICD-10 classification of mental and behavioural disorders: Clinical descriptions and guidelines*. Geneva: World Health Organization.

Yung AR and McGorry PD. (2007). Prediction of psychosis: setting the stage. *The British Journal of Psychiatry*, 191: s1–s8.

Yung AR, Phillips LJ, Yuen HP, and McGorry PD. (2004). Risk factors for psychosis in an ultra high-risk group: psychopathology and clinical features. *Schizophrenia Research*, 67: 131–42.

Zhang Y, Liang W, Yang S, Dai P, Shen L, and Wang C. (2013). Repetitive transcranial magnetic stimulation for hallucination in schizophrenia spectrum disorders: A meta-analysis. *Neural Regeneration Research*, 8: 2666.

Chapter 17

Late-life depression

Fabian Fußer, Tarik Karakaya,
and Johannes Pantel

Introduction to late-life depression

Depressive disorders are a leading cause of disability worldwide leading to more years lived with disability (YLDs) than any other disease (Alexopoulos and Kelly, 2009; Global Burden of Disease Study 2013 Collaborators, 2015). Although major depressive disorder (MDD) is less prevalent among older adults when compared to middle-aged populations, a significant proportion of patients may experience their first depressive episode in old age. Prevalence rates of late life-depression (LLD) vary considerably across studies due to methodological aspects, e.g. sampling and case definition with a significant variation in the definition of 'late-life'. For patients aged 75 years or older, a meta-analysis revealed a pooled prevalence of 7.2% (range 4.6 to 9.3%) for major depression and 17.1% (4.5% to 37.4%) for other depressive disorders, such as minor depression or persistent depressive disorder (dysthymia) (Luppa et al., 2012). In addition, the incidence of clinically relevant depressive symptoms for persons aged ≥70 years is almost twice the incidence of dementia in that age (Büchtemann et al., 2012). Both subsyndromal depression and severe depressive symptoms are associated with a substantial progression of disability in activities of daily living (ADLs). LLD may contribute to an unhealthy lifestyle, and non-adherence to prescribed treatments for somatic comorbidities (including non-pharmacological interventions) can lead to an increase in morbidity and mortality. The general practitioner (GP) should consider that LLD frequently affects patients with other medical or neurological diseases, which may 'hide' a proper diagnosis of depression. For example, depression is a strong risk factor for greater morbidity and mortality in patients with coronary heart disease (CHD). Whereas about half of the patients with CHD and MDD had a previous depressive episode, almost half of the patients after acute myocardial infarction (MI) develop either major depression (20–25%) or minor depression (20–25%), leading to a greater likelihood of rehospitalization, slower recovery, and a three-fold higher risk of death among patients with post-MI MDD (Krishnan et al., 2002; Carney and Freedland, 2003, Alexoupolos, 2005). Evidence also indicates that LLD may adversely impact outcomes in patients with diabetes (Park et al., 2013) or chronic obstructive pulmonary disease (COPD) (Atlantis et al., 2013).

Depression in old age is also a risk factor for incident stroke, and it is even more pronounced in patients with pre-existing cardiac disease (Wouts et al., 2008). In addition, approximately 50% of the patients with stroke develop depressive symptoms within the first year post-stroke. Post-stroke depression is also associated with poorer recovery, greater physical and cognitive impairment, and increased mortality (Robinson and Spaletta, 2010). Another substantial comorbidity of depression is dementia, and depression is both a risk factor and a prodrome of dementia (Enache et al., 2011). During the course of the disease, up to 20% of patients diagnosed with Alzheimer's disease (AD) present a major depressive episode. In subcortical dementias, prevalence rates of depression appear to be even higher (Byers and Yaffe, 2011). Thus, depressive symptoms often accompany an insidious cognitive decline years before the clinical manifestation of dementia.

A large body of evidence indicates that the GP is indeed the primary provider of care for individuals with LLD (Unützer and Park, 2012). Accordingly, this chapter provides a clinical overview of the diagnosis, pathophysiology, and treatment of LLD, with a particular focus on the primary care setting.

Diagnosis

LLD is far from being a unique entity, and likely conveys a wide range of disorders with distinct yet overlapping pathophysiological mechanisms. The clinical manifestation frequently differs from depression appearing in younger adults. This renders a prompt diagnosis challenging not only for the specialist, but particularly for the GP. Patients with LLD less often complain about low mood and/or sadness (Gallo and Rabins, 1999), but often report on multiple and non-specific somatic problems like pain or gastrointestinal symptoms compared to younger depressive patients. Thus, LLD often goes unrecognized in part because of its different (i.e. masked) clinical presentation. Complementary to somatic complaints, LLD often presents with several additional manifestations, including, but not limited to, cognitive impairment, anxiety, sleep disturbances, fatigue, psychomotor retardation, hopelessness, suicidality, and psychotic symptoms. These manifestations seem to be pronounced in patients with LLD compared to younger depressive patients (Fiske et al., 2009).

Notwithstanding its characteristic clinical presentation, there is no specific set of criteria for LLD. Accordingly, LLD depression is diagnosed with the same criteria for MDD applied to younger adults. According to DSM-5 criteria for MDD, depressed mood, loss of interest or pleasure, change in weight or appetite, insomnia or hypersomnia, psychomotor agitation or retardation, fatigue or loss of energy, feelings of worthlessness, impaired concentration, and/or suicidal ideations have to be present most of the day and nearly every day in a two-week period. Further specifications comprise features like anxious distress, melancholic, mixed, atypical, or psychotic features. Severity (mild, moderate, or severe) is based on the number and severity of depressive symptoms and the degree of functional disability (American Psychiatric Association, 2013).

Patients with bipolar disorder typically present with more severe and disabling depressive episodes (Alexopoulos, 2005). Higher clinical depressive severity is also seen in patients with psychotic depression, who exhibit psychotic symptoms like delusions and/or hallucinations during a major depressive episode. Common themes of depressive delusions are guilt, hypochondriasis, nihilism, and persecution. Psychotic depression in old age is often associated with psychomotor disturbances, such as agitation and/or retardation, worse prognosis (e.g. more relapses and recurrences within two years), and more severe executive dysfunction (Gournellis et al., 2014).

Apart from MDD, dysthymia (which is now referred to as persistent depressive disorder in the DSM-5, together with chronic major depression) is characterized by mild to moderate depressive symptoms, lasting for at least two years without meeting criteria for MDD. However, most patients suffering from persistent depressive disorder experience additional severe depressive episodes meeting the criteria for MDD (a condition referred to as double depression). Persistent depressive disorder, as well as minor depression (with at least two but less than five depressive symptoms of MDD), and subsyndromal depression (SSD) are also associated with significant levels of functional impairment compared to non-depressed individuals, which is of clinical importance especially in primary care (Lyness et al., 2007). The DSM-5 criteria for MDD exclude depression due either to another medical condition (e.g. cardiovascular disease, endocrinopathy, diabetes or metabolic disorders) or to the effects of substance abuse. Depressive symptoms may also be induced by a variety of medications (including analgesics, antiepileptic agents, antihypertensive agents, antipsychotics, anxyolytics, anti-parkinsonian drugs, cancer chemotherapeutic agents, hormones, and steroids) (Alexopoulos, 2005).

Medical history should focus on previous psychiatric diagnoses and possible depressive episodes, past suicide attempts or current suicidality, substance abuse, memory complaints, and sleep disturbances. A possible family history of mood disorders, dementia, and/or suicide is of clinical relevance as well as known somatic diseases. Additionally, current use of pharmacological agents (especially polypharmacy) may be relevant for the a etiology and the selection of antidepressant treatment. A social history should focus on exposure to stressors or recent losses, social support, and functional disabilities (Taylor, 2014). The clinician should also seek for collateral sources of information from available family or friends.

To evaluate the presence and severity of depressive symptoms and to characterize the extent of disability, validated assessment scales are available. Self-reported screening instruments, such as the Patient Health Questionnaire 9 (PHQ-9) (Kroenke et al., 2001), the Beck Depression Inventory (Beck et al., 1961), and the Geriatric Depression Scale (GDS) in its 15-item version may aid in the identification of LLD (Sheikh and Yesavage, 1986). All these scales have been validated against the interviewer-based structured diagnostic interviews and may also be used to assess the course and outcome of LLD. Concerning cognitive deficits, a recent systematic review suggests that the Mini-Mental State Examination (MMSE) (Folstein et al., 1975), the Mini-Cog test, and the Addenbrooke's Cognitive Examination-Revised have adequate receiver operating properties for the screening of dementia (Tsoi et al., 2015). However, further neuropsychological testing to identify early dementia should be postponed until depressive symptoms have abated (Taylor, 2014). Differential diagnosis to early dementia and (e.g. apathetic) delirium might be challenging and should be made by the specialist (see Table 17.1 for guidance in the differences between LLD, dementia, and delirium).

Table 17.1 Differential diagnosis of depression, dementia, and delirium

	Depression	Dementia	Delirium
Onset	Slow, variable	Insidious	Acute
Symptoms in the course of a day	Stable, worse mood in the morning	Stable	Fluctuating, often worse at night
Duration	Weeks to months	Months to years	Hours to months
Consciousness	Normal	Normal	Altered
Orientation	Normal	Impaired, inconsistent	Impaired (mostly disorientation in time), fluctuating
Attention	May be impaired	Normal, except in late stages	Impaired
Memory	Unimpaired, subjective complaints after mood changes	Consistent memory impairment for recent events, often unaware of memory deficits, mood changes after memory impairments	Poor short-term memory
Speech	Normal or slow	Mild errors, word finding difficulties	Incoherent
Thought	Normal	Impoverished	Disorganized
Delusion	Rare	Rare	Common
Hallucination	Not usually	Rare until late stages	Common (often visual)
Mood	Depressed or no mood changes reported	Blunted, mood lability	Anxious
Psychomotor changes	Usually reduced, sometimes increased with agitation	No changes or slightly reduced	increased or reduced
Neurological defects	Absent	Often present (agnosia, apraxia, aphasia)	Absent
Disabilities	Highlighted by patient	Concealed by patient	Concealed by patient

Data from *American Family Physician*, 69, 2004, Birrer et al, 'Depression in Later Life: A Diagnostic and Therapeutic Challenge'. pp. 2375–82; data from *Nature Reviews: Neurology*, 5, 2009, Fong et al, 'Delirium in Elderly Adults: Diagnosis, Prevention and Treatment', pp. 210–20.

To rule out other medical issues, a thorough physical examination including a succinct neurological examination should be done. In addition, routine laboratory tests (including complete blood count, liver tests, blood urea, nitrogen, TSH, T3, T4, vitamin B12, folate), an electrocardiogram, and a structural neuroimaging (MRI) are recommended, especially when LLD presents with significant cognitive dysfunction (Blazer, 2003).

Aetiology of late-life depression

Several biological and psychosocial factors may contribute to the development of LLD. Although structural neuroimaging can be completely normal, frequently described structural brain changes in LLD comprise a decline of mesiotemporal volumes (hippocampus, amygdala), or reduced volumes of frontostriatal structures (Alexopoulos, 2005). LLD is also frequently associated with subcortical white matter lesions (WML), which led to the vascular hypothesis of LLD or vascular depression, a possible clinical subtype associated with more pronounced executive dysfunction and poor antidepressant treatment response (Taylor et al., 2013). Therefore, the proper controlling of cardiovascular risk factors may prevent vascular depression (Alexopoulos, 2005). Further biological factors contributing to LLD may include genetic polymorphisms, endocrine abnormalities, and serotonin transported binding changes (Blazer, 2003).

Psychosocial risk factors, especially severe life events such as death of a spouse or a loved one, bereavement, and social isolation have been identified to contribute to LLD (Bruce, 2002). Additionally, frequent and ongoing adverse stressors evolving from medical illness and injuries with consequential disability and functional decline lead to feelings of helplessness and/or hopelessness.

Treatment

Antidepressants have been shown to be more effective compared to placebo in randomized controlled trials (RCTs), although response rates are moderate and variable (Kok et al., 2012; Nelson et al., 2013). Patients with moderate to severe depression and longer illness duration seem to benefit more from a pharmacological treatment compared to patients with mild depression, where psychotherapeutic interventions might be sufficient (Nelson et al., 2013). A recent meta-analysis of 89 controlled studies demonstrated that efficacy of antidepressant treatment of patients with MDD older than 65 years is superior to placebo but less effective than in younger patients (Tedeschini et al., 2011).

Various factors have to be considered in the treatment of LLD. Treatment decisions will be guided by psychopathology, severity, and course of depressive symptoms (e.g. presence of suicidality, psychotic symptoms, insomnia, somatic symptoms, previous depressive episodes, prior antidepressant therapy and outcome, time of remission from a prior episode). Furthermore, medical comorbidities and concomitant medication potentially contributing to depressive symptoms have to be taken into consideration as well as age-related alterations in pharmacokinetics and metabolism. Consented medication lists like the Beers criteria (American Geriatrics Society 2012 Beers Criteria Update Expert Panel, 2012) or the German PRISCUS List (Holt et al.,

2010) register medications that might be inappropriate for older adults help to avoid drug-interactions, adverse drug effects and polypharmacy, and critically evaluate the specific risk-benefit ratio of a given medication.

Pharmacological treatment

The following recommendations for the pharmacological treatment of nonpsychotic major depression are presented with respect to the 2001 United States expert consensus guidelines (Alexopoulos et al., 2001), the 2006 Canadian Coalition for Seniors' Mental Health guideline, and an updated pharmacotherapy algorithm by Mulsant et al. (2014). For the choice of a specific antidepressant, several factors should be considered, including the efficacy, tolerability/safety, and withdrawal rates. A Cochrane systematic review did not reveal clinically significant differences in efficacy between SSRIs, serotonin-norepinephrine reuptake inhibitors (SNRIs), tricyclic antidepressants (TCAs), and agents of other classes (Arroll et al., 2009, Mottram et al., 2006, updated 2009). However, side effects triggered a higher withdrawal rate in TCAs compared to SSRIs. Currently, SSRIs are considered a preferred first-line treatment for older patients because of their efficacy and tolerability. Both the 2001 US expert consensus and the 2006 Canadian guidelines recommend citalopram and sertraline (or venlafaxine) as preferred first-line agents, although due to the association of citalopram with QT-interval prolongation (with a higher risk for torsades de pointes, ventricular tachycardia, or sudden death), Mulsant et al. (2014) proposed to use escitalopram instead of citalopram. Though well tolerated in general, common side effects of SSRIs (or venlafaxine) are gastrointestinal irritation, nausea, or diarrhoea usually resolving after a week. More serious side effects comprise a risk for developing hyponatremia, risk of falls, akathisia, Parkinsonism, the serotonin syndrome (agitation or lethargy, mental confusion, hyperreflexia, high blood pressure, hyperthermia, tachycardia, rhabdomyolysis, renal failure), or gastrointestinal bleeding, especially with concomitant administration of anticoagulants (Blazer, 2003). Alternatives to SSRIs and venlafaxine might include duloxetine, mirtazapine, or bupropion (for a list of common antidepressant agents, starting, target, and maximum dosages, and common and serious side effects, see Taylor, 2014). TCAs are also effective but side effects have to be considered (e.g. cardiotoxicity, anticholinergic, and sedating effects). If TCAs are used (e.g. in the case of a failure of the first line therapy) nortriptyline should be preferred to amitriptyline, doxepin, or imipramine, which are not recommended for older patients.

Treatment protocol

Treatment should be initiated as monotherapy to limit side effects and drug-drug interactions (DDIs). For the starting dose half of the dosage for younger adults is recommended. If well tolerated the dose should be increased gradually up to an average dose within one month ('start low, go slow!'). In case of little or no response after two weeks with an average dosage it should be gradually titrated to the maximum recommended dose. Typically, a clinical effect of the antidepressant medication is expected after four to six weeks, although in older patients a response might not occur until eight to 12 weeks of therapy and a sufficient duration of therapy in an adequate dose is of great importance, especially in the elderly (Espinoza and Unützer, 2015).

Treatment non-response strategies

In case of non-response, a change of the treatment, i.e. a switch of the antidepressant is recommended after at least four to six weeks (Mulsant et al., 2014). The medication might be switched to another SSRI, venlafaxine, duloxetine, or mirtazapine. However, the evidence base for treatment switches following defined multistep treatment algorithms is still limited, and even a class switch might not be beneficial with respect to the long-term outcome. Of agents with dual-mechanisms, duloxetine might be an advantageous option due to its effectiveness in pain syndromes (e.g. neuropathic pain in diabetes, chronic musculoskeletal pain), whereas the sedating effects of mirtazapine might be appropriate in patients with insomnia, agitation, and restlessness.

In case of no or partial response with SSRIs, SNRIs or mirtazapine, Mulsant et al. (2014) suggest another switch of antidepressant medication to bupropion or nortriptyline before the implementation of augmentation strategies. If switching the antidepressant agent again does not lead to clinical improvement, a combination of antidepressant drugs or an augmentation with either lithium or an atypical antipsychotic is recommended. Combination of two antidepressant agents may increase the likelihood of remission due to complementary (and synergic) mechanisms of action. However, RCTs have only been conducted in younger patients and although widely used in clinical practice, increased side effects for combination therapies, e.g. venlafaxine and mirtazapine, SSRI and mirtazapine or bupropion have to be considered.

Another option for refractory depression is an augmentation therapy with lithium or atypical antipsychotics (Cooper et al., 2011). Although the efficacy of lithium augmentation mainly to TCAs is well documented in the elderly (Dew et al., 2007), the treatment requires cautious titration, monitoring of plasma-levels, and timely recognition of potential side effects, which could be more severe in old patients because of decreased renal clearance, dehydration due to lack of thirst, or concomitant diuretics, etc. Augmentation therapy with antipsychotics such as olanzapine, risperidone, and quetiapine is shown to be efficacious for treatment-resistant depression in younger patients. However, RCTs with adjunctive antipsychotics in treatment resistant LLD (TRLLD) are yet sparse. Recently, efficacy and safety have been demonstrated for adjunctive aripiprazole in LLD with incomplete response (Lenze et al., 2015).

An alternative biological treatment strategy for severe nonpsychotic depression with no response to adequate trials (proper dosage and time) of two antidepressant agents is electro-convulsive therapy (ECT), which is also effective in patients with acute suicidality or in the treatment of unipolar psychotic MDD. In unipolar psychotic MDD a combination of antidepressant (e.g. SSRIs or venlafaxine) and atypical antipsychotics is recommended, alternatively ECT can be used (Alexopoulos et al., 2001). The treatment of severe or treatment resistant MDD as well as psychotic MDD or MDD in bipolar disorder, including treatment with ECT, should be reserved for specialized mental institutions and psychiatrists, respectively.

Maintenance treatment

Maintenance treatment is necessary because up to 90% of the patients with LLD have a recurrence within three years (Alexopoulos, 2005). Treatment with the same regimen and dosage is recommended for at least one year in a first episode of depression and full remission; after a second episode antidepressant therapy should be continued for two or even more years, and patients with more than three episodes should receive a continual therapy (Alexopoulos et al., 2001, Blazer, 2003).

Treatment of persistent depressive disorder

In persistent depressive disorders (dysthymia) and mild depression, watchful waiting in combination with psychoeducation or short-term psychotherapeutic interventions alone could be considered. With symptoms persisting longer than two to three months, pharmacotherapy in combination with psychotherapy is recommended as first-line treatment (or pharmacotherapy or psychotherapy alone) (Alexopoulos et al., 2001).

Psychotherapeutic treatment

Often underutilized, psychotherapy for LLD includes short-term treatments delivered over two to four months. RCTs demonstrated that cognitive-behavioural therapy (CBT) and interpersonal therapy (IPT) are effective treatments in older patient with comparable improvement of depressive symptoms (Wilson et al., 2008; Gould et al., 2012). However, IPT could be successfully implemented in general practice leading to significant clinical effects, and satisfactory feedback by patients and physicians (Schulberg et al., 2007; van Schaik et al., 2007). Other psychotherapeutic treatments include problem-solving or supportive therapy. Especially in the primary care sector, psychosocial interventions or community-based programs such as psychoeducation, family counselling, visiting nurses' services, bereavement groups, or senior citizen centres might contribute to the comprehensive management of depression.

Exercise

Significant beneficial effects on depression in older adults have also been found for physical exercise. In particular, cardiovascular (aerobic) (e.g. walking, swimming) and group-based training has been proved to reduce depressive symptoms in LLD (Bridle et al., 2012, Espinoza and Unützer, 2015).

Late-life depression in the primary care setting

Primary care has a special role in the management of depression in the elderly. Ten per cent of older adults in primary care have clinically significant depression (Park and Unützer, 2011), and previous data stated an even higher prevalence, with 17% to 37% of the patients revealing depressive symptoms and approximately 30% of these patients having MDD (Alexopoulos et al., 2001). However, LLD in primary care frequently goes underdetected and underdiagnosed. Patients and physicians tend to consider depressive symptoms like anhedonia, poor energy, or complaints about somatic symptoms as part of 'normal ageing' or comorbid medical issues, and grief as a 'normal' reaction to losses and disability Unützer, 2002). In particular, other medical conditions might be in the focus of the GP's attention during a time-limited office visit. Secondly, the management of LLD might be challenging in primary care, too. According to a study by Luber et al. (2000) approximately 41% of primary care patients with relevant depressive symptoms are not treated and of those who are treated only few patients with LLD receive evidence-based treatment (e.g. sufficient dosage of antidepressants or sufficient time of treatment). Apart from non-treatment, insufficient or non-guideline conform or even harmful treatment, adherence to antidepressant medication might be challenging, and the risk of discontinuation by patients is very high during the first three months (Unützer et al., 2002). Nevertheless, management of LLD is delivered by primary care settings in over 80% in the US (Kessler et al., 2010), and to be effective certain steps are required: detection with screening instruments (e.g. PHQ-9, GDS), diagnosis according to standardized criteria (e.g. DSM 5), patient education, evidence-based treatment (pharmacotherapy and psychotherapy), follow-up visits guaranteeing adherence, and checking treatment-effectiveness and side-effects, respectively (Unützer and Park, 2012) (for a stepped care model for diagnosis and treatment of patients in primary care, see Table 17.2). Although most patients with LLD are treated in primary care, it is important for the GP to identify symptoms requiring a referral to mental health professionals. In particular, MDD in bipolar disorder, double depression, depression with comorbid dementia, inadequate or incomplete response to two or more interventions, recurrent episodes within one year, and self-neglect should be treated by mental health specialists. Furthermore, urgent referral to specialized care is necessary in patients with severe agitation and self-neglect, psychotic depression, and suicidality (Mojtabai, 2014; see also Table 17.2).

Older males have the highest risk for suicide, especially with severe or psychotic depression, recent loss or bereavement, or with recent development of disability due to another medical condition (Alexopoulos et al., 2001). Thus, the detection of suicidal ideations is of special importance because two-thirds or more of older patients who commit suicide contact their GP within one month prior to their death (Luoma et al., 2002). Although there is no item specifically addressing suicidality, the GDS is an easy and effective tool to identify patients with suicidal ideations in primary care (Heisel et al., 2010).

To improve the management of LLD in primary care, collaborative care programs have proved to be effective, an approach successfully applied to the management of chronic diseases. In this collaborative model the GP is supported by a depression care manager (mostly a nurse or a social worker) and a psychiatric consultant (Unützer, Katon et al.2002, Bruce et al., 2004, Alexopoulos et al., 2009).

Having in mind the challenges of managing LLD, recent efforts address primary prevention of depressive symptoms in the elderly. Identifying risk indicators such as medical illness, disability, or spousal loss have been shown to be helpful in predicting the onset of LLD (Schoevers et al., 2006). In patients exhibiting risk factors but with only subsyndromal depressive symptoms, short-term psychotherapeutic interventions applied in a primary care setting are capable of reducing the incidence of LLD by 25–50% over one to two years (Almeida, 2012; Okereke, 2015).

Table 17.2 Stepped-care model for the diagnosis and treatment of patients with depressive symptoms in primary care

Step	Clinical presentation	Practitioner intervention
1	Suspected and known depressive symptoms	Assessment, psychoeducation, support, watchful waiting
2	Persistent subthreshold depressive symptoms, mild-to-moderate depression	Active monitoring, psychosocial interventions (individual guided self-help), medication for moderate depression may be considered in patients with a history of recurrent major depressive episodes
3	Moderate-to-severe depressive symptoms, MDD	Medication and psychotherapy (CBT, IPT), collaborative care
4	Treatment-resistant MDD, major depressive episode in bipolar disorder, recurrent episode within one year, depression with comorbid dementia	Referral to specialized care should be favoured
5	Psychotic MDD, suicidality, severe agitation or self-neglect	Urgent referral to mental health services

Data from *New England Journal of Medicine*, 370, 2014, Mojtabai, Ramin, 'Diagnosing Depression in Older Adults in Primary Care', pp. 1180–82; Kennedy, G J., 2015, *Geriatric Depression: A Clinical Guide*, Guilford Press.

Referral to specialized care for further assessment or more intensive intervention can be considered in step 1–3; CBT = cognitive behavioural therapy, IPT = interpersonal therapy.

Conclusion

In conclusion, primary care plays a key role in the detection and treatment of patients with LLD. This is certainly true, if only because many patients with LLD present with unspecific somatic complaints. Moreover, adequate consideration of mulitmorbidity and polypharmacy plays a key role in the management of LLD. Accordingly, the GP has an important gatekeeper function to initiate the proper diagnostic and therapeutic steps. In turn, overlooking or misdiagnosing symptoms and risk factors for depression in elderly patients may have deleterious consequences for the patients. Nonetheless, the management of LLD in primary care can be critically improved by evidence-based assessment and treatment strategies, including a timely referral to specialized mental care in severe depression. Additionally, increasing evidence indicates that selective prevention strategies reduce the burden of depression in older individuals, their families, and the healthcare system.

References

Alexopoulos GS. (2005). Depression in the elderly. *Lancet*, 365/9475: 1961–70.

Alexopoulos GS, Katz IR, Reynolds CF, Carpenter D, Docherty JP; and Expert Consensus Panel for Pharmacotherapy of Depressive Disorders in Older Patients. (2001). The Expert

Consensus guideline series. pharmacotherapy of depressive disorders in older patients. *Postgrad Med*, Spec No Pharmacotherapy: 1–86.

Alexopoulos GS and Kelly RE. (2009). Research advances in geriatric depression. *World Psychiatry*, 8/3: 140–49.

Alexopoulos GS, Reynolds CF, Bruce ML, Katz IR, Raue PJ, Mulsant BH, Oslin D, and Have TT. (2009). Reducing suicidal ideation and depression in older primary care patients: 24-month outcomes of the PROSPECT study. *The American Journal of Psychiatry*, 166/8: 882–90.

Almeida, OP. (2012). Approaches to decrease the prevalence of depression in later life. *Current Opinion in Psychiatry*, 25/6: 451–56.

American Geriatrics Society 2012 Beers Criteria Update Expert Panel. (2012). American Geriatrics Society updated Beers Criteria for potentially inappropriate medication use in older adults. *Journal of American Geriatric Society*, 60/4: 616–31.

American Psychiatric Association. (2013). *Diagnostic and statistical manual of mental disorders, Fifth Edition (DSM-5)*. Washington, DC: American Psychiatric Association.

Arroll BC, Elley R, Fishman T, Goodyear-Smith FA, Kenealy T, Blashki G, Kerse N, and Macgillivray S. (2009). Antidepressants versus placebo for depression in primary care. *Cochrane Database Syst Reviews*, 3: CD007954.

Atlantis E, Fahey P, Cochrane B, and Smith S. (2013). Bidirectional associations between clinically relevant depression or anxiety and copd: a systematic review and meta-analysis. *Chest*, 144/3: 766–77.

Beck AT, Ward CH, Mendelson M, Mock JE, and Erbaugh JK. (1961). An inventory for measuring depression. *Archives of General Psychiatry*, 4/6: 561–71.

Birrer RB and Vemuri SP. (2004). Depression in later life: a diagnostic and therapeutic challenge. *American Family Physician*, 69/10: 2375–82.

Blazer DG. (2003). Depression in late life: review and commentary. *The Journals of Gerontology. Series A, Biological Sciences and Medical Sciences*, 58/3: 249–65.

Bridle C, Spanjers K, Patel S, Atherton NM, and Lamb SE. (2012). Effect of exercise on depression severity in older people: systematic review and meta-analysis of randomised controlled trials. *The British Journal of Psychiatry*, 201/3: 180–85.

Bruce ML. (2002). Psychosocial risk factors for depressive disorders in late life. *Biological Psychiatry*, 52/3: 175–84.

Bruce ML, Have TRT, Reynolds CF, Katz II, Schulberg HC, Mulsant BH, Brown GK, McAvay GJ, Pearson JL, and Alexopoulos GS. (2004). Reducing suicidal ideation and depressive symptoms in depressed older primary care patients: a randomized controlled trial. *JAMA*, 291/9: 1081–91

Büchtemann D, Luppa M, Bramesfeld B, and Riedel-Heller S. (2012). Incidence of late-life depression: a systematic review. *Journal of Affective Disorders*, 142/1–3: 172–79.

Byers AL and Yaffe K. (2011). Depression and risk of developing dementia. *Nature Reviews. Neurology*, 7/6: 323–31.

Canadian Coalition for Seniors' Mental Health (CCSMH). (2006). *National guidelines for seniors' mental health: the assessment and treatment of depression*. Toronto (ON): CCSMH. Available: http://www.ccsmh.ca/en/projects/depression.cfm. Accessed 05 Aug 2015

Carney RM and Freedland KE. (2003). Depression, mortality, and medical morbidity in patients with coronary heart disease. *Biological Psychiatry*, 54/3: 241–47.

Cooper C, Katona C, Lyketsos K, Blazer D, Brodaty H, Rabins P, de Mendonça Lima CA, and Livingston G. (2011). A systematic review of treatments for refractory depression in older people. *American Journal of Psychiatry*, 168/7: 681–88.

Dew MA, Whyte EM, Lenze EJ, Houck PR, Mulsant PH, Pollock BG, Stack JA, Bensasi S, and Reynolds CF. (2007). Recovery from major depression in older adults receiving augmentation of antidepressant pharmacotherapy. *American Journal of Psychiatry*, 164/6: 892–99.

Enache D, Winblad B, and Aarsland D. (2011). Depression in dementia: epidemiology, mechanisms, and treatment. *Current Opinion in Psychiatry*, 24/6: 461–72.

Espinoza RT and Unützer J. Diagnosis and management of late-life unipolar depression. In: D Solomon, ed. *UpToDate*. Waltham, MA: Wolters Kluwer. Accessed on August 2, 2015.

Fiske A, Wetherell JL, and Gatz M. (2009). Depression in older adults. *Annual Review of Clinical Psychology*, 5: 363–89.

Folstein MF, Folstein SE, and McHugh PR. (1975). Mini-mental state. a practical method for grading the cognitive state of patients for the clinician. *Journal of Psychiatric Research*, 12/3: 189–98.

Fong TG, Tulebaev SR, and Inouye SK. (2009). Delirium in elderly adults: diagnosis, prevention and treatment. *Nature Reviews Neurology*, 5/4: 210–20.

Gallo JJ and Rabins PV. (1999). Depression without sadness: alternative presentations of depression in late life. *American Family Physician*, 60/3: 820–26.

Global Burden of Disease Study 2013 Collaborators. (2015). Global, regional, and national incidence, prevalence, and years lived with disability for 301 acute and chronic diseases and injuries in 188 countries, 1990–2013: a systematic analysis for the Global Burden of Disease Study 2013. *Lancet*, 386/9995: 743–800.

Gould RL, Coulson MC, and Howard RJ. (2012). Cognitive behavioral therapy for depression in older people: a meta-analysis and meta-regression of randomized controlled trials. *Journal of the American Geriatrics Society*, 60/10: 1817–30.

Gournellis R, Oulis P, and Howard R. (2014). Psychotic major depression in older people: a systematic review. *International Journal of Geriatric Psychiatry*, 29/8: 789–96.

Heisel MJ, Duberstein PR, Lyness JM, and Feldman MD. (2010). Screening for suicide ideation among older primary care patients. *Journal of the American Board of Family Medicine*, 23/2: 260–69.

Holt S, Schmiedl S, and Thürmann PA. (2010). Potentially inappropriate medications in the elderly: the PRISCUS list. *Deutsches Ärzteblatt International*, 107/31–32: 543–51.

Kennedy GJ. (2015). *Geriatric depression: A clinical guide*. New York: Guilford Press.

Kessler RC, Birnbaum H, Bromet E, Hwang I, Sampson N, and Shahly V. (2010). Age differences in major depression: results from the National Comorbidity Surveys Replication (NCS-R). *Psychological Medicine*, 40/2: 225.

Kok RM, Nolen WA, and Heeren TJ. (2012). Efficacy of treatment in older depressed patients: a systematic review and meta-analysis of double-blind randomized controlled trials with antidepressants. *Journal of Affective Disorders*, 141/2–3: 103–15.

Krishnan K, Ranga R, Delong M, Kraemer H, Carney R, Spiegel D, Gordon C, McDonald W, Dew M, Alexopoulos G, Buckwalter K, Cohen PD, Evans D, Kaufmann PG, Olin J, Otey E, and Wainscott C. (2002). Comorbidity of depression with other medical diseases in the elderly. *Biological Psychiatry*, 52/6: 559–88.

Kroenke K, Spitzer RL, and Williams JB. (2001). The PHQ-9: Validity of a brief depression severity measure. *Journal of General Internal Medicine*, 16/9: 606–13.

Lenze EJ, Mulsant BH, Blumberger DM, Karp JF, Newcomer JW, Anderson SJ, Dew MA, Butters MA, Stack JA, Begley AE, and Reynolds, CFIII. (2015). Efficacy, safety, and tolerability of augmentation pharmacotherapy with aripiprazole for treatment-resistant depression in late life: a randomised, double-blind, placebo-controlled trial. *Lancet*, **86**/ 10011: 2404–12.

Luber MP, Hollenberg JP, Williams-Russo P, DiDomenico TN, Meyers BS, Alexopoulos GS, and **Charlson ME.** (2000). Diagnosis, treatment, comorbidity, and resource utilization of depressed patients in a general medical practice. *International Journal of Psychiatry in Medicine*, **30**/1: 1–13.

Luoma JB, Martin CE, and **Pearson JL.** (2002a). Contact with mental health and primary care providers before suicide: a review of the evidence. *American Journal of Psychiatry*, **159**/ 6: 909–16.

Luppa M, Sikorski C, Luck T, Ehreke L, Konnopka A, Wiese B, Weyerer S, König HH, and **Riedel-Heller SG.** (2012). Age- and gender-specific prevalence of depression in latest-life- systematic review and meta-analysis. *Journal of Affective Disorders*, **136**/3: 212–21.

Lyness JM, Kim JH, Tang W, Tu X, Conwell Y, King DA, and **Caine ED.** (2007). The clinical significance of subsyndromal depression in older primary care patients. *American Journal of Geriatric Psychiatry*, **15**/3: 214–23.

Mojtabai R. (2014). Diagnosing depression in older adults in primary care. *New England Journal of Medicine*, **370**/13: 1180–82.

Mottram P, Wilson K, and **Strobl J.** (2006). Antidepressants for depressed elderly. *Cochrane Database of Syst Reviews*, **1**: CD003491.

Mulsant, BH, Blumberger DM, Ismail Z, Rabheru K, and **Rapoport MJ.** (2014). A systematic approach to pharmacotherapy for geriatric major depression. *Clinics in Geriatric Medicine*, **30**/3: 517–34.

Craig NJ, Delucchi KL, and **Schneider LS.** (2013). Moderators of outcome in late-life depression: a patient-level meta-analysis. *American Journal of Psychiatry*, **170**/6: 651–59.

Okereke OI., (ed). (2015). *Prevention of late-life depression: current clinical challenges and priorities.* New York: Springer Science + Business Media.

Park M and **Unützer J.** (2011). Geriatric depression in primary care. *Psychiatric Clinics of North America*, **34**/2: 469–510.

Park M, Katon WJ, and **Wolf FM.** (2013). Depression and risk of mortality in individuals with diabetes: a meta-analysis and systematic review. *General Hospital Psychiatry*, **35**/3: 217–25.

Robinson, RG and **Spalletta G.** (2010). Poststroke depression: a review. *Canadian Journal of Psychiatry*, **55**/6: 341–49.

van Schaik D, van Marwijk H, Beekman A, de Haan M, and **van Dyck R.** (2007). Interpersonal psychotherapy (IPT) for late-life depression in general practice: uptake and satisfaction by patients, therapists and physicians. *BMC Family Practice*, **8**: 52.

Schoevers RA, Smit F, Deeg DJH, Cuijpers P, Dekker J, van Tilburg W, and **Beekman ATF.** (2006). Prevention of late-life depression in primary care: do we know where to begin? *American Journal of Psychiatry*, **163**/9: 1611–21.

Schulberg, HC, Post EP, Raue PJ, Have TT, Miller M, and **Martha L. Bruce.** (2007). Treating late-life depression with interpersonal psychotherapy in the primary care sector. *International Journal of Geriatric Psychiatry*, **22**/2: 106–14.

Sheikh JI and **Yesavage JA.** (1986). Geriatric Depression Scale (GDS), Recent evidence and development of a shorter version. In: *Clinical Gerontology: A Guide to Assessment and Intervention*, TL Brink,ed. New York: The Haworth Press, 165–173.

Taylor WD, Aizenstein HJ, and **Alexopoulos GS.** (2013). The vascular depression hypothesis: mechanisms linking vascular disease with depression. *Molecular Psychiatry*, **18**/ 9: 963–74.

Taylor WD. (2014). Clinical practice. depression in the elderly. *New England Journal of Medicine*, 371/13: 1228–36.

Tedeschini E, Levkovitz Y, Iovieno N, Ameral VE, Nelson JC, and Papakostas GI. (2011). Efficacy of antidepressants for late-life depression: a meta-analysis and meta-regression of placebo-controlled randomized trials. *The Journal of Clinical Psychiatry*, 72/12: 1660–68.

Tsoi KKF, Chan JYC, Hirai HW, Wong SYS, and Kwok TCY. (2015). Cognitive tests to detect dementia: a systematic review and meta-analysis. *JAMA Internal Medicine*, 175/9: 1450–58.

Unützer J, Katon W, Callahan CM, Williams JW, Hunkeler E, Harpole L, Hoffing M, Della Penna RD, Noël PH, Lin EH, Areán PA, Hegel MT, Tang L, Belin TR, Oishi S, and Langston C; IMPACT Investigators: Improving Mood-Promoting Access to Collaborative Treatment. (2002). Collaborative care management of late-life depression in the primary care setting: a randomized controlled trial. *JAMA*, 288/22: 2836–45.

Unützer J. (2002). Diagnosis and treatment of older adults with depression in primary care. *Biological Psychiatry*, 52/3: 285–92.

Unützer J and Park M. (2012). Strategies to improve the management of depression in primary care. *Primary Care*, 39/2: 415–31.

Wilson K, Mottram P, and Vassilas CA. (2008). Psychotherapeutic treatments for older depressed people. *Cochrane Database of Syst Reviews*, 1: CD004853.

Wouts L, Oude Voshaar RC, Bremmer MA, Buitelaar JK, Penninx BWJH, and Beekman ATF. (2008). Cardiac disease, depressive symptoms, and incident stroke in an elderly population. *Archives of General Psychiatry*, 65/5: 596–602.

Chapter 18

Psychotherapeutic interventions

Fiammetta Cosci and Giovanni Andrea Fava

Introduction

Primary Care Physicians (PCPs) may offer comprehensive care for patients with prevalent mental disorders. A full appreciation of the patient's medical status is important to determine whether psychiatric symptoms antedate the appearance of a medical disorder (Cosci et al., 2015a), to determine the need for care, and to select psychiatric treatments that do not interact adversely with a somatic illness and/or its treatment.

Pharmacotherapy, psychotherapy, or combined approaches represent first-line therapeutic options for several common mental disorders. The field has witnessed an impressive progress in the development of short-term psychotherapeutic strategies, such as cognitive-behavioural therapy (CBT) and interpersonal therapy (IPT). Furthermore, manual-based psychotherapy may be readily incorporated in the management of mental disorder in primary care settings. These psychotherapies have been found to be effective as alternatives or adjuncts to pharmacotherapy, with enduring benefits following discontinuation of treatment (Roth & Fonagy, 2005). The proper management of patients with psychiatric disorders and the maximization of remission rates require assessment encompassing clinical judgement, repeated evaluation that may entail modification of initial treatment plans, and effective collaboration with psychiatrists or clinical psychologists, when necessary.

Psychotherapeutic intervention: clinical judgment, availability, and patient preference

Selection of treatment according to evidence-based medicine relies primarily on randomized controlled trials (RCTs) and meta-analyses. However, this evidence applies to the 'average' patient and ignores the fact that customary clinical taxonomy does not include patterns of symptoms, effects of comorbid conditions, timing of phenomena, responses to previous treatments, and other clinical distinctions that demarcate major prognostic and therapeutic differences among patients; patients can seem deceptively similar if they share the same diagnosis (Fava et al., 2015a). It is thus important not to simply compare treatment options for the average patient, but also to consider relevant, often neglected, clinical characteristics that could provide valuable insights for treatment formulation. Both pharmacotherapy and psychotherapy entail advantages and disadvantages that should be weighed by clinical judgment (Tomba & Fava, 2012).

We will not discuss the role of psychotherapy for patients with treatment-resistant mental disorders, such as depression (Carvalho et al., 2014).

Unipolar depression

Primary care physicians have emerged as the predominant mental health care providers for the diagnosis and treatment of major depressive disorder (MDD). A considerable proportion of patients go undiagnosed and are consequently not adequately managed. For example, evidence estimates that only about 50% of individuals with MDD receive a first-line treatment. Despite previous efforts toward improving primary care interventions (e.g. American Psychiatric Association, 2010; National Collaborating Centre for Mental Health, 2009) and introducing stepped (i.e. collaborative) care models, these strategies did not yield significant advantages. Therefore, the recognition and treatment of MDD remains a challenge in primary care services.

Current guidelines recommend antidepressants and psychotherapy as options for the acute phase treatment of MDD (American Psychiatric Association, 2010), which should be incorporated in a collaborative care model (National Collaborating Centre for Mental Health, 2009). The severity of depressive symptoms may influence treatment selection (Fava, 2014). Patients with mild depression could be initially managed with brief interventions (e.g. self-help groups or counselling), while patients with moderate to severe MDD should be offered antidepressants and/or evidence-based psychotherapeutic approaches (e.g. CBT or IPT). Evidence suggests that the therapeutic benefits of antidepressants compared to placebo may increase with the severity of depression, a factor that should be considered during treatment decisions.

CBT, problem-solving therapy, and IPT have been shown to be effective in the treatment of depression (Wolf & Hopko, 2008). CBT is a well-established and well-supported treatment for clinical depression in primary care (Wolf & Hopko, 2008), and its effectiveness may not significantly change according to the format of delivery (i.e. guided self-help CBT, telephone-based CBT, computerized CBT and standard one-to-one CBT). Problem-Solving Therapy for Primary Care is a promising intervention (Wolf & Hopko, 2008) designed to attenuate depressive symptoms by assisting patients in generating and developing skills that alleviate the emotional impact of life events or problems which interfere with psychosocial functioning. In primary care, there is little support for IPT (Wolf & Hopko, 2008). Pharmacotherapy remains the most commonly used intervention for the acute treatment of major depressive episodes in primary care, although it is not less expensive than psychological interventions, and not the first choice of treatment for a significant group of patients with MDD. The relative unavailability of psychotherapy resources (e.g. trained therapists) as well as the pressure of pharmaceutical industry marketing (Fava, 2014) may contribute to this scenario.

The acute treatment of MDD is secondary to the main clinical challenges of the prevention of recurrences and the long-term recovery of psychosocial function. Only 51% of the patients treated with an antidepressant experience at least a 50% improvement in depressive symptoms, compared with 32% of the patients in the placebo groups (Sherbourne et al., 2004), and about two-thirds of those treated remain symptomatic

Table 18.1 Steps for implementing a sequential approach in MDD

Step	Action
1.	Identify the major depressive disorder (diagnosis, subtype, stage)
2.	**If the major depressive episode is severe**, administer an antidepressant treatment
3.	Assess carefully the patient three months after starting antidepressant drug treatment, with special reference to residual symptoms
4.	**If remission occurs**, suggest life style, nutrition, and physical activity modifications. **If residual symptoms persist**, refer to a psychotherapist trained in cognitive behavioural therapy to reach full remission
5.	Collaborating with a psychologist in potential tapering of antidepressant drug treatment at the slowest possible pace monitoring for discontinuation syndromes
6.	Suggest life style modifications, if this is the case
7.	Discontinue antidepressants monitoring for withdrawal syndromes
8.	Assess carefully the patient one month after discontinuation

at long-term follow-up (Mulrow et al., 1998). Despite successful response to therapy, residual symptoms are the rule after completion of drug or psychotherapeutic treatment, and their presence correlate with poor outcomes (Fava, 1999) and higher risk of relapse (Cosci & Fava, 2013). Therefore, residual symptoms should be monitored throughout the treatment of MDD. Furthermore, treatment targeting residual depressive symptoms may yield long-term benefits (Fava & Tomba, 2010). At present, the most widely used approach for preventing recurrences is maintenance pharmacotherapy. An operative assumption behind the use of maintenance pharmacotherapy is that patients will continue to take their medication for extended periods or throughout their lives. However, the rate of noncompliance is as high as 40% and the duration of drug treatment does not seem to affect long-term prognosis once the drug is discontinued (Fava, 2014). The alternative is a sequential strategy of integrating pharmacotherapy and psychotherapy for the management of MDD. This strategy relies on the use of pharmacotherapy in the acute phase of depression treatment, and psychotherapy in its residual phase (Guidi et al., 2016). Therefore, monotherapy is unlikely to solve complex (i.e. 'real world') cases of MDD, also because some forms of comorbidity may be masked by the acute manifestations of the disorder, only becoming evident when the most severe symptoms have abated (Fava, 1999). The practical steps for implementing a sequential therapeutic approach for MDD are described in Table 18.1 (for more details please see Fava & Tomba, 2010).

Anxiety disorders

Patients with anxiety disorders often seek treatment in primary care settings, but effective management for each of the anxiety disorders, although available, is currently underused. The primary care setting often lacks adequate provision of psychotherapy or pharmacotherapy as well as structural monitoring and relapse prevention. To improve primary care treatment for these patients, collaborative care models have been implemented to support PCPs in providing evidence-based, continuous care. A few studies found that collaborative care is more effective than usual primary care (Roy-Byrne et al., 2001; Roy-Byrne et al., 2010), although beyond 25 months there were no significant differences in outcomes reported for collaborative care versus usual care. The interventions included in collaborative care studies vary in complexity, from psycho-education with medication provided by a consultant psychiatrist (Roy-Byrne et al., 2001), to computer-supported CBT provided by a care manager and/or antidepressants prescribed by the PCP with supervision from a psychiatrist (Roy-Byrne et al., 2010). Collaborative care has been proposed to follow a stepped care approach, starting with the least intrusive, most effective intervention to enhance self-management and make efficient use of resources. Although still understudied, collaborative stepped care, with guided self-help as a first step, resulted as more effective than care as usual for primary care patients with panic disorder (PD) or generalized anxiety disorder (GAD) (Muntingh et al., 2014).

Current guidelines recommend antidepressants (i.e. selective serotonin reuptake inhibitor—SSRIs—and serotonin noradrenergic reuptake inhibitor—SNRIs), anxiolytics, and psychotherapy as treatment options for anxiety disorders. Among psychological interventions, CBT is efficacious for PD, GAD, and social anxiety disorder (Combs & Markman, 2014). CBT was designed to identify the maladaptive automatic thoughts and behaviours, and then restructure them through therapeutic exercises. It has been shown sufficiently effective for several anxiety disorders, with very limited side effects, so it is often considered the first-line treatment. Disorder-specific and general protocols have been developed. Major drawbacks to therapy include difficulty in engaging the patient and limited or variable availability of well-trained therapists. Although the advent of manualized therapy and computer-based therapy allowed the treatment to be delivered without therapists, this possible resource is still underused.

The literature on long-term follow-up treatment for anxiety disorders suggests differences in terms of duration of effects between psychotherapy and drug treatment (i.e. psychotherapy entails more enduring effects than pharmacotherapy) (Roth & Fonagy, 2005). Evidence indicates that psychotherapy may be associated with a greater likelihood to remain in remission (Roth & Fonagy, 2005). The literature does not substantiate long-term benefits from the sequential use of pharmacotherapy and psychotherapy and the combination of psychotherapy and pharmacotherapy is not superior to pharmacotherapy only or to psychotherapy alone (Roth & Fonagy, 2005). Thus, psychotherapy should be the first choice and pharmacotherapy the second choice to treat anxiety disorders in primary care settings. In this framework, SSRIs and SNRIs should be used with caution since they can induce withdrawal and post-withdrawal disorders, which might persist months after their discontinuation (Chouinard & Chouinard, 2015). Benzodiazepines (BZD), when compared to antidepressants, were found to be more effective and to have fewer treatment withdrawals and adverse events (Offidani et al., 2013), although they need to be specifically selected. Alprazolam and triazolam have been related to continuous and high-dose use, whereas clonazepam

Table 18.2 Steps to treat anxiety disorders in primary care settings

Step	Action
1.	Refer to CBT
2.	If drug treatment appears to be necessary to control anxiety symptoms, use benzodiazepines (i.e. clonazepam and clobazam). Avoid alprazolam and triazolam
3.	If the patient is not responding to benzodiazepines or depression coexists, use antidepressants drugs

and clobazam were not (Cloos et al., 2015). Thus, alprazolam and triazolam should be carefully used or simply avoided (Cosci et al., 2015b). Table 18.2 summarizes the steps to treat anxiety disorders in primary care settings.

Somatic symptom disorders

Primary care providers have a crucial role in the recognition and adequate treatment of patients with multiple somatic symptoms. These patients commonly receive unnecessary and invasive somatic investigations while their psychological aspects are insufficiently explored. Psychosocial factors affecting the individual's vulnerability should be explored (Fava & Sonino, 2005), including 1) early and recent life events; 2) chronic, daily life stress (i.e. allostatic load, conceived as the cost of chronic exposure to fluctuating or heightened neural or neuroendocrine response resulting from repeated or chronic environmental challenges that an individual reacts to as particularly stressful) (Fava et al., 2010); 3) social support; and 4) psychological well-being, which plays a buffering role in coping with stress and has a favourable impact on disease course (Fava & Sonino, 2005). Once the symptoms of a medical disease are experienced by a person, or he/she has been told by a doctor that he/she is ill, even if symptoms are absent, this disease-related information gives rise to psychological responses which are likely to influence the course, therapeutic response, and outcome of a given illness episode. Illness behaviour is one of the factors that demarcate major prognostic and therapeutic differences among patients (Cosci & Fava, 2015). Abnormal illness behaviour may also be associated with psychiatric disorders, for this reason somatic symptom disorders and any other comorbid psychiatric disorders should be thoroughly assessed and diagnosed. The Diagnostic Criteria for Psychosomatic Research (DCPR) Interview is a semi-structured clinical interview widely used to diagnose somatic symptom disorders in medical settings, and has adequate psychometric properties (Porcelli & Sonino, 2007; Porcelli & Guidi, 2015).

Most non-pharmacological interventions focus on addressing cognitions, behaviour, coping styles, and functional consequences of symptoms. These interventions include physical and psychological therapies. Physical therapies usually concern physical activity treatments, which aim to improve physical function by expanding physical activity and thereby reducing symptoms. Psychological therapies are mostly used to target underlying psychological disorders and problems, and aim to change the way patients perceive their symptoms in order to manage them (Kroenke, 2007).

Table 18.3 Steps to treat somatic symptom disorders in primary care settings

Step	Action
1.	Complete a detailed history (including early and recent life events, chronic, daily life, social support, psychological well-being) and physical examination.
2.	Explore illness behaviour.
3.	Educate on how psychosocial stressors and symptoms interact.
4.	Prescribe physical activity treatments, if appropriate.
5.	Treat psychiatric disorders.
6.	In case of non-response OR severe somatic symptom disorder, refer to a psychosomatic specialist trained in CBT and/or explanatory therapy.

In primary care settings, individual treatments such as reattribution techniques (Aiarzaguena et al., 2007) and single-session CBT (Martin et al., 2007) demonstrated some effects on clinical outcomes and showed to reduce doctor visits and somatization severity. Group treatment has promising and beneficial outcomes (Martin et al., 2007), although a specific PCP training based on the reattribution model is needed to improve PCPs' attitudes toward widespread bodily symptoms. New collaborative group interventions have also been proposed. In this model, the PCP and a psychosomatic specialist treat the patient in PCP's office. When compared to pure PCP training, patients in the intervention arm reported significantly greater improvements in mental quality of life than the controls after 12 months (Schaefert et al., 2013). When the PCP needs to refer a patient with somatic symptom disorder to a psychiatrist or a clinical psychologist, a therapist skilled in CBT and/or explanatory therapy may be preferred. CBT has the largest evidence base for the treatment of somatic symptom disorders (Kroenke, 2007). Explanatory therapy promotes significant improvements in illness behaviour, and affective disturbances, while also decreasing health care utilization in patients with hypochondriasis. Such improvement appears to persist at six-month follow-up (Fava et al., 2000). CBT uses a complex mixture of cognitive and behavioural techniques to modify dysfunctional assumptions about health. Explanatory therapy consists in providing accurate information, teaching the principles of selected perception (i.e. attention to one part of the body makes the patient more aware of sensations in that part of the body than in other parts), reassurance, clarification, and repetition.

Table 18.3 shows the steps to treat somatic symptom disorders in primary care settings.

Substance use disorders

Substance use disorders (SUDs) are commonly found in primary care settings and associated with a wide range of medical problems. PCPs may play a role in preventing SUDs through having the opportunity to promote healthy habits, encourage lifestyle modifications, and inform on the effects of health-damaging behaviours. Universal screening, brief intervention, and referral to treatment for substance use are indeed recommended, although there is no evidence addressing the effects on health outcomes of screening and treating opioid, cocaine, or marijuana misuse among asymptomatic individuals in primary care settings (Polen et al., 2008). More promising results have been reported for alcohol use disorders. There is a moderate net benefit to screening for alcohol misuse in the primary care setting for adults 18 years or older (US Preventive Services Task Force, 2014), and brief behavioural counselling interventions are effective in reducing heavy drinking episodes in adults engaging in risky or hazardous drinking. These interventions also reduce weekly alcohol consumption rates and increase adherence to recommended drinking limits (US Preventive Services Task Force, 2014). Behavioural counselling interventions may vary in their specific components, administration, length, and number of interactions. They may include cognitive behavioural strategies, such as action plans, drinking diaries, stress management, or problem solving; they may be delivered in several manners, including face-to-face sessions, written self-help materials, computer- or web-based programmes, or telephone counselling.

Primary care physicians are also ideally placed to treat tobacco use disorders and their clinical practice guidelines support the '5 As' approach of ask, advise, assess, assist, and arrange for tobacco treatment (Fiore et al., 2008). However, only 1–3% of smokers quit smoking in six months after brief counselling by a health professional, while another 2–3% quit smoking with no help at all. Pharmacological treatment with varenicline, nicotine derivatives or certain antidepressants (i.e. bupropion or nortriptyline) is effective and doubles the chances of quitting smoking when used in conjunction with non-pharmacologic methods, which include cognitive-behaviour therapies (Stead et al., 2008) and motivational interview techniques (Soria et al., 2006). The combined use of all these smoking cessation methods, known as multicomponent or intensive intervention, can lead to abstinence rates as high as 30% a year (García -Vera, 2004).

Table 18.4 shows the steps to treat SUD in primary care settings.

Table 18.4 Steps to treat addiction in primary care settings

Substance use disorder SUBTYPE	Action
Substances different from alcohol or tobacco	Refer to secondary and tertiary level integrated treatment.
Alcohol use disorders	Screen for alcohol misuse adults of 18 years of age or older and offer a brief behavioural counselling.
Tobacco use disorders	1. Use the '5 As' approach (i.e. ask, advise, assess, assist, and arrange for tobacco treatment). 2. Consider pharmacological treatment. 3. Refer to a psychotherapist trained in cognitive behaviour therapy AND/OR in motivational interview techniques.

Difficulties in getting off psychotropic medications

Any type of psychotropic drug treatment, particularly after long-term use, may increase the risk of experiencing additional psychopathologic problems or of modifying responsiveness to subsequent treatments (Fava et al., 2013). Negative effects may occur as a result of psychotherapeutic treatment, whether because of techniques, patient or therapist variables, or inappropriate use. These events that affect both pharmacotherapy and psychotherapy constitute iatrogenic comorbidity, which refers to unfavourable modifications in the course, characteristics, and responsiveness of an illness that may be related to treatments administered previously (Fava et al., 2013). Such potential connection should encourage a rational use (and selection) of therapies, i.e. a use which depends on the balance of potential benefits and adverse effects applied to the individual patient, on baseline risk of poor outcomes from an index disorder without treatment, and on expected vulnerability to the adverse effects of treatment (Richardson & Doster, 2014). Unfortunately, the prescribing clinician is often driven by an overestimated consideration of brief-term potential benefits, paying little attention to the likelihood of responsiveness, or to potential vulnerabilities in relation to the adverse effects of treatment (Fava, 2014).

An issue that is frequently overlooked concerns burdensome symptoms that may emerge when the physician attempts to taper and discontinue psychotropic medications. Withdrawal symptoms may occur with all SSRIs and SNRIs (Fava et al., 2015b), similarly to other Central Nervous System (CNS) drugs, including benzodiazepines and antipsychotics (Chouinard & Chouinard, 2008). Withdrawal from CNS drugs produces psychiatric symptoms that can be confounded with true relapse or recurrence of the original illness (Fava et al., 2015b). Different types of syndromes have been described, including: (1) new and rebound symptoms that occur for up to six weeks after drug withdrawal, depending on the drug elimination half-life, and (2) persistent post-withdrawal or tardive disorders associated with long-lasting receptor changes, which may last for more than six weeks after drug discontinuation.

New withdrawal symptoms for CNS drugs are classic withdrawal symptoms that are new (i.e. not part of the patient's original illness presentation), and occur with a decrease in dose or discontinuation of the drug. Rebound symptoms are a rapid return of the patient's original symptoms at a greater intensity than before treatment (Chouinard & Chouinard, 2008). The prevalence of rebound is greater among patients taking benzodiazepines with short to intermediate half-lives (e.g. triazolam, lorazepam, alprazolam) (Cloos et al., 2015) than among those taking agents with long half-lives (e.g. clonazepam) (Cloos et al., 2015). This is also true for short-acting antipsychotics, such as clozapine and quetiapine (Chouinard & Chouinard, 2008), as well as for SSRIs (Chouinard & Chouinard, 2015). Persistent post-withdrawal disorders have been described with different classes of CNS drugs, and even more with specific drugs (e.g. quetiapine and paroxetine) within a drug class. This type of withdrawal consists of the return of the original illness at a greater intensity and/or with additional features of the illness, and/or symptoms related to emerging new disorders. When the previous drug treatment is not restarted after initial withdrawal, these disorders may last for several months to years. Specific diagnostic criteria for SSRIs new withdrawal

Table 18.5 Components of cognitive behavioural therapy for persistent withdrawal disorders induced by antidepressant drugs

Step	Action
1.	Explanatory therapy providing accurate information on withdrawal, giving repeated reassurance and teaching the physiological principles underlying withdrawal phenomena.
2.	Monitoring of emergent symptoms in a diary according to the cognitive behavioural model, followed by cognitive restructuring.
3.	Homework exposure for avoidance patterns.
4.	Lifestyle modifications: avoid alcohol, increase physical exercise, limit caffeine consumption. Do not change smoking habits.
5.	Techniques of decreasing abnormal reactivity to the social environment (i.e. learning ways to cope with stressful situations related to the level of arousal increased by drug withdrawal).
6.	Well-being therapy.

Adapted from *Psychotherapy and Psychosomatics*, 83, Belaise C, et al., 'Persistent postwithdrawal disorders induced by paroxetine, a selective serotonin reuptake inhibitor, and treated with specific cognitive behavioural therapy', pp. 247–8. Copyright (2014) with permission from S. Karger AG

symptoms, for SSRIs rebound symptoms, and for SSRIs post-withdrawal disorders have been proposed (Chouinard & Chouinard 2015). Belaise et al. (2014) illustrated a specific combination of CBT and Well-Being Therapy (Fava, 2016), with protocol of six to 16 weekly one-hour sessions to treat persistent paroxetine post-withdrawal disorders by specifically trained psychotherapists (Table 18.5).

Conclusion

Psychological interventions represent important therapeutic approaches for the management of MDD, anxiety disorder, somatic symptom disorders, and SUD in primary care settings. Psychotherapy also represents a pilot area of intervention to treat withdrawal symptoms and disorders due to dose decreases or discontinuation of psychotropic medications, in particular SSRIs. With the only exception of severe MDD, primary care physicians are thus encouraged to change their prescribing habits with the incorporation of specific psychological interventions as a reflection of their clinical judgement, the availability of the treatment, and patient's preference.

References

Aiarzaguena JM, Grandes G, Gaminde I, Salazar A, Sánchez A, and Ariño J. (2007). A randomized, controlled clinical trial of a psychosocial and communication intervention carried out by GPs for patients with medically unexplained symptoms. *Psychological Medicine* 37: 283–94: doi: 10.1159/000313691.

American Psychiatric Association. (2010). *Practice guideline for the treatment of patients with major depressive disorder*, 3rd ed. Arlington: American Psychiatric Association (APA).

Belaise C, Gatti A, Chouinard VA, and Chouinard G. (2014). Persistent postwithdrawal disorders induced by paroxetine, a selective serotonin reuptake inhibitor, and treated with specific cognitive behavioral therapy. *Psychotherapy and Psychosomatics*, 83/4: 247–8. doi: 10.1159/000362317.

Carvalho AF, Berks M, Hyphantis TN, and McIntyre R. (2014). The integrative management of treatment-resistant depression: a comprehensive review and perspectives. *Psychotherapy and Psychosomatics*, 83: 70–88: doi: 10.1159/000357500.

Chouinard G and Chouinard VA. (2008). Atypical antipsychotics: CATIE study, drug-induced movement disorder and resulting iatrogenic psychiatric-like symptoms, supersensitivity rebound psychosis and withdrawal discontinuation syndromes. *Psychotherapy and Psychosomatics*, 77: 69–77: doi: 10.1159/000112883.

Chouinard G and Chouinard VA. (2015). New classification of selective serotonin reuptake inhibitor withdrawal. *Psychotherapy and Psychosomatics*, 84/2: 63–71. doi:10.1159/000371865.

Cloos JM, Bocquet V, Rolland-Portal I, Koch P, and Chouinard G. (2015). Hypnotics and triazolo benzodiazepines—best predictors of benzodiazepine high-dose use: results from the Luxembourg National Health Insurance Registry. *Psychotherapy and Psychosomatics*, 84/5: 273–83: doi: 10.1159/000434755.

Combs H and Markman J. (2014). Anxiety disorders in primary care. *Medical Clinics of North America*, 98/5: 1007–23: doi: 10.1016/j.mcna.2014.06.003.

Cosci F and Fava GA. (2013). Staging of mental disorders: systematic review. *Psychotherapy and Psychosomatics*, 82/1: 20–34: doi: 10.1159/000342243.

Cosci F, Fava GA, and Sonino N. (2015a). Mood and anxiety disorders as early manifestations of medical illness: a systematic review. *Psychotherapy and Psychosomatics*, 84/1: 22–9: doi: 10.1159/000367913.

Cosci F, Guidi J, and Fava GA. (2015b). Clinical methodology matters in epidemiology: not all benzodiazepines are the same. *Psychotherapy and Psychosomatics*, 84/5: 262–4: doi: 10.1159/000437201.

Cosci F and Fava GA. (2016). The clinical inadequacy of the DSM-5 classification of somatic symptom and related disorders: an alternative trans-diagnostic model. *CNS Spectrums*, 21: 310–7: doi: 10.1017/S1092852915000760.

Fava GA. (1999). Subclinical symptoms in mood disorders: pathophysiological and therapeutic implications. *Psychological Medicine*, 29/1: 47–61: doi: 10.1017/S0033291798007429.

Fava GA. (2014). Rational use of antidepressant drugs. *Psychotherapy and Psychosomatics*, 83: 197–204: doi: 10.1159/000362803.

Fava GA. (2016). *Well-Being Therapy. Treatment manual and clinical applications*. Basel, Karger.

Fava GA and Sonino N. (2005). The clinical domains of psychosomatic medicine. *Journal of Clinical Psychiatry*, 66/7: 849–58: doi: 10.1111/j.1742-1241.2009.02266.x.

Fava GA and Tomba E. (2010). New modalities and treatment planning in depression: the sequential approach. *CNS Drugs*, 24: 453–65: doi: 10.2165/11531580-000000000-00000.

Fava GA, Gatti A, Belaise C, Guidi J, and Offidani E. (2015b). Withdrawal symptoms after selective serotonin reuptake inhibitor discontinuation: a systematic review. *Psychotherapy and Psychosomatics*, 84/2: 72–81: doi: 10.1159/000370338.

Fava GA, Grandi S, Rafanelli C, Fabbri S, and Cazzaro M. (2000). Explanatory therapy in hypochondriasis. *Journal of Clinical Psychiatry*, 61/4: 317–22: doi: 10.4088/JCP.v61n0414.

Fava GA, Guidi J, Rafanelli C, and Sonino N. (2015a). The clinical inadequacy of evidence-based medicine and the need for a conceptual framework based on clinical judgment. *Psychotherapy and Psychosomatics*, **84**/1: 1–3: doi: 10.1159/000366041.

Fava GA, Guidi J, Semprini F, Tomba E, and Sonino N. (2010). Clinical assessment of allostatic load and clinimetric criteria. *Psychotherapy and Psychosomatics*, **79**/5: 280–4: doi: 10.1159/000318294.

Fava GA, Tomba E, and Tossani E. (2013). Innovative trends in the design of therapeutic trials in psychopharmacology and psychotherapy. *Progress in Neuropsychopharmacology and Biological Psychiatry*, **40**: 306–11: doi: 10.1016/j.pnpbp.2012.10.014.

Fiore M, Jaén CR, Baker TB, Bailey WC, Bennett G, Benowitz NL, Christiansen BA, Connell M, Curry SJ, Dorfman SF, Fraser D, Froelicher ES, Goldstein MG, Hasselblad V, Healton CG, Heishman S, Henderson PN, Heyman RB, Husten C, Koh HK, Kottke TE, Lando HA, Leitzke C, Mecklenburg RE, Mermelstein RJ, Morgan G, Mullen PD, Murray EW, Orleans CT, Piper ME, Robinson L, Stitzer ML, Theobald W, Tommasello AC, Villejo L, Wewers ME, and Williams C. (2008). *Clinical practice guideline: treating tobacco use and dependence, 2008 update. A US Public Health Service report. Am J Prev Med*, **35**/2: 158–76: doi: 10.1016/j.amepre.2008.04.009.

García-Vera MP. (2004). Clinical utility of the combination of cognitive-behavioral techniques with nicotina patches as a smoking-cessation treatment: Five-year results of the 'Ex-Moker' program. *Journal of Substance Abuse Treatment*, **27**: 325–33: doi: 10.1016/j.jsat.2004.09.001.

Guidi J, Tomba E, and Fava GA. (2016). The sequential integration of pharmacotherapy and psychotherapy in the treatment of major depressive disorder: A meta-analysis of the sequential model and a critical review of the literature. *American Journal of Psychiatry*, **173**/2: 128–37: doi: 10.1176/appi.ajp.2015.15040476.

Kroenke K. (2007). Efficacy of treatment for somatoform disorders: a review of randomized controlled trials. *Psychosomatic Medicine*, **69**: 881–8: doi: 10.1097/PSY.0b013e31815b00c4.

Martin A, Rauh E, Fichter M, and Rief W. (2007). A one-session treatment for patients suffering from medically unexplained symptoms in primary care: a randomized clinical trial. *Psychosomatics*, **48**/4: 294–303. doi: 10.1017/S003329171400035X.

Mulrow CD, Williams JW Jr, Trivedi M, Chiquette E, Aguilar C, Cornell JE, Badgett R, Noel PH, Lawrence V, Lee S, Luther M, Ramirez G, Richardson WS, and Stamm K. (1998). Treatment of depression—newer pharamacotherapies. *Psychopharamacology Bulletin*, **34**: 409–795.

Muntingh A, van der Feltz-Cornelis C, van Marwijk H, Spinhoven P, Assendelft W, de Waal M, Adèr H, and van Balkom A. (2014). Effectiveness of collaborative stepped care for anxiety disorders in primary care: a pragmatic cluster randomised controlled trial. *Psychotherapy and Psychosomatics*, **83**/1: 37–44: doi: 10.1159/000353682.

National Collaborating Centre for Mental Health. (2009). *Depression: the treatment and management of depression in adults. NICE clinical guideline 90*. London: National Institute for Health and Clinical Excellence.

Offidani E, Guidi J, Tomba E, and Fava GA. (2013). Efficacy and tolerability of benzodiazepines versus antidepressants in anxiety disorders: a systematic review and meta-analysis. *Psychotherapy and Psychosomatics*, **82**/6: 355–62: doi: 10.1159/000353198.

Polen MR, Whitlock EP, Wisdom JP, Nygren P, and Bougatsos C. (2008). *Screening in primary care settings for illicit drug use: staged systematic review for the US Preventive Services Task Force*. Rockville (MD): Agency for Healthcare Research and Quality (US).

Report No.: 08-05108-EF-1. US Preventive Services Task Force Evidence Syntheses, formerly Systematic Evidence Reviews.

Porcelli P and Sonino N. (2007). *Psychological factors affecting medical conditions. a new classification for DSM-V*. Advances in Psychosomatic Medicine. Basel: Karger. doi: 10.1159/000106794.

Porcelli P and Guidi J. (2015). The clinical utility of the Diagnostic Criteria for Psychosomatic Research (DCPR): A review of studies. *Psychotherapy and Psychosomatics*, 84/5: 265–72: doi: 10.1159/000430788.

Richardson WS and Doster LM. (2014). Comorbidity and multimorbidity need to be placed in the context of a framework of risk, responsiveness, and vulnerability. *Journal of Clinical Epidemiology*, 67: 244–6: doi: 10.1016/j.jclinepi.2013.10.020.

Roth A and Fonagy P. (2005). *What works for whom? A critical review of psychotherapy research, 2nd ed*. New York: Guilford.

Roy-Byrne P, Craske MG, Sullivan G, Rose RD, Edlund MJ, Lang AJ, Bystritsky A, Welch SS, Chavira DA, Golinelli D, Campbell-Sills L, Sherbourne CD, and Stein MB. (2010). Delivery of evidence-based treatment for multiple anxiety disorders in primary care: a randomized controlled trial. *JAMA*, 303: 1921–8: doi: 10.1001/jama.2010.608.

Roy-Byrne PP, Katon W, Cowley DS, and Russo J. (2001). A randomized effectiveness trial of collaborative care for patients with panic disorder in primary care. *Archives of General Psychiatry*, 58: 869–76: doi: 10.1001/archpsyc.58.9.869.

Schaefert R, Kaufmann C, Wild B, Schellberg D, Boelter R, Faber R, Szecsenyi J, Sauer N, Guthrie E, and Herzog W. (2013). Specific collaborative group intervention for patients with medically unexplained symptoms in general practice: a cluster randomized controlled trial. *Psychotherapy and Psychosomatics*, 82/2: 106–19: doi: 10.1159/000343652.

Sherbourne C, Schoenbaum M, Wells K, and Croghan T. (2004). Characteristics, treatment patterns, and outcomes of persistent depression despite treatment in primary care. *General Hospital Psychiatry*, 26: 106–114: doi: 10.1016/j.genhosppsych.2003.08.009.

Soria R, Legido A, Escolano C, López-Yeste A, and Montoya J. (2006). A randomized controlled trial of motivational interviewing for smoking cessation. *British Journal of General Practice*, 56/531: 768–74.

Stead F, Bergson G, and Lancaster T. (2008). Physician advice for smoking cessation. *Cochrane Database of Syst Reviews*, 2: CD000165: doi: 10.1002/14651858.CD000165.pub3.

Tomba E and Fava GA. (2012). Treatment selection in depression: the role of clinical judgment. *Psychiatric Clinics of North America*, 35/1: 87–98: doi: 10.1016/j.psc.2011.11.003.

US Preventive Services Task Force. (2014). Screening and behavioral counseling interventions in primary care to reduce alcohol misuse: recommendation statement. *American Family Physician*, 89/12: online.

Wolf NJ and Hopko DR. (2008). Psychosocial and pharmacological interventions for depressed adults in primary care: a critical review. *Clinical Psychology Review*, 28/1: 131–61: doi: 10.1016/j.cpr.2007.04.004.

Chapter 19

Major depressive disorder: how to evaluate and manage patients with psychiatric and medical comorbidities

Sheng-Min Wang and Chi-Un Pae

Introduction

Psychiatric and medical comorbidities occur at a high rate among patients with major depressive disorder (MDD). Both psychiatric and medical comorbidities cause worse outcomes in the treatment of MDD, and they can also lead to more complex disease presentations. Significant symptomatic overlap between MDD with psychiatric and medical conditions generates challenges to correct recognition and treatment of these so-called 'complex' patients in primary care (Smith et al., 2014).

Depression affects approximately 10% of primary care patients. However, MDD frequently goes under-recognized, and evidences suggest that it is recognized in only half of these patients in primary care settings (Cepoiu et al., 2008). Chronic medical conditions are observed in over 50% of depressed patients, and their presence can impede the recognition of depression by primary care providers. Thus, a collaborative care plan can significantly reduce MDD and MDD-related comorbid conditions. The influence of psychiatric and medical comorbidities in evaluation and management of MDD in primary care has increasingly become a topic of main research and clinical interest. In this chapter, we summarize existing evidence on diagnosis and treatment of MDD and co-occurring somatic and mental health conditions in primary care settings (Katon et al., 2010).

Psychiatric comorbidity

A study conducted in a tertiary care showed that more than 64% of MDD patients had at least one comorbid mental disorder, while more than one-third (36.7%, N = 176) had two or more (Zimmerman et al., 2002). Most frequent concurrent comorbid disorders were anxiety disorders (56.8%), and social phobia was the most frequent individual disorder among them. Another study had similar findings, which showed that around 79% of patients having MDD suffered from at least one current comorbid psychiatric disorder, and more than half suffered from two or more. The most common comorbid psychiatric conditions were anxiety disorders (57%), personality disorders (44%), and alcohol use disorders (25%) (Melartin et al., 2002). Such comorbidity was also prevalent in primary care, and 62% of all depressive cases suffered from more than one other current mental disorder (Wittchen et al., 1999). MDD patients having concurrent mental disorders were younger, had earlier onset of MDD, and had a higher suicide risk compared to patients with no comorbidity. Thus, general practitioners (GPs) should diligently investigate and identify psychiatric comorbidities when assessing patients with MDD.

Anxiety Disorders

Overall, more than 62% of patients diagnosed with depression in a primary care setting suffer from a current anxiety disorder (AD). Comorbid MDD and AD is very common, so some even consider that the two are opposite sides of a same coin (Boyer, 2000). Identifying comorbid ADs is critical to the provision of proper care to those patients having the two disorders. Patients with both AD and MDD can require higher antidepressant doses for a longer time with significant higher rates of adverse effects than patients with either disorder alone. Moreover, comorbid AD in patients having MDD increases the severity and chronicity of both illnesses. Patients with comorbid MDD and AD may have higher social and vocational impairment, increased risk of substance use disorders, and a heightened risk of suicide compared to patients with a single diagnosis of MDD (Schaffer et al., 2012).

Many patients not meeting the DSM-5 diagnostic criteria for AD may have subsyndromal but clinically relevant co-occurring anxiety symptoms on top of a diagnosis of MDD. In line with this view, shared neurofunctional and neurochemical alterations are known to play a role in neurobiology of both AD and MDD (Pollack, 2005). Physicians often attempt to demarcate MDD from anxiety and to determine which disorder is the core (i.e. primary) one. This distinction is challenging and of questionable clinical wisdom. Instead, clinicians should focus on investigating whether a patient has any other psychiatric or medical comorbidities in addition to MDD and AD (Schoevers et al., 2008). Since patients having both MDD and AD can have a more pernicious course of illness, a closer assessment of symptom severity, including suicidality, psychotic symptoms, and level of functional impairment, is critical. Severity could be carefully assessed by using diverse validated assessment tools (e.g. Hamilton Depression Rating Scale (HDRS), Hamilton Anxiety Rating Scale (HARS), Beck Depression Inventory (BDI), and the Beck Anxiety Inventory (BAI)) (Aina and Susman, 2006).

Prior to treatment initiation, the clinician should determine which core symptoms should be the initial target of therapy. A treatment guideline suggests targeting depressive symptoms first if the depression is severe and meets full diagnostic threshold for MDD (Schaffer et al., 2012). Importantly, the American Psychiatric Association (APA) practice guidelines suggests that both MDD and AD may satisfactorily respond to antidepressant pharmacotherapy (American Psychiatric Association, 2010).

Combining a benzodiazepine or other sedative/hypnotics to an antidepressant may be effective because this combination may provide rapid anxiolytic effects before any clinical effects of an antidepressant alone can be observed (Pollack, 2005). A buspirone combination may also be helpful in patients having comorbid generalized anxiety disorder (Bech et al., 2012). Beta-blockers can be added in patients having comorbid social anxiety disorder. Atypical antipsychotics may be helpful in treating severe anxious depression, and recent studies suggest positive findings with aripiprazole, olanzapine, risperidone, and quetiapine, but their side effect profile is of concern (Schaffer et al., 2012; Zhou et al., 2015).

Personality disorders

Identification of comorbid personality disorder (PD) in patients with MDD is critical because PD has a clear deleterious effect on the outcome of MDD. For example, a comorbid PD may aggravate MDD-related psychopathology and increase the risk of developing additional comorbid mental disorders; it can also hamper psychosocial and occupational functioning. It may also decrease treatment adherence and increase suicidality in patients with MDD (Rosenbluth et al., 2012; Newton-Howes et al., 2006).

Manifestations of PD occur pervasively throughout an individual's life, but the course of symptoms may vary across a lifetime. It may be difficult to separate a manifestation of PD from depressive symptoms, so an accurate diagnosis of comorbid PD could be difficult in the first few consultations. Depressive symptoms in PD could also wax and wane at least in part as a result of varying degrees of psycho-social stress. Among all PDs, the most frequently encountered and most troublesome clinical presentation is comorbidity between borderline PD and MDD (Rosenbluth et al., 2012; Beatson and Rao, 2013). The following 'red flag' patient behaviour could suggest the presence of borderline PD in those with established diagnosis of MDD:

- After a brief therapeutic honeymoon period, clinician becomes overwhelmed by patient transference and counter-transference issues
- Shows recurrent suicidal gestures, which prompt a careful evaluation, but are also used as means to manipulate the therapeutic relationship
- Presents 'dramatic' emotional expressions during consultations
- Extremely demanding and may attempt to cross therapeutic boundaries
- Presents seductive appearances and behaviours
- Is very resistant to antidepressants, or shows a rapid response to antidepressants (i.e. < two weeks)

Several psychotropic medications, either alone or in combination with each other, including mood stabilizers, anticonvulsants, atypical or typical antipsychotics, and antidepressants, could be helpful in treating patients having both MDD and borderline PD. Nevertheless, because these patients have higher risk of developing dependence, it is important to be very cautious when using benzodiazepines. Additionally, these pharmacological treatments must be provided with psychotherapy, such as psychodynamic or dialectical cognitive-behavioural therapies. The management of borderline PD is very complex, so a referral to specialist should be considered (Silk, 2015).

Substance use disorders

Substance use disorders (SUDs) are highly prevalent among patients with MDD. The Sequential Treatment Alternative to Relieve Depression (STAR-D) study showed that one-third of patients with MDD presented a concurrent SUD. Lifetime prevalence of SUDs among patients with MDD ranged from 30–42.8%. STAR-D showed that patients with MDD who had comorbid SUD were significantly more impaired, had a greater current suicide risk with a higher number of prior suicide attempts, an earlier age of onset of MDD, and showed more severe depressive symptomatology with more frequent concurrent AD. Substances such as alcohol, hallucinogens, opioids, sedatives, and psychostimulants could also induce depression, which further complicates diagnostic assessment and therapeutic management of these patients (Davis et al., 2006).

A study showed that among those with MDD and co-occurring SUD, alcohol was the most commonly used substance, with a rate of 78%. According to National Epidemiologic Survey on Alcohol and Related Conditions, a general population study, more than 40% of individuals with MDD also had a comorbid alcohol use disorder (AUD) (Grant et al., 2004). Comorbid AUD was associated with treatment resistance in MDD, while the presence of MDD also resulted in worse treatment response and higher rates of relapse among patients with AUD. More importantly, patients having both AUD and MDD had higher suicide rates than those patients having either disorder alone (Aharonovich et al., 2002).

The complex relationship between AUD and MDD is a clinical challenge as patients' depressive symptoms could result either from MDD or from chronic alcohol use. Thus, a clear anamnesis is necessary. There are three possible relationships between AUD and MDD: 1) MDD leading AUD; 2) AUD leading MDD, and; 3) a reciprocal, synergistic, deleterious relationship between AUD and MDD. Due to the complex relationships between AUD and MDD, Table 19.1 proposes three important conceptual approaches to treating comorbid AUD/MDD: sequential, parallel, and integrated. Treating both disorders simultaneously appears ideal, but this may not be possible in 'real' clinical situations. For example, when a patient is acutely suicidal due to MDD, a clinician must first focus on the management of MDD. In contrast, severe alcohol intoxication, Wernicke's encephalopathy, or alcohol withdrawal delirium could be more urgent issues if depressive symptoms are not severe (DeVido and Weiss, 2012).

When considering pharmacotherapy, one must first determine whether hospitalization for detoxification or psychiatric instability (e.g. suicidality) is necessary. Thereafter, clinician should observe the patient for at least a two-week period of abstinence from alcohol for diagnostic clarification. Studies supported that patients who received naltrexone, an opioid antagonist, with selective serotonin re-uptake inhibitors (SSRIs) showed higher rates of abstinence from alcohol and improvement of depressive symptoms than those who received either placebo, antidepressant, or AUD pharmacologic interventions alone (Beaulieu et al., 2012). Naltrexone is contraindicated in patients with hepatic dysfunction. Acamprosate can replace naltrexone if the hepatic dysfunction is not severe, but it must be used cautiously in patients with renal impairment (Plosker, 2015). Mirtazapine, with or without anti-craving agent naltrexone, is recommended as a first-line treatment option for AUD comorbid with MDD. Sertraline (an SSRI) + naltrexone is also a first option. Clinicians should also be aware of any possible drug-drug interactions. For example, benzodiazepines should be used cautiously because simultaneous intake of alcohol and benzodiazepines can result in

Table 19.1 Three different conceptual approaches in treatment of MDD patient with co-occurring AUD

Type		Advantage	Challenge
Sequential	MDD symptoms not addressed until a period of abstinence (around two weeks) from alcohol has been achieved	More useful when patient hospitalized due to an acute exacerbation of MDD or AUD	Trying to sequentially address co-occurring MDD and AUD may jeopardize timely intervention of both disorders
Parallel	Both disorders are addressed simultaneously by two teams	Can overcome disadvantage encountered with Sequential approach	Confusion may occur because two teams can provide different recommendations
Integrated	Both disorders are addressed simultaneously by one team	Can prevent disadvantages of both Sequential and Parallel approach	Finding or collaborating a team competent in providing expert care for AUD and MDD simultaneously.

Data from *Current Psychiatry Reports*, 14, 2012, DeVido, J.J. and R.D. Weiss, 'Treatment of the depressed alcoholic patient', pp. 610–8.

cross-tolerance. Patients with co-occurring MDD and AUD are also more prone to developing multiple SUDs (Beaulieu et al., 2012).

Attention deficit hyperactivity disorder

Attention deficit hyperactivity disorder (ADHD) is a common debilitating mental disorder which is highly prevalent in both children and adults. Around 5.4~12.1% of patients with MDD have comorbid ADHD (McIntyre et al., 2010). Comorbid ADHD has a negative impact on MDD outcomes. It is associated with an earlier age of MDD onset, more severe mood symptoms, and more suicide attempts. Even after patients achieve remission of MDD symptoms, they may continuously experience social and occupational impairment because of their ADHD symptoms, which could lead to MDD recurrence. Moreover, adult ADHD often goes unrecognized and untreated among patients with MDD (McIntyre et al., 2010; Bond et al., 2012). Hyperactive symptoms diminish with age, so ADHD may not be obvious to family and friends. Moreover, these patients often use coping strategies to compensate functional impairment and mask their ADHD symptoms. ADHD and MDD can also have symptom overlap, such as difficulty concentrating and psychomotor agitation, making the diagnosis even more difficult. Bupropion is recommended as a first-line antidepressant because it is proven to be effective in treating ADHD. Additional treatment options include other antidepressants (i.e. SSRI) + long-acting stimulant, or cognitive-behavioural therapy.

Medical comorbidity

Studies have shown that medical comorbidity is associated with worse outcomes among patients with MDD. A study showed that the prevalence of significant medical comorbidity was approximately 53% among patients with MDD, whereas prevalence of MDD was also elevated among patients with various chronic somatic illnesses (Fig. 19.1) (Evans et al., 2005).

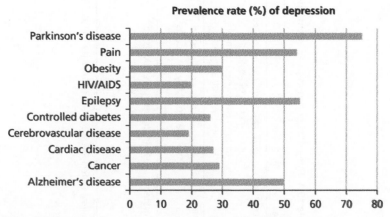

Fig. 19.1 Prevalence of depression in patients with medical illness

The relationship between MDD and medical disorders is bidirectional in nature. For example, medications used to treat medical conditions may induce depression, whereas MDD may increase mortality among patients with medical illnesses (Table 19.2) (Iosifescu et al., 2003; Ramasubbu et al., 2012).

Table 19.2 Reciprocal relationships between of major depressive disorder and medical conditions

1. Systemic medications inducing major depressive disorder

Analgesics and anti-inflammatory drugs
Antibacterial and antifungal agents
Anticholinesterase drugs
Antineoplastic drugs
Benzodiazepines and other sedative-hypnotic agents
Cardiac and antihypertensive drugs (i.e., calcium channel blockers)
Nonsteroidal anti-inflammatory drugs (NSAIDs)
Opiates
Statins
Steroids, hormones, interleukins, and interferons

2. Impact of MDD on medical illness

Medical illness	MDD increases risk of developing medical illness	MDD causes poor outcomes in medical illness
Alzheimer's disease	2 times by depression	Decreased compliance and faster functional decline
Cancer	1.35 ~ 1.88 times by depression	Mortality increased by 2.6 times
Coronary artery disease	1.5 ~ 2 times by depression	Mortality increased by 3.5 to 4 times
Diabetes mellitus type II	1.6 times by depression	Greater risk of developing early onset vascular complication, functional disability, and death
Epilepsy	4 ~ 6 times by depression	Burden of disease and quality of worsened
Ischemic stroke	1.8 times by depression	Mortality increased by 3.4 times and poor functional recovery

Data from *American Journal of Psychiatry*, 160, 2003, Iosifescu, D.V., et al., 'The impact of medical comorbidity on acute treatment in major depressive disorder', p. 2122–7; data from *Annals of Clinical Psychiatry*, 24, 2012, Ramasubbu, R., et al., 'The CANMAT task force recommendations for the management of patients with mood disorders and comorbid medical conditions: diagnostic, assessment, and treatment principles', pp. 82–90.

Diagnostic considerations

Clinicians sometimes wrongly consider that all somatic symptoms complained by patients having MDD as a part of their depressive symptoms. However, symptoms of MDD such as loss of appetite, pain, loss of energy, and insomnia presented could be due to underlying medical conditions. Thus, essential first step in management of patient having both MDD and medical illness rests on a precise diagnostic assessment (Rackley and Bostwick, 2012). Clinicians must understand unique clinical challenge of assessing depression among medically ill patients (Table 19.3). Among four possible approaches in diagnosing MDD in medically ill, inclusive approach seems

Table 19.3 Unique challenges of assessing depression in medically ill patients

1. Understanding the cause and effect	
Depression as a results of psychological impact of medical illness	Example: Depression after a patient was informed about stage IV lung cancer
Depression as a result of physiological impact of medical illness	Example: Depression from hypothyroidism
Depression as a cause of medical illness	Example: Hypothalamic–pituitary–adrenal (HPA) axis dysfunction from depression increases risk of developing metabolic disorder
Pseudo-depression: appearance of 'depression' without this being the appropriate diagnosis	Example: Hypoactive delirium mimicking depression
Masked presentation of depression: Somatic symptoms as a symptom presentation of depression	Example: A patient with MDD presenting with physical pain, low energy, and memory decline with no overt objective mood symptoms
2. Four different approaches to assess depression in the medically ill	
Inclusive approach	All depressive symptoms are counted, irrespective of whether they are related to medical illness
Exclusive approach	Only depression-specific mood and cognitive symptoms (i.e. anhedonia, feelings of guilt, hopelessness, worthlessness, and suicidal ideation) considered in diagnosis of depression
Etiological approach	A symptom is counted only if it is determined not to be caused by the medical illness
Substitutive approach	Psychological symptoms, mood, and cognitive symptoms replace the vegetative symptoms

Data from *American Journal of Psychiatry,* 160, 2003, Iosifescu, D.V., et al., 'The impact of medical comorbidity on acute treatment in major depressive disorder', p. 2122–7; data from *Annals of Clinical Psychiatry,* 24, 2012, Ramasubbu, R., et al., 'The CANMAT task force recommendations for the management of patients with mood disorders and comorbid medical conditions: diagnostic, assessment, and treatment principles', pp. 82–90.

to be the most appropriate in clinical settings. Although inclusive approach carries an inherent risk of over-diagnosing depression, this risk is evidently less troublesome compared to the risks associated with under-diagnosing depression. Use of depression screening instruments has been advocated in several guidelines, but no high level evidence has yet indicated that an active screening strategy of MDD improved outcomes among primary care patients (Thombs et al., 2014).

Treatment of MDD in specific populations with medical disorders

Cardiovascular disease

Tricyclic antidepressants (TCA), due to their type 'A' anti-arrhythmic effect, have long been contraindicated in MDD patients having comorbid cardiovascular disorder (CVD). Notwithstanding, both SSRIs and serotonin–norepinephrine reuptake inhibitors (SNRIs) have been shown to be beneficial and safe for the treatment of depression after a cardiac event, although clinicians have preferred SSRIs due to their higher receptor selectivity (Ramasubbu et al., 2012). However, recent studies showed that SSRIs, although to a lesser extent than TCAs, may be associated with a modest but significant prolongation of QTc interval. Citalopram was associated with a more significant QTc prolongation than other SSRIs, so the FDA alerted health care professionals a warning about QTc prolongation with citalopram use in 2011 (US FDA, 2012). Unfortunately, non-SSRI agents are not safer either. SNRIs, such as venlafaxine, showed dose-dependent increases in blood pressure and decreases in heart rate variability. Mirtazapine may cause weight gain and increase body fat mass, which are known risk factors for negative cardiac outcomes. Therefore, SSRIs are still considered to be the safest agent for treatment of MDD in patients with CVD. Choice within SSRIs should be based on individual risk factors for arrhythmias and other patient-specific factors (e.g., drug interactions). Bupropion could also be considered if sexual dysfunction of SSRI is not tolerated or concurrent smoking cessation is a target of therapy (Nemeroff and Goldschmidt-Clermont, 2012; Mavrides and Nemeroff, 2013).

Diabetes

MDD has a detrimental effect on psychological well-being and outcomes of diabetes mellitus (DM). Evidence indicated that successful treatment outcomes may be expected for both DM and MDD. Targeting both depressive symptoms and glycaemic control simultaneously is the best treatment approach (McIntyre et al., 2012). Nevertheless, this approach is not always clinically possible. For example, MDD has a significant deleterious impact on treatment adherence among individuals with type II DM. Thus, rapid improvement MDD is often recommended as the first priority because treatment of depression may be a prerequisite for good self-management of glycaemic control. In terms of pharmacotherapy, antidepressants (i.e. mirtazapine) and atypical antipsychotics (olanzapine) may disrupt glucose homeostasis. SNRIs, duloxetine and venlafaxine, could be helpful in both depressive symptoms and diabetic neuropathy. Bupropion, again, can be considered for those experiencing sexual dysfunction. Treatment tactics could be different depending on severity of depression (Petrak and Herpertz, 2009):

♦ DM with mild depression:
  ♦ Psycho-education about depression and bidirectional links between depression with DM.
  ♦ SSRI and/or psychotherapy if a patient has a history of severe, recurrent MDD.
♦ DM with moderate depression or not responding to step 1:
  ♦ Initiate treatment for depression either with SSRI or psychotherapy
  ♦ SSRI + psychotherapy if a patient has a history of severe, recurrent MDD
♦ DM with severe depression or not responding to step 2:
  ♦ SSRI + psychotherapy
  ♦ Increase SSRI dosage if no response is observed
  ♦ Consider inpatient setting

Cancer

A meta-analytic review suggested that MDD may contribute to increased mortality of patients having cancer (Schneider and Moyer, 2010). Both psychosocial interventions and pharmacotherapy may be effective in treating depression in patients having cancer. In terms of pharmacotherapy, it is difficult to derive clinically relevant first-line treatment recommendations. The clinician must be aware of possible drug-drug interaction when prescribing antidepressants in patients having cancer. For example, numerous studies support paroxetine, but its anticholinergic activity and strong inhibitory action on cytochrome P450 2D6 (CYP 2D6) enzymes are important limitations (Ramasubbu et al., 2012). Tamoxifen, which is an important chemotherapeutic agent for breast cancer, undergoes metabolism via CYP 2D6 to its active metabolite. SSRIs may significantly inhibit CYP 2D6 reducing the effectiveness of tamoxifen and increasing the risk of breast cancer relapse. Thus, CYP 2D6 inhibitors should be avoided in women taking tamoxifen, and clinicians should use alternative treatment options (such as venlafaxine) (Henry et al., 2008).

Treatment of cancer with chemotherapeutic agents may frequently aggravate depressive symptoms (e.g. loss of appetite and insomnia). Mirtazapine could be a good option because of its anti-emetic effect resulting from blockade of 5-HT3 receptors and sleep improvement effect resulting from blockade of H1 receptors. However, no evidence showed that any particular antidepressant is more efficacious than others in management of patients having depression and cancer. Thus, choice of an antidepressant such patients is not a straightforward decision and may be influenced by following issues (Torta and Ieraci, 2013):

1) Type of cancer and its clinical dimensions
2) Stage of cancer
3) Risks-benefit ratio of administering an antidepressant
4) Drug-drug interactions, pharmacodynamics, and pharmacokinetics of an antidepressant
5) Antidepressants must be started at their lowest dosage and doses should be titrated slowly

Thyroid disorder

Countless studies showed relationship between thyroid dysfunction and MDD. Classically, hypothyroidism has a strong association with depression whereas hyperthyroidism is acknowledged to be associated with both depression and mania. More accurately, the relationship is bidirectional and spans within entire spectrum of thyroid dysfunctions (Bunevicius and Prange, 2010).

Treatment of patient having both MDD and thyroid disease is difficult. Lithium, which is an effective augmenting agent for treatment–resistant depression, may induce subclinical or clinical hypothyroidism. Hypothyroidism and depression may also share similar clinical manifestations (e.g. low energy), which may hinder clinicians from accurately detecting thyroid dysfunctions among patients having MDD or vice-versa. Hormonal dysregulation, such as decreased levels of T3 and T4 and increased level of thyroid stimulating hormone (TSH), could also decrease efficacy of antidepressants (Ragson et al., 2009). The following principles may be considered when treating patient having depression with hypothyroidism:

◆ MDD + Lithium induced hypothyroidism: Start replacement (or augmentation) with thyroid hormone and consider stopping lithium

◆ MDD + subclinical hypothyroidism: Initiate thyroid supplementation for at least 6 weeks before considering antidepressant

◆ MDD + hypothyroidism: Monotherapy with thyroxin. If MDD is severe or patient has a positive history of depression during euthyroid state, concomitant antidepressant (e.g. SSRI) with thyroid hormone is recommended.

Other medical disorders

Comorbidity of MDD in patients having chronic painful conditions was also common (approximately 43%). Chronic pain increased severity of fatigue, insomnia, psychomotor retardation, weight gain, low mood, and concentration difficulties. It can also prolong duration and recurrence of depressive episodes (Ohayon, 2004). Comorbidity of these 2 chronic conditions has bidirectional and potentially causative influence on one another. In such patients, SNRIs are considered as the first-line pharmacotherapy. Among SNRIs, duloxetine received US FDA approval for treatment of fibromyalgia and chronic musculoskeletal pain (including osteoarthritis and chronic lower back pain) (Pergolizzi et al., 2013). Migraine and MDD have long been noted to co-occur, but treating the co-occurrence can be complicated because pharmacotherapy for one disorder may worsen the other. For example, SSRIs may worsen migraine whereas topiramate used for migraine may worsen depression. In contrast, TCAs such as amitriptyline have shown a significant effect in reducing the frequency of migraine attacks with prophylactic efficacy. SNRIs, venlafaxine and duloxetine, may also be effective with a better side effect profile than TCAs (Torta and Ieraci, 2012).

Depression is also common in patients having respiratory disorders such as asthma or chronic obstructive pulmonary disease (COPD). Antidepressants, usually SSRIs, are the best choice for not only the depressive symptoms but also for anxiety symptoms which frequently co-occur. Benzodiazepines may be problematic because of its potential negative effect in respiration and CO2 retention (Panagioti et al., 2014).

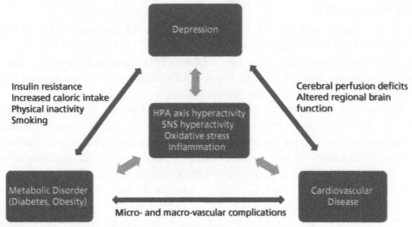

Fig. 19.2 Potential multi-directional mechanism among depression with cardio-metabolic conditions
HPA, hypothalamus–pituitary–adrenal axis; SNS, sympathetic nervous system

Treating obese patient with MDD is difficult. Many antidepressants including paroxetine and mirtazapine can cause weight gain. Most atypical antipsychotics also result in varying degrees of weight gain. Among antidepressants, bupropion is the only approved agent for both MDD and weight loss. Bupropion, in combination with naltrexone, marketed as Contrave® (Naltrexone/bupropion 32 mg/360 mg), is FDA approved for chronic weight management as an adjunct to a reduced-calorie diet and increased physical activity. Fluoxetine was also shown to decrease weight and reduce fasting plasma glucose, glycated haemoglobin A1c (HbA1c) and triglyceride (TG) in type 2 DM. However, life style modification such as proper diet, appropriate activities, and reducing stress must be accompanied with pharmacotherapy (McIntyre et al., 2012; Ramasubbu et al., 2012).

Please see Fig. 19.2 for potential shared mechanisms implicated in depression with comorbid cardio-metabolic conditions.

Collaborative care

Collaborative care model was developed in the 1990s to improve the quality of depression management in patients having comorbid medical conditions at primary care setting (Katon et al., 1995). The central objective of collaborative care is to provide empirically supported treatment for depression in a form acceptable to primary care settings. It is a multicomponent, healthcare system–level intervention that uses case managers to link patients, primary care physicians, and mental health specialists. Its main advantages include psycho-education to support treatment adherence, systematic monitoring of treatment adherence and outcomes, and as-needed consultation with psychiatrists and/or psychologists (see Fig. 19.3 for an example) (Gilbody et al., 2006).

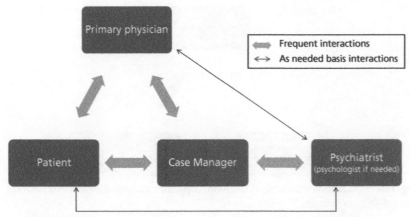

Fig. 19.3 An example of collaborative care system for patients having depression

Numerous clinical trials strongly supported the effectiveness of collaborative care programs for depression across a broad range of primary care settings. A meta-analysis showed effectiveness of collaborative care in improving depression symptoms (adherence to treatment (OR = 2.22); response to treatment (OR = 1.78); remission of symptoms (OR = 1.74); recovery from symptoms (OR = 1.75)) (Thota et al., 2012). In addition, collaborative care was shown to significantly improve depression outcome, as well as adherence to antidepressant medication and oral hypoglycemic agents in patients having comorbid depression and diabetes. Thus, collaborative care models might have beneficial effect in treatment for both depression and of comorbid medial disorders at the primary care level (Huang et al., 2013).

Conclusion

Presence of psychiatric and medical comorbidities considerably worsens the prognosis of both MDD and its associated comorbidities in a bidirectional and reciprocal fashion. For example, patients with MDD could be comorbid with an eating disorder (anorexia nervosa). Poor appetite could result from MDD and anorexia nervosa may decrease thyroid functions and metabolism. Hypothyroidism in turn may aggravate depressive symptoms leading to a potential a vicious cycle among MDD, anorexia nervosa, and hypothyroidism (Fig. 19.4).

Patients often seek treatment for MDD in primary care settings. Identification of depression and its associated comorbidities is a challenging issue. Notwithstanding collaborative models hold promise as a strategy for the diagnosis and management of MDD and comorbid diseases in the primary care, there are several barriers to its effective implementation. The diagnosis of comorbidities in patients having MDD should be 'simple and positive initial diagnosis with comprehensive examinations during the course of treatment'. The selection of the appropriate treatment for patients with MDD and complex medical and psychiatric comorbidities is a challenging issue. For selection of antidepressant, the GP must consider the propensity of an antidepressant to

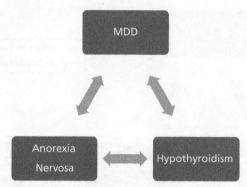

Fig. 19.4 Vicious cycle created by depression, psychiatric comorbidity (anorexia nervosa), and medical comorbidity (hypothyroidism)

cause metabolic derangements in a patient with comorbid obesity. Furthermore, drug-drug interactions may emerge as significant issues.

Evidence-based psychotherapeutic intervention including cognitive-behavioral therapy and interpersonal therapy should be considered. Some randomized clinical trials have established the effectiveness of these interventions for the management of MDD in primary care. However, these important therapeutic approaches are not universally available throughout different medical service settings.

Acknowledgements

This work was supported by a grant of the Korean Health Technology R&D Project, Ministry of Health & Welfare, Republic of Korea (HI12C0003).

References

Aharonovich E, Liu X, Nunes E, and Hasin DS. (2002). Suicide attempts in substance abusers: effects of major depression in relation to substance use disorders. *Am J Psychiatry*, 159/ 9: 1600–2.

Aina Y and Susman JL. (2006). Understanding comorbidity with depression and anxiety disorders. *J Am Osteopath Assoc*, 106/ 5 Suppl 2: S9–14.

American Psychiatric Association. (2010). *Practice guideline for the treatment of patients with major depressive disorder*, 3rd edn. Arlington: American Psychiatric Association Publishing.

Beatson JA and Rao S. (2013). Depression and borderline personality disorder. *Med J Aust*, 199/ 6 Suppl: S24–7.

Beaulieu S, Saury S, Sareen J, Tremblay J, Schütz CG, McIntyre RS, Schaffer A; Canadian Network for Mood and Anxiety Treatments (CANMAT) Task Force. (2012). The Canadian Network for Mood and Anxiety Treatments (CANMAT) task force recommendations for the management of patients with mood disorders and comorbid substance use disorders. *Ann Clin Psychiatry*, 24/ 1: 38–55.

Bech P, Fava M, Trivedi MH, Wisniewski SR, and Rush AJ. (2012). Outcomes on the pharmacopsychometric triangle in bupropion- SR vs. buspirone augmentation of citalopram in the STAR*D trial. *Acta Psychiatr Scand*, 125/ 4: 342–8.

Bond DJ, Hadjipavlou G, Lam RW, McIntyre RS, Beaulieu S, Schaffer A, Weiss M; Canadian Network for Mood and Anxiety Treatments (CANMAT) Task Force. (2012). The Canadian Network for Mood and Anxiety Treatments (CANMAT) task force recommendations for the management of patients with mood disorders and comorbid attention- deficit/ hyperactivity disorder. *Ann Clin Psychiatry*, 24/ 1: 23–37.

Boyer P. (2000). Do anxiety and depression have a common pathophysiological mechanism? *Acta Psychiatr Scand Suppl*, 406: 24–9.

Bunevicius R and PrangeJr AJ. (2010). Thyroid disease and mental disorders: cause and effect or only comorbidity? *Curr Opin Psychiatry*, 23/ 4: 363–8.

Cepoiu M, McCusker J, Cole MG, Sewitch M, Belzile E, and Ciampi A. (2008). Recognition of depression by non- psychiatric physicians—a systematic literature review and meta-analysis. *J Gen Intern Med*, 23/ 1: 25–36.

Davis LL, Frazier E, Husain MM, Warden D, Trivedi M, Fava M, Cassano P, McGrath PJ, Balasubramani GK, Wisniewski SR, and Rush AJ. (2006). Substance use disorder comorbidity in major depressive disorder: a confirmatory analysis of the STAR*D cohort. *Am J Addict*, 15/ 4: 278–85.

DeVido JJ and Weiss RD. (2012). Treatment of the depressed alcoholic patient. *Curr Psychiatry Rep*, 14/ 6: 610–8.

Evans DL, Charney DS, Lewis L, Golden RN, Gorman JM, Krishnan KR, Nemeroff CB, Bremner JD, Carney RM, Coyne JC, Delong MR, Frasure- Smith N, Glassman AH, Gold PW, Grant I, Gwyther L, Ironson G, Johnson RL, Kanner AM, Katon WJ, Kaufmann PG, Keefe FJ, Ketter T, Laughren TP, Leserman J, Lyketsos CG, McDonald WM, McEwen BS, Miller AH, Musselman D, O'Connor C, Petitto JM, Pollock BG, Robinson RG, Roose SP, Rowland J, Sheline Y, Sheps DS, Simon G, Spiegel D, Stunkard A, Sunderland T, Tibbits PJr, Valvo WJ. (2005). Mood disorders in the medically ill: scientific review and recommendations. *Biol Psychiatry*, 58/ 3: 175–89.

Gilbody S, Bower P, Fletcher J, Richards D, and Sutton AJ. (2006). Collaborative care for depression: a cumulative meta- analysis and review of longer- term outcomes. *Arch Intern Med*, 166/ 21: 2314–21.

Grant BF, Stinson FS, Dawson DA, Chou SP, Dufour MC, Compton W, Pickering RP, and Kaplan K. (2004). Prevalence and co- occurrence of substance use disorders and independent mood and anxiety disorders: results from the National Epidemiologic Survey on Alcohol and Related Conditions. *Arch Gen Psychiatry*, 61/ 8: 807–16.

Henry NL, Stearns V, Flockhart DA, Hayes DF, and Riba M. (2008). Drug interactions and pharmacogenomics in the treatment of breast cancer and depression. *Am J Psychiatry*, 2008. 165/ 10: 1251–5.

Huang Y, Wei X, Wu T, Chen R, and Guo A. (2013). Collaborative care for patients with depression and diabetes mellitus: a systematic review and meta- analysis. *BMC Psychiatry*, 13: 260.

Iosifescu DV, Nierenberg AA, Alpert JE, Smith M, Bitran S, Dording C, and Fava M. (2003). The impact of medical comorbidity on acute treatment in major depressive disorder. *Am J Psychiatry*, 160/ 12: 2122–7.

Katon W, Von Korff M, Lin E, Walker E, Simon GE, Bush T, Robinson P, and Russo J. (1995). Collaborative management to achieve treatment guidelines. Impact on depression in primary care. *JAMA*, 273/ 13: 1026–31.

Katon WJ, Lin EHB, Von Korff M, Ciechanowski P, Ludman EJ, Young B, Peterson D, Rutter CM, McGregor M, and McCulloch D. (2010). Collaborative care for patients with depression and chronic illnesses. *N Engl J Med*, 363/ 27: 2611–20.

Mavrides N and Nemeroff C. (2013). Treatment of depression in cardiovascular disease. *Depress Anxiety*, 30/ 4: 328–41.

McIntyre RS, Alsuwaidan M, Goldstein BI, Taylor VH, Schaffer A, Beaulieu S, Kemp DE; Canadian Network for Mood and Anxiety Treatments (CANMAT) Task Force. (2012). The Canadian Network for Mood and Anxiety Treatments (CANMAT) task force recommendations for the management of patients with mood disorders and comorbid metabolic disorders. *Ann Clin Psychiatry*, 24/ 1: 69–81.

McIntyre RS, Kennedy SH, Soczynska JK, Nguyen HT, Bilkey TS, Woldeyohannes HO, Nathanson JA, Joshi S, Cheng JS, Benson KM, and Muzina DJ. (2010). Attention- deficit/ hyperactivity disorder in adults with bipolar disorder or major depressive disorder: results from the international mood disorders collaborative project. *Prim Care Companion J Clin Psychiatry*, 12/ 3: doi: 10.4088/ PCC.09m00861gry.

Melartin TK, Rytsälä HJ, Leskelä US, Lestelä- Mielonen PS, Sokero TP, and Isometsä ET. (2002). Current comorbidity of psychiatric disorders among DSM- IV major depressive disorder patients in psychiatric care in the Vantaa Depression Study. *J Clin Psychiatry*, 63/ 2: 126–34.

Natalie Ragson N, Hendrick VC, and Garrick T. (2009). Psychosomatic medicine: endocrine and metabolic disorder. In: *Comprehensive Textbook of Psychiatry*, 9th edn, VA Sadock, BJ Sadock, and P Ruiz, eds. Philadelphia: Lippincott Williams and Wilkins, 2303–14.

Nemeroff CB and Goldschmidt- Clermont PJ. (2012). Heartache and heartbreak- - the link between depression and cardiovascular disease. *Nat Rev Cardiol*, 9/ 9: 526–39.

Newton- Howes G, Tyrer P, and Johnson T. (2006). Personality disorder and the outcome of depression: meta- analysis of published studies. *Br J Psychiatry*, 188: 13–20.

Ohayon MM. (2004). Specific characteristics of the pain/ depression association in the general population. *J Clin Psychiatry*, 65/ Suppl 12: 5–9.

Panagioti M, Scott C, Blakemore A, and Coventry PA. (2014). Overview of the prevalence, impact, and management of depression and anxiety in chronic obstructive pulmonary disease. *Int J Chron Obstruct Pulmon Dis*, 9: 1289–306.

Pergolizzi JVJr, Raffa RB, Taylor RJr, Rodriguez G, Nalamachu S, and Langley P. (2013). A review of duloxetine 60 mg once- daily dosing for the management of diabetic peripheral neuropathic pain, fibromyalgia, and chronic musculoskeletal pain due to chronic osteoarthritis pain and low back pain. *Pain Pract*, 13/ 3: 239–52.

Petrak F and Herpertz S. (2009). Treatment of depression in diabetes: an update. *Curr Opin Psychiatry*, 22/ 2: 211–7.

Plosker GL. (2015). Acamprosate: A Review of Its Use in Alcohol Dependence. *Drugs*, 75/ 11: 1255–68.

Pollack MH. (2005). Comorbid anxiety and depression. *J Clin Psychiatry*, 66/ Suppl 8: 22–9.

Rackley S and Bostwick JM. (2012). Depression in medically ill patients. *Psychiatr Clin North Am*, 35/ 1: 231–47.

Ramasubbu R, Beaulieu S, Taylor VH, Schaffer A, McIntyre RS; Canadian Network for Mood and Anxiety Treatments (CANMAT) Task Force. (2012). The CANMAT task force recommendations for the management of patients with mood disorders and comorbid medical conditions: diagnostic, assessment, and treatment principles. *Ann Clin Psychiatry*, 24/ 1: 82–90.

Ramasubbu, R, Taylor VH, Samaan Z, Sockalingham S, Li M, Patten S, Rodin G, Schaffer A, Beaulieu S, and McIntyre RS; Canadian Network for Mood and Anxiety Treatments (CANMAT) Task Force. (2012). The Canadian Network for Mood and Anxiety Treatments

(CANMAT) task force recommendations for the management of patients with mood disorders and select comorbid medical conditions. *Ann Clin Psychiatry*, 24/ 1: 91–109.

Rosenbluth M, Macqueen G, McIntyre RS, Beaulieu S, and Schaffer A; Canadian Network for Mood and Anxiety Treatments (CANMAT) Task Force. (2012). The Canadian Network for Mood and Anxiety Treatments (CANMAT) task force recommendations for the management of patients with mood disorders and comorbid personality disorders. *Ann Clin Psychiatry*, 24/ 1: 56–68.

Schaffer A, McIntosh D, Goldstein BI, Rector NA, McIntyre RS, Beaulieu S, Swinson R, and Yatham LN; Canadian Network for Mood and Anxiety Treatments (CANMAT) Task Force. (2012). The CANMAT task force recommendations for the management of patients with mood disorders and comorbid anxiety disorders. *Ann Clin Psychiatry*, 2012. 24/ 1: 6–22.

Schneider S and Moyer A. (2010). Depression as a predictor of disease progression and mortality in cancer patients: a meta- analysis. *Cancer*, 116/ 13: 3304; author reply 3304–5.

Schoevers RA, Van HL, Koppelmans V, Kool S, and Dekker JJ. (2008). Managing the patient with comorbid depression and an anxiety disorder. *Drugs*, 68/ 12: 1621–34.

Silk KR. (2015). Management and effectiveness of psychopharmacology in emotionally unstable and borderline personality disorder. *J Clin Psychiatry*, 76/ 4: e524–5.

Smith SM, Soubhi H, Fortin M, Hudon C, and O'Dowd T. (2012). Interventions for improving outcomes in patients with multimorbidity in primary care and community settings. *Cochrane Database Syst Rev*, 4: CD006560.

Thombs BD, Ziegelstein RC, Roseman M, Kloda LA, and Ioannidis JP. (2014). There are no randomized controlled trials that support the United States Preventive Services Task Force Guideline on screening for depression in primary care: a systematic review. *BMC Med*, 12: 13.

Thota AB, Sipe TA, Byard GJ, Zometa CS, Hahn RA, McKnight- Eily LR, Chapman DP, Abraido- Lanza AF, Pearson JL, Anderson CW, Gelenberg AJ, Hennessy KD, Duffy FF, Vernon- Smiley ME, Nease DEJr, Williams SP; Community Preventive Services Task Force. (2012). Collaborative care to improve the management of depressive disorders: a community guide systematic review and meta- analysis. *Am J Prev Med*, 42/ 5: 525–38.

Torta R and Ieraci V. (2012). Migraine and depression comorbidity: antidepressant options. *Neurol Sci*, 33/ Suppl 1: S117–8.

Torta RG and Ieraci V. (2013). Pharmacological management of depression in patients with cancer: practical considerations. *Drugs*, 2013. 73/ 11: 1131–45.

US Food and Drug Administration. (2012). *FDA drug safety communication: abnormal heart rhythms associated with high doses of Celexa (citalopram hydrobromide).* http:// www. fda. gov/ Drugs/ DrugSafety/ ucm297391.htm. Accessed November 18, 2012.

Wittchen HU, Lieb R, Wunderlich U, and Schuster P. (1999). Comorbidity in primary care: presentation and consequences. *J Clin Psychiatry*, 60/ Suppl 7: 29–36; discussion 37–8.

Zhou XP, Keitner GI, Qin B, Ravindran AV, Bauer M, Del Giovane C, Zhao J, Liu Y, Fang Y, Zhang Y, and Xie P. (2015). Atypical Antipsychotic Augmentation for Treatment-Resistant Depression: A Systematic Review and Network Meta- Analysis. *Int J Neuropsychopharmacol*, 18/ 11: doi: 10.1093/ ijnp/ pyv060.

Zimmerman M, Chelminski I, and McDermut W. (2002). Major depressive disorder and axis I diagnostic comorbidity. *J Clin Psychiatry*, 63/ 3: 187–93.

Chapter 20

Untoward side effects of psychiatric drugs

Manu S. Sharma, Ives Cavalcante Passos, and André F. Carvalho

Introduction

Adverse effects are an unavoidable risk of medication treatment. Although it is impossible to have an encyclopaedic knowledge of all adverse effects of psychiatric drugs, clinicians should be aware of the most frequent side effects, including those with significant medical consequences. It is known that psychotropic medications are some of the most commonly prescribed drugs in medical practice. For instance, between 2005–2008 among people aged 18–44 years, antidepressants were the third most commonly prescribed medications (US Department of Health and Human Services, 2011) and atypical antipsychotics accounted for almost 5% of all drug expenditure in the US (Alexander et al., 2012). Consequently, more and more primary care physicians find themselves treating psychiatric illnesses. In a survey conducted by the WHO in 17 countries, primary care physicians (PCPs) were found to provide the majority of mental health care (Wang et al., 2010).

It is important to have a low threshold for suspecting adverse drug reactions because clinical trials often do not have the necessary power to detect rare adverse reactions (O'Neill et al., 1996; Sills et al., 1986). Clinical trials often do not follow its participants for extended periods of time, and may miss adverse reactions associated with long-term drug use. Additionally, clinical trials carefully select their participants and often exclude special populations like pregnant women and children, who may experience a unique set of side effects in comparison to the general population (Sills et al., 1986). Thus it is important to be vigilant for post-marketing surveillance reports for a more comprehensive understanding of drug side effects.

In the following sections we cover some of the most common and serious side effects of widely prescribed psychotropic medications. This information should enable a PCP in early identification and appropriate management of the side effects.

Gastrointestinal side effects

Some of the most common gastrointestinal (GI) side effects are result of the action of psychotropic medications on the autonomic system and the serotonin receptors in the GI tract. The tricyclic antidepressants (TCA) block the muscarinic receptors, which in turn cause dry mouth and constipation. Some of the low potency first generation antipsychotics (like chlorpromazine, thioridazine) can also cause dry mouth and constipation through similar mechanisms (Leucht et al., 2013). It is important to remember that there is an abundance of serotonin receptors in the GI tract and that these receptors play an important role in the motility of the GI tract (Borman et al., 2002). The selective serotonin reuptake inhibitors (SSRIs) act on these receptors, which in turn cause the GI side effects, including diarrhoea, dyspepsia, GI bleeding, and abdominal pain (Goldstein and Goodnick, 1998). Among the SSRIs, fluvoxamine is the most notorious for these side effects, and escitalopram was the best tolerated (Spigset, 1999). Similarly, nausea caused by taking SSRIs is a result of their action on the central 5HT-3 receptors (Goldstein and Goodnick, 1998). At the time of initiation of therapy, it is important to counsel the patient about these side effects as they are the some of the leading causes that patients discontinue treatment. Also, more than half of patients experience one of the GI side effects within the first few weeks of starting treatment. Reassuring patients that these side effects wear off over time might be an important factor in helping them continue treatment (Uher et al., 2009).

Blurred vision and ocular side effects

The muscles in the pupil that control its size are innervated by both sympathetic and parasympathetic nerve fibres. Since many of the psychotropic medications act on the autonomic system, they can have adverse effects on vision. TCAs and some antipsychotics, mainly the phenothiazines, have strong anticholinergic action and cause mydriasis (dilatation of the pupils), which can cause increased sensitivity to light (Moeller and Maxner, 2007). In some cases, they can also cause cyclopegia (paralysis of ciliary muscles), which can affect accommodation and cause blurred vision (Malone et al., 1992;, Edler et al., 1971). SSRIs have similar effects on vision, but these side effects are extremely rare (Costagliola et al., 2004). Most of these effects are transient but may warrant lowering of doses of the medications if they persist (Richa and Yazbek, 2010)

Clinicians must be careful while prescribing TCAs, phenothiazines and, rarely, topirmate in patients who might have an established diagnosis or pre-disposition for angle closure glaucoma (Oshika, 1995; Lowe, 1966; Fraunfelder et al., 2004). Any drug which causes pupillary dilatation can precipitate an episode of angle closure glaucoma. Thus patients at increased risk, such as Asians, Hispanics, Inuits, those with a positive family history of angle closure glaucoma, nanopthalmos, and the elderly should be warned about this possible side effect and educated about the symptoms of angle closure glaucoma for early identification (Tripathi et al., 2003).

Long-term use of phenothiazines, especially chlorpromazine and thioridazine, has been associated with increased risk of cataracts and corneal opacities (Li et al., 2008Hansen et al., 1997). Studies suggest that almost one-third of the patients receiving long-term treatment with chlorpromazine had corneal or lens deposits (Siddall, 1968). This effect appears to be dose dependent and is more common among individuals treated with higher doses for a longer time (Satanove, 1965). Unlike other side effects, these happen after prolonged exposure and are irreversible. Some other rare side effects include defects in colour vision due to valproic acid and myopia secondary to use of topiramate (Richa and Yazbek, 2010).

Urinary retention and urinary incontinence

Drug-induced urinary retention is caused by drugs blocking parasympathetic input to the urinary bladder, affecting central D1 dopaminergic pathways, or affecting central serotonergic activity (Verhamme et al., 2008; Ouslander, 2004). Some of the first-generation antipsychotics, especially phenothiazine and thioxanthines (chlorprotixen) can cause urinary retention mainly because of their strong anticholinergic nature (Tueth, 1994). Among second-generation antipsychotics, risperidone and ziprasidone can cause urinary retention because of their action on central $5HT_2$ receptors (Xomalis et al., 2006). The risk of retention is higher when risperidone is used in combination with fluoxetine (Bozikas et al., 2001). Anti-muscarinic action of the TCA can also cause urinary retention. There have been numerous case reports which suggest the possibility of urinary retention with the use of SSRIs, especially fluvoxamine, although such incidences are rare (Verhamme et al., 2008). Special care should be taken while prescribing drugs in the elderly and patients with benign prostate hypertrophy, as they are more prone to the side effects of these drugs. In an acute setting, bladder catheterization can be used to relive the retention. In the long run, alternative pharmacological agents should be used to avoid side effects.

Urinary incontinence may occur in patients taking clozapine, risperidone, olanzapine, and gabapentin (Schneider et al., 2006). It is speculated that these medications block the adrenergic receptors responsible for containing urine flow which are located in the lower region of the bladder. In the management, it is necessary to exclude other hypothesis, such as diabetes, seizures, benign hyperplasia, prostate cancer, and neurogenic bladder. The use of ephedrine (up to 150mg/day) may be useful in urinary incontinence caused by olanzapine or clozapine. Moreover, oxybutynin 5mg, two to three times a day can also help (Schneider et al., 2006).

Sexual side effects

Sexual side effects are some of the most under-reported side effects experienced by those who use psychotropic drugs. Studies show that spontaneous self-report is not a reliable way to assess these symptoms and clinicians should use sexual dysfunction questionnaires to better assess these symptoms (Reichenpfader et al., 2014). Almost 50–70% of patients who take psychotropic medications will experience at least one sexual side effect. It is important to remember that psychotropic medications can affect almost all aspects of sexual functions, including libido, orgasm, and arousal functioning (erection in males and vaginal lubrication in females) in both males and females (Montejo et al., 2015).

It is difficult to assess the incidence of drug-induced sexual dysfunction in individuals with depression because it can, in itself, be a symptom of depression and not a consequence of the medications. Most studies have found that antidepressants where the primary action is serotonergic (SSRIs and lower doses of venlafaxine) have high rates of sexual dysfunction ranging from 26% (for fluvoxamine) to 80% (for sertraline)

Table 20.1 Management of sexual side effects

Drug group	Management strategies
SSRI	◆ Change the antidepressants to agents with known lower side effects like bupropion, nefazodone. ◆ Use phosphodiesterase inhibitors like sildenafil, tadalfil
Antipsychotics	◆ Lower the dose of the drug ◆ Use phosphodiesterase inhibitors like Sildenafil, tadalfil ◆ Can use bromocriptine, cabergoline or amantadine (supported by open label trials and case studies.)

(Bella and Shamloul, 2013). Antidepressants like bupropion, nefazodone, mirtazapine, and agomelatine did not have statistically significant differences in the incidence of sexual side effects when compared to a placebo. Men are more likely to experience dysfunction in desire and orgasm phases where as women are more likely to experience dysfunction in the arousal phase (Angst, 1998). Although the exact mechanism behind SSRI-induced sexual dysfunction is unknown, some studies have shown the possible involvement of reduced dopaminergic transmission through serotonergic receptors in the mesolimbic region (Bella and Shamloul, 2013).

Patients with diagnosis of schizophrenia have a higher incidence of sexual dysfunction as compared to the general population (McGahuey et al., 2000). Among the antipsychotics some of the highest rates of sexual dysfunction were associated with olanzapine (50%) and risperidone (60–70%) (La Torre et al., 2013). Clozapine has been associated with high rates of both erectile and ejaculation dysfunction. Like antidepressants, antipsychotics can affect all aspects sexual functions (Bella and Shamloul, 2013). A possible mechanism of sexual dysfunction includes increased prolactin levels because of D2 antagonism, and peripheral anticholinergic effects.

Benzodiazepines have also been associated with increased incidence of erectile dysfunction and decreased libido, but available evidence is often conflicting secondary to multiple confounding factors. However, when benzodiazepines are used along with lithium the rates of sexual dysfunction increase to as high as 49% (38). See Table 20.1 for management strategies.

Skin reactions

Overall, the incidence of adverse skin reactions secondary to psychotropic medications is as low as 0.1%. Among all psychotropics, mood stabilizers like carbamazepine and lamotrigine are by far the most notorious for skin reactions (Lange-Asschenfeldt et al., 2009). Almost any drug can result in hypersensitivity reactions, which present with urticaria characterized by pruritic papules or plaques. These lesions can emerge on any part of the body and can start appearing from minutes to hours after taking the medications and generally do not last for more than 24 hours after the last dose. These can be early signs of an allergic reaction and can proceed to life-threatening anaphylaxis (Garnis-Jones, 1996).

Adverse skin reactions are more common during summer when the exposure to UV rays increases and women are more prone to these side effects as compared to men. Certain individuals with specific HLA types, like HLA-B1502 (Han Chinese and Indians) or HLA-A3101 (Japanese and Northern European ethnicities) increase the risk of drug reaction to carbamazepine. Although not routinely practised, it may benefit clinicians to genotype patients of at risk ethnicities before starting treatment with offending agents (Mitkov et al., 2014).

Among mood stabilizers, carbamazepine and lamotrigine are associated with the highest incidence of adverse skin reaction (Lange-Asschenfeldt et al., 2009). It is important to remember that both these drugs can cause life-threatening Steven Johnson's Syndrome (SJS) and Toxic Epidermal Necrolysis (TEN). When the lesions involve less than 10% of the body surface it is classified as SJS and when they involve greater than 30% it is classified as TEN. These syndromes are characterized initially by flu-like symptoms, dusky red macules which progress to bullaes, and eventually end with necrosis and detachment of the epidermis and mucous membranes. Such reactions are common at the time of treatment initiation, particularly with higher initial doses and quick titration. However, the risk reduces with longer treatment durations (Mitkov et al., 2014). Use of depakote and lamotrigine should be avoided as it increases the risk of adverse skin reactions.

Photosensitivity reaction is common with benzodiazepines and chlorpromazine whereas alopecia can be seen with patients using TCAs and lithium. Lithium use is also associated with higher incidence of acne and psoriasis because of the possible action of lithium on adenylate cyclase in keratocytes (Orwin, 1983). Most antipsychotics have been associated with skin pigmentation changes. Additionally, olanzapine and seroquel have been associated with seborrhoeic dermatitis. Hyperhidrosis is common with bupropion use (Bliss and Warnock, 2013).

Blood dyscrasias

Neutropenia and agranulocytosis are some of the most serious adverse reactions secondary to the use of psychotropic medications. Although the association of agranulocytosis and clozapine use is common knowledge, it is also important to remember that other psychotropic medications also have the potential to cause neutropenia and agranulocytosis (Duggal and Singh, 2005). The incidence of neutropenia is highest with clozapine (one in 30 patients), whereas with olanzapine and phenothiazine it is much lower (one in 10,000). Among the mood stabilizers carbamazepine is associated with the highest incidence of neutropenia, with one in every 200 patients experiencing these side effects (Flanagan and Dunk, 2008).

Neutropenia and agranulocytosis can present with fever, sore throat, or the first presentation may be similar to an infection. If a patient taking a drug known to cause agranulocytosis presents with fever, the clinician should order a complete blood count immediately and stop the medications till the results are available. In Europe, WBC and neutrophil counts are monitored every week for first 18 weeks and then once every four weeks as long as the patient is taking clozapine. In the US, WBC and neutrophil counts are monitored every week for the first 26 weeks, followed by every two weeks for the next 26 weeks and every four weeks after that. If the patient misses a dose he can be restarted on the same dose within 48 hours of the last dose (Cohen and Monden, 2013). If the time elapsed between two doses is greater than 48 hours, the titration is similar to a clozapine-naïve patient. As evidenced by the more frequent monitoring, the risk of agranulocytosis is the highest within the first 6–18 weeks after beginning the treatment. Agranulocytosis is completely reversible and the WBC and neutrophil counts reach normal levels within two weeks after treatment cessation. The risk of agranulocytosis increases if clozapine is used with other drugs, which can cause neutropenia, like valproate and carbamazepine. Among all the antipsychotics, sulpiride and fluphenazine have been associated with the lowest risk of agranulocytosis (Delieu et al., 2006).

It is important to remember that patients being treated with clozapine can have a transient fall in their WBC and neutrophil counts. Close monitoring and more frequent blood draws are warranted in such patients. Another strategy involves using adjunctive lithium along with clozapine to try and increase the WBC count. It is important to keep in mind that although lithium helps increase neutrophil count it cannot prevent agranulocytosis. Patients with history of clozapine-induced agranulocytosis are at increased risk of developing the same side effect again if rechallenged with clozapine. If the risks of not starting clozapine outweigh the risks of side effects a rechallenge can be considered, but it requires closer monitoring and treatment with concomitant lithium or colony stimulating factors (Whiskey and Taylor, 2007).

SSRIs are a class of drug that can affect platelet function. Serotonin helps in platelet aggregation and, more importantly, it is responsible for potentiating platelet aggregation induced by ADP, epinephrine, and collagen. SSRIs can affect this function and have been associated with increased risk of bleeding. Thus the use of SSRIs with other drugs like NSAIDS, aspirin, and blood thinners should be avoided (de Abajo, 2011). The more potent SSRIs like fluoxetine and paroxetine are more likely to cause these side effects (Halperin and Reber, 2007).

Hypothyroidism

Most of the psychotropic drugs can have an effect on thyroid functions through a variety of mechanisms. Phenothiazines can affect uptake of iodine by cells in the thyroid gland and form protein bound complexes which can deactivate thyroid iodine and result in the formation of anti-thyroid antibodies. The D2 antagonists (antipsychotics) can result in the increase in the TSH levels secondary to stimulation of TRH. Whereas the TCAs can cause deactivation of thyroid peroxidases, most of these drugs do not result in clinically significant dysfunction of the thyroid gland. The effects can be manifested in individuals who already have a pre-existing dysfunction of the thyroid gland or who may be at increased risk of developing one (Bou Khalil and Richa, 2007).

Lithium is known to cause clinically significant dysfunction of the thyroid gland. Lithium can disrupt iodine uptake by the thyroid glands and also inhibit the release of T4 into the blood (Pfeifer et al., 1976). Studies have suggested that lithium can inhibit deiodinase activity, which can result in reduction in activation of the thyroid hormone (Spaulding et al., 1972). Clinically significant effects are generally noted after prolonged therapy but almost 40–50% of patients have been known to develop hypothyroidism with chronic use of lithium. Women are more prone to these effects as compared to men but women are also generally more likely to have thyroid dysfunction (Perrild et al., 1990). It is also important to remember that lithium use can also cause hyperparathyroidism, which can manifest as an increase in blood calcium levels. It is important to have baseline thyroid function tests and calcium levels in patients on initiation of lithium therapy, and follow up monitoring is also recommended, especially in women and at-risk individuals.

Nephrotoxicity

Nephrogenic diabetes insipidus is one of the most common adverse effects associated with lithium use and can occur in 20–40% of the patients on lithium treatment (Pauzé and Brooks, 2007). The underlying mechanism involves development of resistance to anti-diuretic hormone (ADH) (Dupuis et al., 1996). Lithium can accumulate in the cells of the collecting duct and reduce the ability of ADH to increase the water permeability in these cells. It is important to identify early signs, e.g. increased frequency of nocturnal micturition, because with chronic use the changes might be irreversible. Early symptoms, like polydipsia and polyuria can be treated using potassium-sparing and thiazide diuretics, although, if possible, discontinuation of lithium treatment is suggested. Continued use of lithium can lead to the development of interstitial nephropathy, which can in turn lead to end-stage renal disease, although this is very rare (McKnight et al., 2012). Around 1% of patients taking lithium over 15 years develop end-stage renal disease (Tredget et al., 2010). In most individuals some reduction in glomerular filtration rate (GFR) is observed but these changes are not clinically significant. Comorbid conditions like diabetes mellitus and hypertension can increase the risk of impairment of renal functions among patients using lithium. There is a direct correlation between the duration and the dose of lithium used and impairment of renal function. Clinicians should avoid using ACE inhibitors in patients using lithium as it has a potential for causing renal insufficiency by increasing lithium levels. On very rare occasions lithium has been associated with nephrotic syndrome (Wills et al., 2006).

Clinicians should be aware that SSRIs have been known to cause hyponatremia and the incidence varies from between 0.5% to 32% in different studies. The exact mechanism by which the SSRIs can cause hyponatremia is unknown, but studies have proposed that SSRIs can either increase the release of ADH, through its inhibition of norepinephrine uptake, or by increasing ADH sensitivity, which in turn can result in a SIADH-like syndrome. Elderly females and individuals using diuretics are at increased risk of developing hyponatremia. Treatment includes stopping the SSRIs, fluid restriction, and aggressive diuresis depending on the severity of the hyponatremia (Jacob, 2006).

Liver toxicity

There are generally three patterns of acute drug-induced liver injury (DILI): hepatocellular, cholestasis, and mixed pattern. DILI is considered clinically significant when the ALT levels rise to greater than three times the upper normal limit. Hepatocellular type changes are associated with raised ALT (greater than three times the upper limit) and can be seen with certain SSRIs, risperidone and valproic acid. Cholestasis is associated with raised alkaline phosphatase levels (two times greater than the upper normal limit) and can be seen with use of chlorpromazine and amitriptyline. In mixed pattern (DILI), elevation is seen in the levels of both alkaline phosphatase and ALT, and can occur with carbamazepine use. Individuals who develop jaundice have been known to have poorer prognosis as compared to patients with asymptomatic increase in liver enzymes (Chang and Schiano, 2007).

All classes of antidepressants have been associated with risk of liver injury. The incidence is lower (0.5%–1%) among individuals using SSRIs and SNRIs but higher in individuals using TCAs and MAOI (up to 3%). Among the antidepressants, citalopram, escitalopram, paroxetine and fluvoxamine have been associated with lower risk of liver toxicity, whereas TCAs and MAOIs, along with nefazodone, venlafaxine, duloxetine and agomelatine, have been reported to cause life-threatening liver toxicity. Polypharmacy is one of the biggest risk factors for antidepressant-induced liver toxicity, especially if the drugs being used are metabolized through the same CYP enzymes (Voican et al., 2014). It is also important to be aware of the possibility of liver toxicity because the symptoms, e.g. fatigue, loss of appetite, can be confused with the symptoms of depression.

Almost all antipsychotics can cause a transient rise in liver enzymes, but this does not warrant discontinuation of treatment. It is important to follow up on the liver enzymes, which generally returns to baseline. Various trials have shown that about 0.1–0.8% of cases can develop serious liver toxicity. Phenothiazines, risperidone and clozapine are commonly associated with liver dysfunction (Sedky et al., 2012).

Among mood stabilizers, carbamazepine and valproic acid are notorious for their liver toxicity. Carbamazepine is metabolized through the CYP P450 3A4 enzyme and can induce its own metabolism, affect the metabolism of several other drugs, and lead to severe liver damage. Similarly, valproic acid can lead to steatosis in up to 60% of the individuals with long-term treatment (Luef et al., 2009). Among the stimulants, atomoxetine has been associated with severe liver toxicity, with liver enzyme levels rising up to 20 times the baseline (Sedky et al., 2012).

Hyperprolactinemia

Psychotropic medications are the leading cause of drug-induced hyperprolactinemia. Dopamine binds to D2 receptors on the lactotroph cells in the anterior pituitary and inhibits release of prolactin. On the other hand, serotonin plays an important role in increasing the prolactin secretion at night as well as release of prolactin in response to mammary stimulation. These two mechanisms are affected in patients taking antipsychotics and antidepressant medications, thus causing hyperprolactinemia (La Torre and Falorni, 2007). In men, increased prolactin levels can cause gynecomastia, hypogonadism, reduced libido, and rarely, galactorrhoea. In females, it generally presents with menstrual abnormalities and galactorrhoea.

Antipsychotics block D2 receptors and remove the inhibitory effect of dopamine, thus causing raised prolactin levels. Almost all typical antipsychotics can cause an increase in prolactin levels because of their strong D2 blockade (Goodnick et al., 2002). Among the newer antipsychotics, risperidone is by far the worst offender. Almost 1–10% of patients treated with risperidone developed clinically significant increases in prolactin level. In fact, some studies have shown that risperidone can cause a larger increase in prolactin levels when compared with typical antipsychotics (Kinon et al., 2003). Another atypical antipsychotic, amisulpiride, is also notorious for causing significant rises in prolactin levels (Wetzel et al., 1994).

Clozapine, olanzapine, and some of the newer atypical antipsychotics like aripiprazole and quetiapine, do not cause clinically significant increases in prolactin levels. Several investigators have tried to use dopamine agonists like bromocriptine and cabergoline to try and counteract the prolactin increasing effect of antipsychotics, but with mixed results. In some cases, use of these drugs was associated with a worsening of psychotic symptoms. Therefore, the best way of treating antipsychotic-induced hyperprolactinemia is by switching from risperidone or typical antipsychotics to drugs like olanzapine, aripiprazole or quetiapine (La Torre and Falorni, 2007).

Through their action on serotonin, antidepressants can also cause increased prolactin levels. The prolactin level increase with antidepressants rarely reaches levels high enough to cause clinical symptoms. Clinically significant elevations are generally caused when they are used together with antipsychotics. Among SSRIs, fluoxetine, paroxetine, and sertraline are most commonly associated with raised prolactin levels (Petit et al., 2003), whereas among TCAs, clomipramine, amoxapine, desipramine, and amitriptyline can cause significant increase in prolactin levels.

When faced with symptoms of hyperprolactinemia it is always important to rule out pregnancy and CNS tumours like prolactinomas before attributing it to a drug. Other endocrine abnormalities such as Cushing's disease and severe hypothyroidism should also be ruled out. Patients with increased prolactin levels warrant a thorough medical examination, which should include, but not be limited to, brain imaging and serum hormone levels.

Extrapyramidal side effects

The most common extrapyramidal side effects (EPS) include akathisia, dystonia, parkinsonian features, and tardive dyskinesia. Akathisia can be described as a constant urge to move and restlessness. Quick titration of antipsychotics has been associated with increased risk of akathisia. Dystonia can be described as painful involuntary contraction of muscles and are commonly seen in younger individuals possible because of the stronger dopamine response. Parkinsonian features include resting tremors, a mask-like face, and bradykinesia, and are commonly seen in the elderly because of the lower concentration of dopamine receptors in the striatum (Marsden and Jenner, 1980). Tardive dyskinesia is a set of peculiar involuntary movements such as lip smacking, lateral jaw movement, grimacing, and choreoathetoid movements, and these are more commonly seen in the elderly and with chronic antipsychotic treatment (Kane et al., 1982).

Antipsychotics cause EPS by blocking the dopamine receptors in the striatal region of the basal ganglia. PET studies have suggested that the risk of EPS is higher when medications block more than 80% of the dopamine receptors (Weiden, 2007). Antagonism of 5HT2A receptors increases the availability of dopamine in the basal ganglia and thus antipsychotics that act on the 5HT2-A receptors have reduced risk of EPS (Ichikawa and Meltzer, 1999). Almost all typical antipsychotics have been associated with EPS when given at therapeutic doses. The risk of EPS is higher with high potency typical antipsychotics (like Haldol) and decreases as the potency decreases (lower in chlorpromazine). Among the newer or atypical antipsychotics, the difference in the dose needed to control symptoms and the dose needed to cause EPS varies widely. On one hand, risperidone can cause EPS even at therapeutic doses whereas, on the other hand, this difference is highest with clozapine (EPS being very rare), followed by quetiapine, olanzapine, and ziprasidone in decreasing order (Jibson and Tandon, 1998).

Some antidepressants such as duloxetine, sertraline, escitalopram and bupropion have been associated with very rare cases of EPS (Madhusoodanan et al., 2010).

Strategies that can be used to prevent or manage EPS are as follows.

- Start with a low dose and titrate slowly
- Use antipsychotics with lower risk of EPS like quetiapine, olanzapine, or aripiprazole.
- For pure akathisia, beta blockers like propranolol can be used
- Anti-cholinergic drugs like benztropine and diphenhydramine can be along given along with the antipsychotics to prevent EPS.

Withdrawal/discontinuation syndromes

Often clinicians have to make a decision to discontinue a medication because of side effects, interactions, or patient requests. We must be aware of the possible effects of abrupt discontinuation of a therapeutic agent. In animal models, chronic reduction in dopamine levels in the brain results in hyper-sensitization of the dopamine receptors in the substantia nigra (Ungerstedt, 1971). Thus it is often observed that abrupt discontinuation of antipsychotics, especially those of high potency, results in development of akathisia, dyskinesia, and parkinsonian symptoms (Fallon and Dursun, 2011). It is also important to remember that most antipsychotics (chlorpromazine, clozapine, and olanzapine) have anti-cholinergic actions and abrupt discontinuation can result in cholinergic rebound, characterized by nausea, vomiting, abdominal cramping, sweating, headache, and muscle spasms. There is an increased risk of relapse of psychotic symptoms once an antipsychotic is discontinued (Cerovecki et al., 2013).

Discontinuation of almost all SSRIs has been noted to cause withdrawal symptoms which can include flu-like symptoms, tremors, tachycardia, shock-like sensation, paresthesia, myalgia, tinnitus, neuralgia, ataxia, vertigo, sexual dysfunction, sleep disturbances, vivid dreams, nausea and vomiting, diarrhoea, worsening anxiety, and mood instability. Paroxetine is the most notorious for withdrawal symptoms because of its short half-life. Interestingly, although tapering has some advantages, it does not completely eliminate the risk of developing withdrawal symptoms. These symptoms generally appear few days after stopping the medications and can last for a few weeks (Fava et al., 2015). Along with the above mentioned symptoms, venlafaxine discontinuation has been associated with blood pressure irregularities. Discontinuation of TCAs has been associated with symptoms similar to discontinuation of SSRIs. Desipramine and amineptine have been associated with parkinsonian symptoms and tremors of the jaw and tongue. Some case reports also suggest that neonates born to mothers who were taking TCAs during pregnancy can display signs such as irritability, respiratory difficulty, and poor feeding. Similar symptoms have also been reported in infants when breastfeeding mothers abruptly discontinue treatment with SSRIs (Harrison, 2001).

If the patient suffers from the withdrawal symptoms and needs continuation of antidepressant therapy, merely restarting the antidepressant medications helps resolve the withdrawal symptoms. If continuation of the antidepressant medication is needed, the patient can be managed symptomatically depending on the severity of symptoms.

Metabolic side effects

For most psychiatric disorders the biggest aim is optimum control of symptoms with eventual hope of remission. Like most other chronic diseases, this means that the patients have to keep taking medications for a long duration. One of the biggest concerns with chronic treatment with psychotropic medications is development of metabolic side effects such as weight gain, type 2 diabetes mellitus (T2DM), and dyslipidaemia.

Increased weight gain and increased risk of developing T2DM are commonly seen with the use of antipsychotic medications (Table 20.2). Studies show that the maximum increase in weight happens between four and 12 weeks of initiation of treatment, after which the rate of weight gain slows down. On average, the weight gain associated with clozapine was about 4.45 kg, olanzapine (4.15 kg), risperidone (2.10 kg) and ziprasidone (0.04 kg) (Tschoner et al., 2007). Increased central obesity plays in important role in the subsequent development of insulin resistance and dyslipidaemia.

Table 20.2 Metabolic side effects of antipsychotics

Antipsychotic	Weight gain	Risk for T2DM	Dyslipidaemia
Clozapine	+++	+	+
Olanzapine	+++	+	+
Risperidone	++	IR	IR
Quetiapine	++	IR	IR
Aripiprazole	+/–	–	–
Ziprasidone	+/–	–	–
Amisulpiride	–	–	–

+, increasing effect; –, no effect; IR, inconclusive results.

Reproduced from Tschoner A, et al. Metabolic side effects of antipsychotic medication, *International Journal of Clinical Practice*; 61, pp. 1356–70. Copyright (2007) with permission from John Wiley and Sons.

Among TCAs, amitriptyline is associated with weight gain more consistently as compared to imipramine and desipramine. Weight gain of around 0.6–1.4 kg was observed over 6–9 months of treatment. SSRIs have been shown to cause some weight loss but this effect is limited to the initial part of the therapy. In studies with long-term follow up, patients invariably showed an increase in weight when compared to baseline. Fluoxetine appears to be associated with more weight gain when compared to sertraline and paroxetine. Mirtazepine is notorious for causing increase in appetite and subsequent weight gain (Zimmermann et al., 2003). Mood stabilizers such as lithium, carbamazepine, and valproate have been consistently shown to cause weight gain among patients who have taken these medications over long periods.

Some of the strategies that can be used to treat metabolic syndromes secondary to psychotropic medication use are:

- Switching the patient to a weight-neutral drug. For example, using ziprasidone, lurasidone or aripiprazole in lieu of olanzapine or quetiapine, using bupropion in place of SSRI, etc.
- Educating the patient about the potential risk of weight gain and metabolic syndrome and encouraging patient to make lifestyle changes and to seek help of a nutritionist to help make any necessary dietary changes.

Cardiac side effects

Most common cardiac side effects associated with psychotropic medications are a result of their anti-cholinergic action. Low potency first generation antipsychotics like chlorpromazine and thioridazine, along with second generation antipsychotics like clozapine, olanzapine, and seroquel, have been associated with reports of dizziness and orthostatic hypotension as a result of their strong anti-cholinergic profiles. Individuals with pre-existing cardiac disease, poor renal function, and the elderly are at increased risk of developing dizziness/hypotension (Mackin, 2008).

Classically, all TCAs have been associated with prolongation of the QT interval by action on the sodium channels. Among the TCAs, amitriptyline was most commonly associated with reports of QT prolongation, whereas clomipramine was the TCA least likely to cause the same effect (Vieweg and Wood, 2004). Among the SSRIs, citalopram is the most notorious for causing QT prolongation. There have been some reports that suggest that fluoxetine and sertraline can cause a prolonged QT interval but this is generally observed in individuals with pre-existing risk factors for the same. Paroxetine appears to be the safest SSRI when it comes to it effect on the QT interval. Interestingly, escitalopram, which is an enantiomer of citalopram, has a lower effect on the QT interval when compared to citalopram (Beach et al., 2013). Among the antipsychotics, thirodazine, ziparsidone and intravenous formulation of haloperidol are associated with the highest risk of QT prolongation and torsades de pointes (TdP), whereas fluphenazine, haloperidol (intra-muscular and oral), paliperidone, and risperidone are associated with moderate risk of QT prolongation and TdP. Asenapine, olanzapine, quetiapine, lurasidone, and aripiprazole are associated with minimal risk of QT prolongation and TdP. Female sex, advanced age, and electrolyte dysfunction, along with renal and liver dysfunction, increases the risk of clinically significant QT prolongation. Care should be taken to get baseline EKGs followed by EKGs with every dose increase to keep a track of the QT interval (Beach et al., 2013).

Clozapine has repeatedly been associated with development of myocarditis. It is hypothesized that clozapine-induced myocarditis is a type 1 IgE-mediated hypersensitivity reaction. Clinically these cases present with tachycardia, chest pain, flu-like symptoms, eosinophilia, and elevated cardiac enzymes and inflammatory markers (Kilian et al., 1999). In rare cases, clozapine-induced myocarditis progresses into dilated cardiomyopathy (Merrill et al., 2006).

Conclusion

We conclude where we started: *'Adverse effects are an unavoidable risk of medication treatment. Although it is impossible to have an encyclopaedic knowledge of all adverse effects of psychiatric drugs, clinicians should be aware of the most frequent side effects, including those with significant medical consequences'.*

Some of the important ways to avoid medications side effects are as follows:

♦ Clinicians should try and establish a good timeline to assess the possibility that the presenting complaint is a medication side effect.

♦ Good baseline medical work up will go a long way in choosing an appropriate medication and avoiding side effects. This could include measuring liver functions, renal functions, BMI, performing a lipid panel, and EKG.

♦ Start at a low dose and titrate slowly, as per guidelines.

♦ Always think about possible drug-drug interaction

♦ If medication adverse reaction is suspected, stop the offending agent immediately, and follow with a proper evaluation of presenting symptoms. The decision to re-challenge the patient with the medication should be made by taking into account the clinical necessity and available guidelines.

♦ Always consult specialists.

References

de Abajo FJ. (2011). Effects of selective serotonin reuptake inhibitors on platelet function: mechanisms, clinical outcomes and implications for use in elderly patients. *Drugs Aging*, 28/5: 345–67. Available from: http://www.ncbi.nlm.nih.gov/pubmed/21542658

Alexander GC, Gallagher SA, Mascola A, Moloney RM, and Stafford RS. (2012). Increasing off-label use of antipsychotic medications in the United States, 1995–2008. *Pharmacoepidemiol Drug Saf*, 20/2:177–84.

Angst J. (1998). Sexual problems in healthy and depressed persons. *Int Clin Psychopharmacol*, 13/Suppl 6: S1–4. Available from: http://www.ncbi.nlm.nih.gov/pubmed/9728667

Beach SR, Celano CM, Noseworthy PA, Januzzi JL, and Huffman JC. (2013). QTc prolongation, Torsades de Pointes, and psychotropic medications. *Psychosomatics*, 54/1: 1–13. Available from: http://dx.doi.org/10.1016/j.psym.2012.11.001

Bella AJ and Shamloul R. (2013). Psychotropics and sexual dysfunction. *Cent Eur J Urol*, 66: 466–71.

Bliss SA and Warnock JK. (2013). Psychiatric medications: adverse cutaneous drug reactions. *Clin Dermatol*, 31/1: 101–9. Available from: http://www.ncbi.nlm.nih.gov/pubmed/23245981

Borman RA, Tilford NS, Harmer DW, Day N, Ellis ES, Sheldrick RL, Carey J, Coleman RA, and Baxter GS. (2002). 5-HT(2B) receptors play a key role in mediating the excitatory effects of 5-HT in human colon in vitro. *Br J Pharmacol*, 135/5: 1144–51. Available from: http://www.ncbi.nlm.nih.gov/pubmed/11877320

Bou Khalil R and Richa S. (2011). Thyroid adverse effects of psychotropic drugs: a review. *Clin Neuropharmacol*, 34/6: 248–55. Available from: http://www.ncbi.nlm.nih.gov/pubmed/21996646

Bozikas V, Petrikis P, and Karavatos A. (2001). Urinary retention caused after fluoxetine-risperidone combination. *J Psychopharmacol*, 15/2: 142–3. Available from: http://www.ncbi.nlm.nih.gov/pubmed/11448089

Cerovecki A, Musil R, Klimke A, Seemüller F, Haen E, Schennach R, Kühn KU, Volz HP, and Riedel M. (2013). Withdrawal symptoms and rebound syndromes associated with switching and discontinuing atypical antipsychotics: Theoretical background and practical recommendations. *CNS Drugs*, 27: 545–72.

Chang CY and Schiano TD. (2007). Review article: drug hepatotoxicity. *Aliment Pharmacol Ther*, 25/10: 1135–51. Available from: http://doi.wiley.com/10.1111/j.1365-2036.2007.03307.x

Cohen D and Monden M. (2013). White blood cell monitoring during long-term clozapine treatment. *Am J Psychiatry*, 170/4: 366–9.

Costagliola C, Parmeggiani F, and Sebastiani A. (2004). SSRIs and intraocular pressure modifications: evidence, therapeutic implications and possible mechanisms. *CNS Drugs*, 18/8: 475–84. Available from: http://www.ncbi.nlm.nih.gov/pubmed/15182218

Delieu JM, Horobin RW, and Duguid JK. (2006). Formation of immature neutrophil leucocytes in schizophrenic patients treated with various antipsychotic drugs: comparisons and predictions. *J Psychopharmacol*, 20/6: 824–8. Available from: http://jop.sagepub.com/cgi/doi/10.1177/0269881106061112

Duggal HS and Singh I. (2005). Psychotropic drug-induced neutropenia. *Drugs Today (Barc)*, 41/8: 517–26. Available from: http://www.ncbi.nlm.nih.gov/pubmed/16234875

Dupuis RE, Cooper AA, Rosamond LJ, and Campbell-Bright S. (1996). Multiple delayed peak lithium concentrations following acute intoxication with an extended-release product. *Ann Pharmacother*, 30/4: 356–60. Available from: http://www.ncbi.nlm.nih.gov/pubmed/8729888

Edler K, Gottfries CG, Haslund J, and Ravn J. (1971). Eye changes in connection with neuroleptic treatment especially concerning phenothiazines and thioxanthenes. *Acta Psychiatr Scand*, 47/4: 377–84. Available from: http://www.ncbi.nlm.nih.gov/pubmed/5146713

Fallon P and Dursun SM. (2011). A naturalistic controlled study of relapsing schizophrenic patients with tardive dyskinesia and supersensitivity psychosis. *J Psychopharmacol*, 25/6: 755–62. Available from: http://www.ncbi.nlm.nih.gov/pubmed/20147573

Fava GA, Gatti A, Belaise C, Guidi J, and Offidani E. (2015). Withdrawal symptoms after selective serotonin reuptake inhibitor discontinuation: a systematic review. *Psychother Psychosom*, 84/2: 72–81. Available from: http://www.ncbi.nlm.nih.gov/pubmed/25721705

Flanagan RJ and Dunk L. (2008). Haematological toxicity of drugs used in psychiatry. *Hum Psychopharmacol Clin Exp*, 23/S1: S27–41. Available from: http://doi.wiley.com/10.1002/hup.917

Fraunfelder FW, Fraunfelder FT, and Keates EU. (2004). Topiramate-associated acute, bilateral, secondary angle-closure glaucoma. *Ophthalmology*, 111/1: 109–11. Available from: http://www.ncbi.nlm.nih.gov/pubmed/14711721

Garnis-Jones S. (1996). Dermatologic side effects of psychopharmacologic agents. *Dermatol Clin*, 14/3: 503–8. Available from: http://linkinghub.elsevier.com/retrieve/pii/S0733863505703788

Georgiadis JR and Holstege G. (2005). Human brain activation during sexual stimulation of the penis. *J Comp Neurol*, 493/1: 33–8. Available from: http://doi.wiley.com/10.1002/cne.20735

Goldstein BJ and Goodnick PJ. (1998). Selective serotonin reuptake inhibitors in the treatment of affective disorders--III. Tolerability, safety and pharmacoeconomics. *J Psychopharmacol*, 12/3 Suppl B: S55–87. Available from: http://www.ncbi.nlm.nih.gov/pubmed/9808079

Goodnick PJ, Rodriguez L, and Santana O. (2002). Antipsychotics: impact on prolactin levels. *Expert Opin Pharmacother*, 3/10: 1381–91. Available from: http://www.ncbi.nlm.nih.gov/pubmed/12387684

Halperin D and Reber G. (2007). Influence of antidepressants on hemostasis. *Dialogues Clin Neurosci*, 9/1: 47–59. Available from: http://www.ncbi.nlm.nih.gov/pubmed/17506225

Hansen TE, Casey DE, and Hoffman WF. (1997). Neuroleptic intolerance. *Schizophr Bull*, 23/4: 567–82. Available from: http://www.ncbi.nlm.nih.gov/pubmed/9365996

Harrison Y. (2001). Antidepressant discontinuation syndromes—Clinical relevance, prevention and management. *Drug Saf*, 24/3: 183–97.

Ichikawa J and Meltzer HY. (1999). Relationship between dopaminergic and serotonergic neuronal activity in the frontal cortex and the action of typical and atypical antipsychotic drugs. *Eur Arch Psychiatry Clin Neurosci*, 249/ Suppl: 90–8. Available from: http://www.ncbi.nlm.nih.gov/pubmed/10654114

Jacob S. (2006). Hyponatremia associated with selective serotonin-reuptake inhibitors in older adults. *Ann Pharmacother*, 40/9: 1618–22. Available from: http://aop.sagepub.com/lookup/doi/10.1345/aph.1G293

Jibson MD and Tandon R. (1998). New atypical antipsychotic medications. *J Psychiatr Res*, 323–4: 215–28. Available from: http://www.ncbi.nlm.nih.gov/pubmed/9793875

Kane JM, Woerner M, Weinhold P, Wegner J, and Kinon B. (1982). A prospective study of tardive dyskinesia development: preliminary results. *J Clin Psychopharmacol*, 2/5: 345–9. Available from: http://www.ncbi.nlm.nih.gov/pubmed/6127353

Kilian JG, Kerr K, Lawrence C, and Celermajer DS. (1999). Myocarditis and cardiomyopathy associated with clozapine. *Lancet*, 354/9193: 1841–5. Available from: http://www.ncbi.nlm.nih.gov/pubmed/10584719

Kinon BJ, Gilmore JA, Liu H, and Halbreich UM. (2003). Prevalence of hyperprolactinemia in schizophrenic patients treated with conventional antipsychotic medications or risperidone. *Psychoneuroendocrinology*, 28/Suppl 2: 55–68. Available from: http://www.ncbi.nlm.nih.gov/pubmed/12650681

Lange-Asschenfeldt C, Grohmann R, Lange-Asschenfeldt B, Engel RR, Rüther E, and Cordes J. (2009). Cutaneous Adverse Reactions to Psychotropic Drugs. *J Clin Psychiatry*, 70/9: 1258–65. Available from: http://article.psychiatrist.com/?ContentType=START&ID=10004654

La Torre A, Conca A, Duffy D, Giupponi G, Pompili M, and Grözinger M. (2013). Sexual dysfunction related to psychotropic drugs: a critical review part II: antipsychotics.

Pharmacopsychiatry, 46/6: 201–8. Available from: http://www.ncbi.nlm.nih.gov/pubmed/23737244

La Torre D and Falorni A. (2007). Pharmacological causes of hyperprolactinemia. *Ther Clin Risk Manag*, 3/5: 929–51.

Leucht S, Cipriani A, Spineli L, Mavridis D, Orey D, Richter F, Samara M, Barbui C, Engel RR, Geddes JR, Kissling W, Stapf MP, Lässig B, Salanti G, and Davis JM. (2013). Comparative efficacy and tolerability of 15 antipsychotic drugs in schizophrenia: a multiple-treatments meta-analysis. *Lancet*, 382/9896: 951–62. Available from: http://dx.doi.org/10.1016/S0140-6736(13)60733-3

Li J, Tripathi RC, and Tripathi BJ. (2008). Drug-induced ocular disorders. *Drug Saf*, 31/2: 127–41. Available from: http://www.ncbi.nlm.nih.gov/pubmed/18217789

Lowe RF. (1966). Amitriptyline and glaucoma. *Med J Aust*, 2/11: 509–10. Available from: http://www.ncbi.nlm.nih.gov/pubmed/5923732

Luef G, Rauchenzauner M, Waldmann M, Sturm W, Sandhofer A, Seppi K, Trinka E, Unterberger I, Ebenbichler CF, Joannidis M, Walser G, Bauer G, Hoppichler F, and Lechleitner M. (2009). Non-alcoholic fatty liver disease (NAFLD), insulin resistance and lipid profile in antiepileptic drug treatment. *Epilepsy Res*, 86/1: 42–7. Available from: http://www.epires-journal.com/article/S0920-1211(09)00118-1/abstract

Mackin P. (2008). Cardiac side effects of psychiatric drugs. *Hum Psychopharmacol Clin Exp*, 23/S1: S3–14. Available from: http://doi.wiley.com/10.1002/hup.915

Madhusoodanan S, Alexeenko L, Sanders R, and Brenner R. (2010). Extrapyramidal symptoms associated with antidepressants—a review of the literature and an analysis of spontaneous reports. *Ann Clin Psychiatry*, 22/3: 148–56.

Malone DA, Camara EG, and Krug JH. (1992). Ophthalmologic effects of psychotropic medications. *Psychosomatics*, 33/3: 271–7. Available from: http://www.ncbi.nlm.nih.gov/pubmed/1410200

Marsden CD and Jenner P. (1980). The pathophysiology of extrapyramidal side-effects of neuroleptic drugs. *Psychol Med*, 10/1: 55–72. Available from: http://www.ncbi.nlm.nih.gov/pubmed/6104342

McGahuey CA, Gelenberg AJ, Laukes CA, Moreno FA, Delgado PL, McKnight KM, and Manber R. (2000). The Arizona Sexual Experience Scale (ASEX): reliability and validity. *J Sex Marital Ther*, 26/1: 25–40. Available from: http://www.ncbi.nlm.nih.gov/pubmed/10693114

McKnight RF, Adida M, Budge K, Stockton S, Goodwin GM, and Geddes JR. (2012). Lithium toxicity profile: a systematic review and meta-analysis. *Lancet*, 379/9817: 721–8. Available from: http://linkinghub.elsevier.com/retrieve/pii/S014067361161516X

Merrill DB, Ahmari SE, Bradford JM, and Lieberman JA. (2006). Myocarditis during clozapine treatment. *Am J Psychiatry*, 163/2: 204–8. Available from: http://www.ncbi.nlm.nih.gov/pubmed/16449471

Mitkov MV, Trowbridge RM, Lockshin BN, and Caplan JP. (2014). Dermatologic side effects of psychotropic medications. *Psychosomatics*, 55/1: 1–20. Available from: http://dx.doi.org/10.1016/j.psym.2013.07.003

Moeller JJ and Maxner CE. (2007). The dilated pupil: an update. *Curr Neurol Neurosci Rep*, 7/5: 417–22. Available from: http://www.ncbi.nlm.nih.gov/pubmed/17764632

Montejo AL, Montejo L, and Navarro-Cremades F. (2015). Sexual side-effects of antidepressant and antipsychotic drugs. *Curr Opin Psychiatry*, 28/6: 418–23. Available from: http://content.wkhealth.com/linkback/openurl?sid=WKPTLP:landingpage &an=00001504-201511000-00004

O'Neill RT and Anello C. (1996). Does research synthesis have a place in drug regulatory policy? Synopsis of issues: assessment of efficacy and drug approval. *Clin Res Regul Aff*, 13/ 1: 23–9. Available from: http://www.tandfonline.com/doi/full/10.3109/10601339609019626

Orwin A. (1983). Hair loss following lithium therapy. *Br J Dermatol*, 108/4: 503–4. Available from: http://doi.wiley.com/10.1111/j.1365-2133.1983.tb04607.x

Oshika T. (1995). Ocular adverse effects of neuropsychiatric agents. Incidence and management. *Drug Saf*, 12/4: 256–63. Available from: http://www.ncbi.nlm.nih.gov/ pubmed/7646824

Ouslander JG. (2004). Management of overactive bladder. *N Engl J Med*, 350/8: 786–99. Available from: http://www.ncbi.nlm.nih.gov/pubmed/14973214

Pauzé DK and Brooks DE. (2007). Lithium toxicity from an Internet dietary supplement. *J Med Toxicol*, 3/2: 61–2. Available from: http://www.ncbi.nlm.nih.gov/pubmed/18072162

Perrild H, Hegedüs L, Baastrup PC, Kayser L, and Kastberg S. (1990). Thyroid function and ultrasonically determined thyroid size in patients receiving long-term lithium treatment. *Am J Psychiatry*, 147/11: 1518–21. Available from: http://www.ncbi.nlm.nih.gov/pubmed/ 2221166

Petit A, Piednoir D, Germain M-L, and Trenque T. (2003). [Drug-induced hyperprolactinemia: a case-non-case study from the national pharmacovigilance database]. *Therapie*, 58/2: 159–63. Available from: http://www.ncbi.nlm.nih.gov/pubmed/12942857

Pfeifer WD, Davis LC, and van der Velde CD. (1976). Lithium accumulation in some endocrine tissues. *Acta Biol Med Ger*, 35/11: 1519–23. Available from: http://www.ncbi.nlm. nih.gov/pubmed/1022135

Reichenpfader U, Gartlehner G, Morgan LC, Greenblatt A, Nussbaumer B, Hansen RA, Van Noord M, Lux L, and Gaynes BN. (2014). Sexual dysfunction associated with second-generation antidepressants in patients with major depressive disorder: results from a systematic review with network meta-analysis. *Drug Saf*, 37/1: 19–31. Available from: http://www.ncbi.nlm.nih.gov/pubmed/24338044

Richa S and Yazbek JC. (2010). Ocular adverse effects of common psychotropic agents: a review. *CNS Drugs*, 24/6: 501–26. Available from: http://www.ncbi.nlm.nih.gov/pubmed/ 20443647

Satanove A. (1965). Pigmentation due to phenothiazines in high and prolonged dosage. *JAMA*, 191/4: 263–8. Available from: http://www.ncbi.nlm.nih.gov/pubmed/5899740

Schneider LS, Dagerman K, and Insel PS. (2006). Efficacy and adverse effects of atypical antipsychotics for dementia: meta-analysis of randomized, placebo-controlled trials. *Am J Geriatr Psychiatry*, 14/3: 191–210. Available from: http://www.ncbi.nlm.nih.gov/pubmed/ 16505124

Sedky K, Nazir R, Joshi A, Kaur G, and Lippmann S. (2012). Which psychotropic medications induce hepatotoxicity? *Gen Hosp Psychiatry*, 34/1: 53–61. Available from: http://www.ncbi. nlm.nih.gov/pubmed/22133982

Siddall JR. (1968). Ocular complications related to phenothiazines. *Dis Nerv Syst*, 29/3 Suppl: 10–3. Available from: http://www.ncbi.nlm.nih.gov/pubmed/4876740

Sills JM, Tanner LA, and Milstien JB. (1986). Food and Drug Administration monitoring of adverse drug reactions. *Am J Hosp Pharm*, 43/11: 2764–70. Available from: http://www. ncbi.nlm.nih.gov/pubmed/3799612

Spaulding SW, Burrow GN, Bermudez F, and Himmelhoch JM. (1972). The inhibitory effect of lithium on thyroid hormone release in both euthyroid and thyrotoxic patients. *J Clin Endocrinol Metab*, 35/6: 905–11. Available from: http://www.ncbi.nlm.nih.gov/pubmed/4634489

Spigset O. (1999). Adverse reactions of selective serotonin reuptake inhibitors: reports from a spontaneous reporting system. *Drug Saf*, 20/3: 277–87. Available from: http://www.ncbi.nlm.nih.gov/pubmed/10221856

Tredget J, Kirov A, and Kirov G. (2010). Effects of chronic lithium treatment on renal function. *J Affect Disord*, 126/3: 436–40. Available from: http://www.ncbi.nlm.nih.gov/pubmed/20483164

Tripathi RC, Tripathi BJ, and Haggerty C. (2003). Drug-induced glaucomas: mechanism and management. *Drug Saf*, 26/11: 749–67. Available from: http://www.ncbi.nlm.nih.gov/pubmed/12908846

Tschoner A, Engl J, Laimer M, Kaser S, Rettenbacher M, Fleischhacker WW, Patsch JR, and Ebenbichler CF. (2007). Metabolic side effects of antipsychotic medication. *Int J Clin Pract*, 61: 1356–70.

Tueth MJ. (1994). Emergencies caused by side effects of psychiatric medications. *Am J Emerg Med*, 12/2: 212–6. Available from: http://www.ncbi.nlm.nih.gov/pubmed/8161398

Uher R, Farmer A, Henigsberg N, Rietschel M, Mors O, Maier W, Kozel D, Hauser J, Souery D, Placentino A, Strohmaier J, Perroud N, Zobel A, Rajewska-Rager A, Dernovsek MZ, Larsen ER, Kalember P, Giovannini C, Barreto M, McGuffin P, and Aitchison KJ. (2009). Adverse reactions to antidepressants. *Br J Psychiatry*, 195/3: 202–10.

Ungerstedt U. (1971). Postsynaptic supersensitivity after 6-hydroxy-dopamine induced degeneration of the nigro-striatal dopamine system. *Acta Physiol Scand*, S367: 69–93. Available from: http://www.ncbi.nlm.nih.gov/pubmed/4332693

US Department of Health and Human Services. (2011). *Health, United States, 2010: With special feature on death and dying*. Hyattsville, MD: National Center for Health Statistics.

Verhamme KMC, Sturkenboom MCJM, Stricker BHC, and Bosch R. (2008). Drug-induced urinary retention: incidence, management and prevention. *Drug Saf*, 31/5: 373–88. Available from: http://www.ncbi.nlm.nih.gov/pubmed/18422378

Vieweg WVR and Wood MA. (2004). Tricyclic antidepressants, QT interval prolongation, and torsade de pointes. *Psychosomatics*, 45/5: 371–7. Available from: http://linkinghub.elsevier.com/retrieve/pii/S0033318204701504

Voican CS, Corruble E, Naveau S, and Perlemuter G. (2014). Antidepressant-induced liver injury: a review for clinicians. *Am J Psychiatry*, 171/4: 404–15. Available from: http://www.ncbi.nlm.nih.gov/pubmed/24362450

Wang PS, Aguilar-Gaxiola S, Alonso J, Angermeyer MC, Borges G, Bromet EJ, Bruffaerts R, de Girolamo G, de Graaf R, Gureje O, Haro JM, Karam EG, Kessler RC, Kovess V, Lane MC, Lee S, Levinson D, Ono Y, Petukhova M, Posada-Villa J, Seedat S, Wells JE. (2010). Use of mental health services for anxiety, mood, and substance disorders in 17 Countries in the WHO world mental health surveys. *Lancet*, 370/9590 : 841–50.

Weiden PJ. (2007). EPS profiles: the atypical antipsychotics are not all the same. *J Psychiatr Pract*, 13/1: 13–24. Available from: http://www.ncbi.nlm.nih.gov/pubmed/17242588

Wetzel H, Wiesner J, Hiemke C, and Benkert O. (1994). Acute antagonism of dopamine D2-like receptors by amisulpride: effects on hormone secretion in healthy volunteers. *J Psychiatr Res*, 285: 461–73. Available from: http://www.ncbi.nlm.nih.gov/pubmed/7897617

Whiskey E and Taylor D. (2007). Restarting clozapine after neutropenia: evaluating the possibilities and practicalities. *CNS Drugs*, 21/1: 25–35. Available from: http://www.ncbi.nlm.nih.gov/pubmed/17190527

Wills BK, Mycyk MB, Mazor S, Zell-Kanter M, Brace L, and Erickson T. (2006). Factitious lithium toxicity secondary to lithium heparin-containing blood tubes. *J Med Toxicol*, 2/2: 61–3. Available from: http://www.ncbi.nlm.nih.gov/pubmed/18072115

Xomalis D, Bozikas VP, Garyfallos G, Nikolaidis N, Giouzepas J, and Fokas K. (2006). Urinary hesitancy and retention caused by ziprasidone. *Int Clin Psychopharmacol*, 21/1: 71–2. Available from: http://www.ncbi.nlm.nih.gov/pubmed/16317320

Zimmermann U, Kraus T, Himmerich H, Schuld A, and Pollmächer T. (2003). Epidemiology, implications and mechanisms underlying drug-induced weight gain in psychiatric patients. *J Psychiatr Res*, 37/3: 193–220. Available from: http://linkinghub.elsevier.com/retrieve/pii/S0022395603000189

Chapter 21

Drug interactions involving psychotropic drugs

Subramoniam Madhusoodanan,
Marina Tsoy-Podosenin, Leah R. Steinberg,
and Nitin Tandan

Introduction to psychotropic drug interactions

Psychiatric patients often present with a number of comorbidities, requiring concurrent non-psychotropic pharmacological treatment, which may increase the risk for drug interactions (Short et al., 2009). Drug interactions may include, but are not limited to drug-drug interactions (DDIs), including over-the-counter (OTC) medications and smoking, drug-food interactions, drug-beverage interactions, drug-alcohol interactions, and drug-disease interactions (Gardiner et al., 2008; Hussar, 2013). Clinically significant DDIs occur when a patient concurrently takes two or more medications, resulting in changes of the effectiveness, tolerability, and/or toxicity of one drug (Ereshefsky et al., 2005; Labos et al., 2011; Muscatello et al., 2012; English et al., 2012; Burger et al., 2013). The two major types of DDIs include pharmacokinetic and pharmacodynamic interactions. Drug interactions may also be related to aging and/or certain disease states due to pathophysiological changes.

Metabolic drug interactions constitute a major portion of the spectrum of drug interactions. Many psychotropics, OTC medications, and dietary supplements undergo hepatic metabolism via cytochrome P450 (CYP).

Physicians should be aware of potential changes in drugs' concentrations to prevent toxicity and maximize the efficacy of prescribed treatments. Treatment-emergent adverse events are responsible for approximately 700,000 emergency department visits each year in the US, one-sixth of which require hospitalization for further treatment (CDC, 2012). Older adults are twice as likely to visit emergency departments for adverse drug events compared to younger adults. Close to two-thirds of hospitalizations for the elderly are due to unintentional overdoses, highlighting the importance of recognition and prevention of drug interactions (Budnitz et al., 2011).

This chapter provides an overview of common pharmacokinetic and pharmacodynamic interactions involving psychotropic drugs. We have classified the types of drug interactions according to their anticipated severity in order to provide clinical guidance (Madhusoodanan et al., 2014). The understanding of DDIs involving psychotropics is imperative for the provision of adequate care for psychiatric patients attending diverse treatment settings, including primary care practices.

Pharmacokinetic interactions

Absorption

Most psychotropic medications are administered orally. Interactions during the absorption phase affect the influx of drugs from the gut into the bloodstream. Factors affecting absorption include changes in gastrointestinal (GI) pH and/or motility. Some drugs (e.g. erythromycin and metoclopramide) may speed gastric emptying, potentially increasing initial absorption, but at the same time reducing total drug bioavailability. Factors that diminish intestinal motility (e.g. opiates, marijuana) may either reduce or increase absorption. For example, the anticholinergic effect of marijuana slows gut motility and may dramatically increase lithium levels, leading to lithium toxicity. Antacids, charcoal, kaolin-pectin, cholestyramine, and iron salts bind to drugs, forming complexes that pass unabsorbed through the GI lumen. Antacids may also decrease the rate of absorption of certain benzodiazepines (e.g. chlordiazepoxide). Proton pump inhibitors and histaminic H2 blockers may increase the absorption of midazolam and methadone by increasing gastric pH. Food may also affect the absorption of some psychotropic drugs like ziprasidone and lurasidone, which are recommended to be administered concurrently with food. However, drug interactions during the absorption phase have little relevance for psychotropic drugs because these compounds are mainly absorbed through passive diffusion (Wilkinson, 2001).

Transporter proteins regulate the transport of a large number of drugs across the intestinal epithelium. P-glycoprotein (P-gp), the most important of these transporters, is involved in the absorption, distribution, and elimination of drugs (Akamine et al., 2012). This carrier may substantially influence peripheral concentrations and bioavailability of certain drugs. P-gp regulates the permeability at several sites, including but not limited to the intestinal epithelia, lymphocytes, renal tubules, biliary tract epithelia, as well as capillary endothelial cells in the brain. As a part of the blood-brain barrier, P-gp ejects drugs back into the bloodstream, limiting drug availability to the central nervous system (CNS). Verapamil and quinidine inhibit P-gp, but their effect on the pharmacological activity of psychotropics is unclear (Akamine et al., 2012). Carbamazepine and St John's wort, which are inducers of P-gp, may reduce peripheral levels of risperidone and paliperidone. St John's wort was also shown to lower blood levels of cyclosporine and indinavir (Thompson et al., 2006).

Distribution

In the body, lipophilic antipsychotic drugs are bound to plasma proteins and distributed via the circulation. Most psychotropic drugs are more than 80% protein bound. Fluoxetine, aripiprazole, lorazepam, diazepam, and valproic acid are examples of highly protein bound psychotropic drugs. In contrast, venlafaxine, lithium, topiramate, gabapentin, pregabalin, and memantine are examples of drugs with minimal protein binding, and, therefore, fewer DDIs related to protein binding. Competition by two or more drugs for protein binding sites may result in displacement of a previously bound drug, potentially increasing free (i.e. pharmacologically active) peripheral levels of a given drug. Reduced concentrations of plasma proteins in patients with lower levels of serum proteins (e.g. patients with liver disease, nephrotic syndrome, severe malnourishment, and elderly patients) also may be associated with an increase in the fraction of the unbound drug. However, clinical impact of these interactions is limited since displacement from binding proteins results in an increase of metabolism and clearance of the displaced drug. Significant changes in drug concentration due to displacement from binding proteins may occur when a drug with high clearance is administered intravenously. Changes in the relative distribution of body fat and water alter the distribution of drugs, leading to changes in drug levels and toxicity.

Metabolism

Metabolism is an enzyme-mediated process of biotransformation of a drug to another form called the metabolite that may or may not be pharmacologically active. Phase I reactions include oxidation, reduction, and hydrolysis. Metabolic reactions convert lipophilic drugs into more polar metabolites, which then undergo phase II metabolic reactions (including conjugation and acetylation), leading to the formation of water-soluble products, which are readily excreted by the kidney. Most psychotropic drugs undergo both phase I and phase II metabolic reactions. Important exceptions include some benzodiazepines (lorazepam, oxazepam, and temazepam), which skip phase I metabolism, and thus are exclusively metabolized via phase II reactions. Most pharmacokinetic DDIs involve alterations in phase I metabolism. Most phase I reactions are catalysed by CYP enzymes, predominantly expressed in the hepatocytes (CYP3A4 isoenzyme is also expressed in the gut wall). CYPs comprise a group of approximately 50 oxidative heterogeneous isoenzymes classified into families by numbers (CYP1, CYP2 and CYP3) and subfamilies by a capital letter, based on shared amino acid sequences (Nebert et al., 1987). CYP isoenzymes play a pivotal role in the metabolism of over 80% of all prescribed drugs. The synthesis or activity of hepatic microsomal enzymes is affected by metabolic inhibitors and inducers, as well as genetic polymorphisms which determine the bioactivity of particular isoenzymes. Most psychotropics are metabolized by CYP2D6, 3A4, 1A2, 2C9, and 2C19 isoforms. Drugs that inhibit or induce the metabolic activity of CYP450 isoenzymes may affect the metabolism of psychotropics, resulting in changes of their efficacy and/or incidence of adverse effects (Huang, 2011; Nadkarni et al., 2012; Sockalingam et al., 2013).

Drugs that are metabolized by a particular CYP enzyme are referred to as *substrates*. Enzyme *inhibitors* impair the ability of the specific CYPs to metabolize their target substrates by competing for the same enzyme-binding site (competitive) or by binding to an allosteric site (noncompetitive). The common denominator of both mechanisms is a decreased rate of hepatic biotransformation of the substrate, leading to increments in serum concentrations and toxicity (if the substrate is an active drug). Inhibition of CYP isoenzymes may be either reversible or irreversible. When enzymes are reversibly inhibited, CYP function may be restored following the elimination of the inhibitory agent from the body, whereas with irreversible inhibition, the liver must synthesize a new enzyme before the re-establishment of full CYP activity. Inhibition is usually immediate, occurring via one or more of a variety of mechanisms (including competitive inhibition or inactivation of the enzyme). Although the majority of interactions caused by inhibition of CYP isoenzymes may increase the potential for side effects and/or toxicity, there are a few interactions where CYP inhibition may actually diminish the therapeutic efficacy of a drug. Prodrugs that require CYP-mediated activation include codeine, tamoxifen, and clopidogrel. Both codeine and tamoxifen are converted into their active metabolites—morphine and endoxifen, respectively—by CYP2D6, while clopidogrel is converted to its active form by either CYP2C19 (major) or CYP3A4 (minor), depending on the concentration of the drug. Inhibitors of CYP2D6—such as fluoxetine, paroxetine, and others—can reduce the effectiveness of codeine or tamoxifen, which is a concern in breast cancer chemotherapy (Spina et al., 2008; Caraci et al., 2011; English et al., 2012). The concurrent use of some selective serotonin reuptake inhibitors (SSRIs) in women taking tamoxifen may even result in higher cancer recurrence and mortality (Kelly et al., 2010).

Enzyme *inducers* increase the metabolism of CYP substrates, thereby reducing the peripheral concentration of the drug. The chronic use of ethanol induces the CYP2E1 isoenzyme, which converts acetaminophen into its toxic metabolite, N-acetyl-p-benzoquinone imine (NAPQI), with resultant hepatic damage even at normal therapeutic doses. The phenomenon of enzymatic induction is a gradual process, requiring enhanced synthesis of the metabolic enzyme. The time required for CYP to reach a new, elevated steady state level following the introduction of an inducer may range from a few days to a few weeks, depending on the half-life of the drug and the degradation half-life of the enzyme. Furthermore, the induction phenomenon is reversible. Upon discontinuation of an inducer, it may take approximately two to four weeks for the return of overall CYP activity to baseline rates. A fall in plasma levels of a substrate may not be apparent for days to weeks following the addition of an inducer. On the contrary, an elevation in plasma drug concentrations could suggest the previous discontinuation of an inducer or the addition of an inhibitor to the therapeutic regimen (Kalgutkar et al., 2007).

Phase I metabolism can also be mediated by non-CYP enzymes, the most significant of which are flavin-containing monooxygenase, monoamine oxidase (MAO), alcohol dehydrogenase, aldehyde dehydrogenase, aldehyde oxidase, and xanthine oxidase. The clinically significant interactions are between MAO inhibitors (MAOIs) and a vast array of noradrenergic, dopaminergic, and serotonergic drugs, as well as with dietary tyramine (e.g. certain types of cheese). Another DDI of clinical significance is the inhibition of aldehyde dehydrogenase by disulfiram (and possibly metronidazole).

Phase II metabolism, which also occurs in the liver, usually follows phase I metabolism. The most significant enzymatic family that carries out phase II reactions is the uridine 5'-diphosphate glucuronosyltransferase (UGT). Several drugs, including olanzapine, lamotrigine, and many narcotic analgesics, are primarily metabolized by UGTs (Liston et al., 2001). Phase II interactions do not cause any clinically significant DDIs.

Excretion

Most psychotropic medications are largely eliminated by hepatic metabolism, and factors that affect renal excretion (glomerular filtration, tubular reabsorption, active tubular secretion) are generally far less important to the pharmacokinetics of these drugs except lithium, for which such factors may have clinically significant consequences.

Lithium competes with sodium for reabsorption, mainly in the proximal tubules. Since lithium has a low therapeutic window, conditions resulting in decreased sodium (dehydration due to vomiting or polyuria, sodium restriction, use of thiazide diuretics) are likely to cause an increased proximal reabsorption of lithium, leading to increased lithium level and potential toxicity. Hypokalaemia could also enhance toxicity of lithium. Factors associated with an increased glomerular filtration rate (GFR), particularly pregnancy, may lead to an increase in lithium clearance and a decrease in lithium levels (English et al., 2012). In certain circumstances, an increment in renal excretion may be a therapeutic strategy for treatment of drug overdose. Urine acidification after administration of ascorbic acid, ammonium chloride, or methenamine mandelate enhances renal clearance of weak bases (e.g. amphetamines and phencyclidine). Alkalinization of the urine following the administration of sodium bicarbonate or acetazolamide may hasten the excretion of weak acids (including long-acting barbiturates, such as phenobarbital).

Genetic polymorphism

Several CYP isoenzymes involved in antidepressant metabolism have genetic variants referred to as single nucleotide polymorphisms (SNPs), which may affect enzymatic activity. For example, polymorphisms in the gene encoding CYP2D6 enzymes, which are responsible for the metabolism of approximately 25% of psychotropic drugs, have been reported. Inter-individual differences in metabolic capacity for these particular enzyme pathways (phenotype), which match closely with the underlying genetic polymorphism (genotype), have been demonstrated in human studies. The polymorphism of the CYP2D6 enzyme results in poor, intermediate, efficient, or ultra-rapid metabolizers (Ingelman-Sundberg, 2005). Evidence indicates that polymorphisms in the CYP2D6 may even contribute to treatment resistance and treatment intolerance in patients treated with SSRIs (Rasmussen-Torvik and McAlpine, 2007). For instance, ultra-rapid metabolizers that occur in approximately 5.5% of Western European populations would rapidly remove SSRIs metabolized by CYP2D6 (e.g. paroxetine), and may result in treatment non-response. Conversely, poor metabolizers could have a higher rate of treatment-emergent side effects. Similarly, polymorphisms in CYP2D6 enzymes may also influence the propensity for clinically significant DDIs (Ereshefsky et al., 2005). For example, individuals with intermediate or efficient phenotypes could be more prone to have significant interactions with the co-administration of fluoxetine and a potent inhibitor of CYP2D6 (e.g. quinidine), whereas this type of interaction would not be particularly relevant for ultra-rapid metabolizers. Ethnicity and the widely varying predominant polymorphism frequencies observed on CYP isoenzymes across the world have important implications for drug safety and dosage. For example, poor metabolizers of the CYP2D6 isoenzyme occur in 6–10% of Caucasians and 1–2% of Asians. About 1–2% of Caucasians and over 25% of Ethiopians are ultra-rapid metabolizers (Fleeman et al., 2011).

Pharmacodynamic interactions

Pharmacodynamics refers to 'what a drug does to the body', and includes effects on receptors and neurotransmitters, post-receptor effects, and neurochemical

interactions. While a drug's pharmacodynamics could be affected by the use of concomitant drugs, medical comorbidities and aging may also contribute to pharmacodynamic interactions (Turnheim, 2003). Pharmacodynamic drug interactions may be
agonistic or antagonistic. If target receptors are known, one can predict whether the
drug will act as an agonist or antagonist.

In this section, pharmacodynamic drug interactions involving psychotropics will be
reviewed, with a focus on moderate and severe interactions. Severe interactions should
be avoided, while moderate interactions should be closely monitored. In certain clinical scenarios, the concomitant use of drugs with potential for interactions may be necessary. In these situations, treatment should be initiated at lower doses, and adverse
effects closely monitored (see Tables 21.1–3).

SSRIs are potent inhibitors of serotonin (5-HT) reuptake. When SSRIs are concomitantly administered with drugs that increase the synthesis and/or release of 5-HT
(e.g. MAOIs), or inhibit the reuptake of this monoamine from the synaptic cleft into
the presynaptic neuron (e.g. serotonin norepinephrine reuptake inhibitors (SNRIs),
an additive DDI is anticipated. Direct 5-HT agonists, such as atypical antipsychotics,
or drugs that increase the sensitivity of postsynaptic receptor (e.g. lithium, valproate)
may cause interactions when combined with SSRIs. These DDIs could result in serotonin syndrome, which may be severe (Sternbach, 1991). Moderate interactions occur
when SSRIs are given concomitantly with opioids, antiemetics (5-HT3 antagonist,
e.g. ondansetron), and antipsychotics. Combination of dextromethorphan, which
is a weak 5-HT reuptake inhibitor and SSRIs, especially fluoxetine and paroxetine,
may increase serum concentrations of dextromethorphan, possibly leading to serotonin syndrome. SNRIs inhibit serotonin and NE transporters (NET). They include
venlafaxine and desvenlafaxine, duloxetine, and milnacipran (not approved in the
US for depression, but approved for fibromyalgia). Bupropion is a norepinephrine-
dopamine reuptake inhibitor (NDRI). Norepinephrine reuptake inhibitors (NRIs) are
not very selective since they also block other receptors. They include atomoxetine,
reboxetine, and edivoxetine. NRIs given with beta2-agonists and sympathomimetics
may cause tachycardia and/or hypertension. Trazodone is referred to as serotonin
antagonist-reuptake inhibitor (SARI), and when concurrently used with other drugs
that alter serotonin metabolism/concentration, may also lead to DDIs.

Monoamine oxidase inhibitors (MAOIs) are mostly irreversible enzyme inhibitors,
which significantly increase concentrations of norepinephrine (NE), dopamine (DA),
and 5-HT. Patients taking any of the MAOIs, like phenelzine, tranylcypromine, or isocarboxazid should be counselled to avoid tyramine-rich foods, which may significantly
increase NE release, leading to potentially fatal hypertensive crisis, and even stroke.
The concomitant use of sympathomimetics, like decongestants (e.g. ephedrine), may
also elevate blood pressure through adrenergic stimulation. Antihistamine decongest-
ant drugs may not cause this type of DDI. Brompheniramine and chlorpheniramine
are 5-HT reuptake inhibitors, which may cause serotonin syndrome when combined
with MAOIs through an increment in 5-HT levels (Sternbach 1991). Cough medicines
with expectorants and codeine are generally safe, with the exception of dextrometho-
phan. For local anaesthesia, an agent that does not contain vasoconstrictor drugs may
be preferred. For elective surgeries, MAOIs should be discontinued ten days prior to
the procedure (Stahl, 2013).

Table 21.1 Outcome-based classification of **severe** drug-drug interactions

Involved drugs	Mechanism	Outcome	Clinical management
Beta-blockers: carvedilol, metoprolol, propranolol	fluoxetine, paroxetine Strong CYP2D6 inhibition	Increased (↑) level of beta-blockers. Severe bradycardia, hypotension, atrioventricular block	Avoid combination. Consider atenolol, nadolol, sotalol as a beta-blocker or citalopram as an antidepressant
	chlorpromazine, thioridazine, thiothixene CYP2D6 inhibition	↑ level of beta-blockers. Severe bradycardia, hypotension, atrioventricular block	Avoid combination. Consider atenolol, nadolol, sotalol as a beta-blocker
Calcium channel blockers: nicardipine, nimodipine, verapamil	fluoxetine, fluvoxamine, nefazodone Strong CYP3A4 inhibition	↑ level of CCB. Pathologic bradycardia, hypotension, cardiac arrhythmias	Consider dose adjustment (decrease dose of CCB by 50%)
Antiarrhythmics: encainide, flecainide, mexiletine, propafenone	duloxetine, fluoxetine, paroxetine Strong CYP2D6 inhibition	↑ level of antiarrhythmics. Rebound arrhythmias, ataxia, nausea, vomiting, heartburn	Avoid combination. Consider citalopram as an antidepressant
Antiarrhythmics: amiodarone, disopyramide, procainamide, quinidine, sotalol **Antimicrobials:** gatifloxacin, moxifloxacin	amisulpride, chlorpromazine, haloperidol, pimozide, quetiapine, sertindole, thioridazine, ziprasidone Additive or potentiating effect	QTc prolongation: arrhythmias, ventricular fibrillation, torsades de pointes, sudden death	Avoid combination
TCAs: amitriptyline, clomipramine, desipramine imipramine	terbinafine CYP2D6 inhibition	Potential TCA toxicity	Consider dose adjustment, monitor for CNS and CV effects

(continued)

Table 21.1 Continued

Involved drugs	Mechanism	Outcome	Clinical management
TCAs: amitriptyline, clomipramine, desipramine, imipramine	amisulpride, chlorpromazine, pimozide, sotalol, thioridazine, trifluoperazine, ziprasidone	Additive or potentiating effect	QTc prolongation	Avoid combination or closely monitored for CV effects
warfarin	disulfiram, fluoxetine, fluvoxamine, paroxetine, quetiapine, sertraline, valproic acid	CYP3A4, 2C9, 2C19 inhibition, protein binding displacement	↑INR, risk of bleeding	Monitor INR, PT, dose adjustment
MAOIs: isocarboxazid, moclobemide, phenelzine, selegiline, tranylcypromine	**Antidepressants:** buspirone, SNRIs, SSRIs, St John's wort, TCAs, trazodone **Opioids:** fentanyl, meperidine, methadone, tramadol sympathomimetics cold/allergy/sinus medications containing brompheniramine, chlorpheniramine, dextromethorphan, linezolid	Excessive serotonergic central and peripheral synergism. Increased serotonin production, neuronal release and decreased reuptake.	Serotonin Syndrome*	Avoid combination

	Interacting drugs	Mechanism	Effect	Management
	lithium, maprotiline, procarbazine, pseudoephedrine, non-subcutaneous sumatriptan			
SSRIs	**Antiemetics:** 5-HT3 antagonists, dextromethorphan, linezolid, St John's wort	Increase in serotonin levels	Serotonin Syndrome*	Avoid combination; taper off St John's wort before initiating SSRI
linezolid	SNRIs, TCAs, and mirtazapine	Increase in serotonin levels	Serotonin Syndrome*	Avoid combination
Antiemetics: 5-HT3 antagonists, e.g. metoclopramide	lithium, mirtazapine, SNRIs, TCAs, trazodone	Increase in serotonin levels	Serotonin Syndrome*	Avoid combination
TCAs	**Antihypertensives:** alpha2-agonist, like alpha-methyldopa, clonidine, guanabenz	TCAs may diminish the antihypertensive effect of alpha2-agonist	Hypertensive crisis°	Discontinue if blood pressure starts rising
	ephedra	Increase in NE		
MAOIs	Dietary amines (tyramine), ephedra, methyldopa	Increase in catecholamines	Hypertensive crisis°	Discontinue if blood pressure starts rising
	buspirone	Mechanism unknown		

(continued)

Table 21.1 Continued

Involved drugs	Mechanism	Outcome	Clinical management
beta-adrenergic blockers	Possible beta-blockade in the presence of unopposed alpha-adrenergic activity		

Notes: CCB—Calcium channel blockers; CNS—Central nervous system; CV—Cardiovascular; INR—International normalized ratio; MAOIs- monoamine oxidase inhibitors; PT—Prothrombin time; SNRIs—Serotonin norepinephrine reuptake inhibitors; SSRIs—Selective serotonin reuptake inhibitors; TCAs—Tricyclic antidepressants

*Serotonin Syndrome:

- *Mental status changes*: anxiety, agitation, delirium, restlessness, and disorientation
- *Autonomic manifestations*: diaphoresis, tachycardia, hyperthermia, shivering, hypertension (rapid fluctuations of vital signs), vomiting, and diarrhoea
- *Neuromuscular hyperactivity*: tremor, muscle rigidity, myoclonus, hyperreflexia, and bilateral Babinski sign;
- *Death*

°Hypertensive crisis:

- *Hypertensive urgency* (BP > 180 systolic OR > 110 diastolic) with no associated acute end-organ damage: headache, nosebleed, anxiety, shortness of breath
- *Hypertensive emergency* (BP > 180 systolic OR > 120 diastolic) with associated acute end-organ damage: hypertensive encephalopathy, retinal haemorrhages, papilledema, stroke, loss of consciousness, aortic dissection, pulmonary edema, acute and subacute kidney injury.

Table 21.2 Outcome-based classification of **moderate** drug-drug interactions

Involved drugs	Mechanism	Outcome	Clinical Management
Antidepressants: bupropion, duloxetine, fluoxetine, fluvoxamine, paroxetine, sertraline	CYP2D6 inhibition prevents opioids from conversion into an active metabolite	Reduction of analgesic effect of opioids	Dose adjustment, consider fentanyl
Antidepressants: fluoxetine, fluvoxamine, nefazodone	CYP3A4 inhibition by antidepressants. CYP2D6 inhibition by antiarrhythmics.	Increased (↑) level of antidepressants and antiarrhythmics.	Monitor closely, consider dose adjustment or alternative drugs
Class III antiarrhythmics: amiodarone, sotalol			
TCAs: amitriptyline, clomipramine, imipramine	CYP3A4 inhibition	↑ TCA plasma level	Monitor for side effects, dose reduction, consider azithromycin
Antimicrobials: clarithromycin, erythromycin, troleandomycin **Antifungals:** fluconazole, itraconazole, ketoconazole, **Antiretrovirals:** indinavir, ritonavir **Calcium channel blockers:** diltiazem, verapamil			
Others: carbamazepine, chronic alcohol use, isoniazid, phenobarbital, rifampin, tobacco products	CYP3A4 induction	DecreasedTCA plasma level	Dose adjustment
Oral contraceptives (OCP)	CYP3A4 induction	Accelerated clearance of OCP, compromised contraceptive efficacy	Consider use of an additional method of birth control
carbamazepine, St John's wort			

(continued)

Table 21.2 Continued

Involved drugs		Mechanism	Outcome	Clinical Management
Cyclosporine A, tacrolimus	St John's wort	CYP3A4 induction	Subtherapeutic levels of cyclosporine A/ tacrolimus, transplant rejection	Consider an SSRI
Warfarin	carbamazepine, St John's wort, tobacco products, trazodone	CYP3A4, 1A2 and 2C9 induction	Decreased INR Decreased anticoagulant effect	Monitor INR, dose adjustment
HCV protease inhibitors: boceprevir, telaprevir	desipramine, imipramine, trazodone	HCV protease inhibitors inhibit CYP2D6, 1A2, 2C19, 3A and P-gp	Potential for ↑ concentration of antidepressants: dizziness, hypotension, syncope	Use with caution, low doses recommended
	aripiprazole, clozapine, paliperidone, quetiapine, risperidone, ziprasidone	HCV protease inhibitors inhibit CYP2D6, 1A2, 2C19, 3A and P-gp	Potential for ↑ concentration of antipsychotic. EPS, sedation, weight gain.	Use with caution, monitor for toxicity, low doses recommended
Tamoxifen	bupropion, fluoxetine, paroxetine	Strong CYP2D6 inhibition prevents tamoxifen from conversion into an active metabolite	Failure of breast cancer therapy	Avoid combining with tamoxifen
	duloxetine, fluvoxamine, sertraline	Moderate CYP2D6 inhibition decreases the conversion into an active metabolite	Reduced bioactivation of tamoxifen	Consider venlafaxine, mirtazapine (minimal CYP2D6 inhibition) citalopram, escitalopram (minimal CYP2D6 inhibition)

Loperamide	Quinidine	Quinidine is a P-gp inhibitor	Respiratory depression (increased loperamide concentration in the brain)	Monitor closely, use alternatives
ARBs (losartan)	fluoxetine, fluvoxamine, nefazodone	CYP2C9, CYP3A4 inhibition	Decreased losartan metabolism. May cause hypotension, dizziness	Consider dose adjustment
Itraconazole, ketoconazole	paroxetine, risperidone	Itraconazole and ketoconazole are P-gp and CYP3A4 inhibitors	Increased level of psychotropics	Monitor side effects, consider dose adjustment
Lithium	ACE inhibitors, ARBs, COX-2 inhibitors, metronidazole, NSAIDs, tetracycline, thiazide diuretics	Inhibition of lithium clearance	Increased lithium level, potential lithium toxicity	Lithium dose reduction and level monitoring. Beta-blocker instead of ACEI
	Methylxanthines: theophylline, aminophylline Osmotic diuretics: mannitol Others: sodium bicarbonate, sodium chloride load	Increase renal clearance	Decreased lithium level	Lithium level monitoring
	Urine alkalinizing agents: acetazolamide, sodium bicarbonate, Osmotic diuretics: mannitol, urea Others: sodium chloride ingestion	Increases lithium secretion	Decreased lithium level	Lithium level monitoring
Primidone	Fluvoxamine	CYP2C19 inhibition prevents primidone from conversion into an active metabolite	Failure of anticonvulsant therapy	Consider citalopram, escitalopram
Citalopram, escitalopram	Prednisone and rifampin	CYP2C19 inducers	Failure of antidepressive treatment	Consider dose adjustment. Consider an alternative agent

(continued)

Table 21.2 Continued

Involved drugs		Mechanism	Outcome	Clinical Management
HCV protease inhibitors: boceprevir, telaprevir	Duloxetine	CYP1A2, CYP2D6 inhibition	Risk of hepatotoxicity	Avoid combination
Fluoxetine	Ritonavir	Strong CYP2D6 inhibition	Side effects of fluoxetine, serotonin syndrome	Consider sertraline, citalopram, escitalopram as a safer choice
Efavirenz, lopinavir, nevirapine, ritonavir	Methadone	CYP3A4 inhibitors	Increased methadone level can cause respiratory depression and cardiac arrhythmias	Monitor for side effects, adjust methadone dosage
Valproic acid	Lamotrigine	Unknown mechanism	Increased level of lamotrigine, including hypersensitivity reactions (Stevens-Johnson syndrome)	Monitor for side effects, consider dosage adjustment
Carbamazepine	Furosemide, thiazide diuretics	Unknown mechanism	Severe hyponatremia	Monitoring of electrolytes
	Clarithromycin, danazol, diltiazem erythromycin, fluconazole, fluoxetine, fluvoxamine, isoniazid, itraconazole, ketoconazole, nefazodone, propoxyphene, valproic acid, verapamil	CYP3A4 inhibitors	Increased risk of carbamazepine toxicity (ataxia, drowsiness, slurred speech, nausea, vomiting, tremors, seizures, blurred vision)	Monitor for side effects, consider dosage adjustment

Phenytoin, phenobarbital	Microsomal enzyme inducers	Subtherapeutic carbamazepine level	Dose adjustment
Clozapine	Unknown mechanism	Bone marrow suppression	Monitor cell blood count, avoid combination
Levetiracetam	Additive effect of CNS depression	Sedation, blurred vision, slurred speech, impaired perception of time and space, slowed reflexes and breathin, psychomotor impairment	Monitor for side effects, consider dosage adjustment
Aspirin, clopidogrel	Antiplatelet activity, increased gastric acidity	Increased risk of abnormal bleeding	Monitor coagulation, consider alternative antidepressant
Clopidogrel	CYP2C19 inhibition	Impaired efficacy of clopidogrel	Consider alternative antidepressant

Notes: ACE—Angiotensin-converting enzyme; ARBs—Angiotensin II receptor antagonists; CNS—Central nervous system; EPS—Extrapyramidal side effects; GI—Gastrointestinal; HCV—Hepatitis C virus; MAOIs—monoamine oxidase inhibitors; SNRIs—Serotonin norepinephrine-reuptake inhibitors; SSRIs—selective serotonin-reuptake inhibitors; TCAs—Tricyclic antidepressants

*Lithium toxicity may include:

- *GI symptoms:* nausea, vomiting, and diarrhoea;
- *Neurologic symptoms:* sluggishness, ataxia, dysarthria, delirium;
- *Neuromuscular excitability:* irregular coarse tremors, fasciculations, or myoclonic jerks

Table 21.3 Outcome-based classification of **mild** drug-drug interactions

Involved drugs		Mechanism	Outcome	Clinical management
HCV protease inhibitors: Boceprevir, telaprevir	Desvenlafaxine, mirtazapine, sertraline, venlafaxine	CYP 2B6, 3A4, 2D6, UGT inhibition by HCV protease inhibitors	Potential increase in antidepressant concentration, clinical significance unknown	Monitor patient for adverse reactions, use with caution
Tamoxifen	Mirtazapine, venlafaxine	Minimal CYP2D6 inhibition	Unknown	Safest choice; monitor patient
	Citalopram, escitalopram	Slight CYP2D6 inhibition	Unknown	Secondary choice
Hypnotic sedatives	Erythromycin	CYP3A4 inhibitor	Somnolence, headache and nausea	Monitor patient for neurological signs
Caffeine	Fluvoxamine	CYP1A2 inhibitor	Anxiety and palpitation	Monitor patient
Morphine	Clomipramine, nefazodone, nialamide, pargyline	Interaction(s) unidentified	Enhanced analgesic effects	Monitor patient for increased sedation
Antipsychotics	Acetylcholinesterase inhibitors (central)	Possibly due to a relative acetylcholine/ dopamine imbalance	Increased EPS	Monitor patient for new, abnormal movements
SSRIs	Cyproheptadine	Antagonistic action	May diminish the therapeutic effect of SSRIs	Monitor patient for adverse reactions
TCAs	Acetylcholinesterase inhibitors (e.g: donepezil, galantamine, rivastigmine)	Antagonistic action	May diminish the therapeutic effect of Acetylcholinesterase inhibitors	Monitor patient for adverse reactions
Mirtazapine, SNRIs, TCAs	Alpha-2 agonist (exception: apraclonidine)	Interaction(s) unidentified	May diminish the antihypertensive effect of alpha-2 agonist.	Monitor changes in blood pressure
Antipsychotics, lithium	Amphetamines	Interaction(s) unidentified	May diminish the stimulatory effect of amphetamines	Monitor patient for adverse reactions

Notes: EPS—Extrapyramidal side effects; HCV—Hepatitis C nirus; SNRIs—Serotonin norepinephrine-reuptake inhibitors; SSRIs—Selective serotonin-reuptake inhibitors; TCAs—Tricyclic antidepressants.

Tricyclic antidepressants (TCAs) that block reuptake pumps of both NE and 5-HT also have varying antagonistic effects on histaminergic, muscarinic, and alpha-1 adrenergic receptors. TCAs, when combined with ipratropium or tiotropium, may cause additive anticholinergic side effects, including worsening dry mouth, constipation, and urinary retention (Lexicomp Online®, 2015).

Antipsychotics bind to numerous receptors, including serotonergic, dopaminergic, muscarinic, histaminergic, and alpha-adrenergic receptors. These drugs also may act on 5-HT and NE transporters (SERT and NET). Antipsychotics, when combined with anticholinergic drugs like benztropine, trihexyphenidyl hydrochloride, or diphenhydramine, may cause additive anticholinergic side effects. Atropine may potentially interact with all classes of antipsychotics (Ciraulo, 2006). When combined with CNS depressants, such as alcohol or doxylamine, atropine may have additive effects, including excessive sedation.

Intensity-based classification of clinically significant drug-drug interactions

Based on the intensity of clinical outcome, we have classified DDIs into severe, moderate, and mild (Madhusoodanan et al., 2014).

Severe interactions (see Table 21.1) may be acutely life threatening. These interactions are more often inhibitory interactions with cardiovascular drugs, or DDIs between MAOIs and SSRIs, other antidepressants, or a tyramine-rich diet, leading to serotonin syndrome or hypertensive crisis (Ereshefsky, 2009).

Moderate interactions (see Table 21.2) include toxic side effects due to increased levels or lowered efficacy due to decreased plasma levels of the substrate. The list is not all-inclusive because it is beyond the scope of this chapter. Since many antipsychotics may prolong the QTc interval (e.g. thioridazine, ziprasidone, amisulpride, flupenthixol, fluphenazine, haloperidol, levomepromazine, melperone, perphenazine, pimozide, pipamperone, quetiapine, risperidone, sertindole, and sulpiride), their combination with drugs known to increase the QTc interval, or those which cause electrolyte imbalances (e.g. amiodarone, disopyramide, mefloquine, procainamide, quinidine, erythromycin, sotalol) should be avoided. Use of carbamazepine, a potent 3A4 inducer, with quetiapine, which is a substrate for 3A4, may decrease quetiapine plasma concentrations up to 90%. This could lead to a lack of efficacy of the antipsychotic drug (Castberg et al., 2007).

Mild interactions (see Table 21.3) may lead to minor reductions in efficacy and/or non-significant side effects. For example, fluvoxamine, a potent CYP1A2 inhibitor, may increase caffeine plasma concentrations, leading to anxiety and tachycardia.

Age-related pharmacokinetic and pharmacodynamic changes and their implications in the elderly

Elderly patients are at high risk for DDIs due to age-related pharmacokinetic and pharmacodynamic changes, comorbidities, and concurrent medications (Devane, 1998). DDIs have been shown to be a significant factor for increased hospitalizations due to drug toxicity in this population. Therefore, the use of psychotropics in the elderly should follow the rule 'start low, go slow' (i.e. starting doses should generally be about 25–50% of the initial dose for a young adult), and titrating to maintenance doses should be slower (final maintenance doses between 30–50% of young adult's doses are usually advised) (American Psychiatric Association, 1997; Sajatovic et al., 2000).

Total body water and lean body mass decrease with a relative increase in the body fat. The prolonged half-life of lipid soluble drugs (e.g. benzodiazepines) is secondary to a higher volume of distribution (Devane, 1998; Klotz et al., 1975), which leads to higher rates of side effects, some of which may be serious (e.g. falls). Water-soluble drugs (e.g. lithium) have a lower volume of distribution, which may result in higher serum levels (and toxicity) in the elderly unless appropriate dose adjustments are made (Mangoni and Jackson, 2004).

Age-related changes in liver enzymes are not uniform (i.e. the level of some CYP isoenzymes decreases while the level of others remain unchanged). Thus, differential drug effects depending on the mechanisms of the interactions and the CYP system primarily involved ensue. Hepatic clearance of drugs metabolized by phase I reactions is more likely to be prolonged in the elderly. Usually, age does not greatly affect clearance of drugs that are metabolized by conjugation (phase II reactions). The amount of a drug that will be metabolized by the liver depends on hepatic blood flow. Hepatic clearance would, therefore, be influenced by the extraction ratio and portal blood flow. The former depends on how capable the liver is of metabolizing drugs. Drugs are usually classified depending on their ratio of extraction as high, intermediate, or low. When the extraction ratio is high, clearance will be rate-limited by perfusion. In the elderly, liver size and blood flow are decreased. Therefore, when the extraction rate is low, clearance is not substantially affected by blood flow, and drugs with a high extraction rate only will be affected by aging (Mangoni and Jackson, 2004).

Older people have a decrease in renal function, especially the GFR. This change will affect the clearance of water-soluble drugs. Small changes in renal excretion may cause lithium toxicity, which may be serious considering its narrow therapeutic index (Hewick et al., 1977). Similar to the liver, kidney mass also decreases with age (Dunnill and Halley, 1973). The number of nephrons decreases and blood flow is reduced. Serum creatinine levels often remain within reference range despite a decrease in GFR due to the lower muscle mass and the relatively limited physical activity of the elderly compared to younger adults, which limits the synthesis of creatinine. Normal serum creatinine levels in the elderly may mislead clinicians to assume normal kidney function. Decreases in tubular function with age are similar to changes in GFR. The daily dose of drugs that rely heavily on renal elimination should be lower and/or the frequency of dosing be decreased in elderly populations. As renal function is dynamic, maintenance doses of drugs may need adjustment when patients become ill or dehydrated, or if they have recently recovered from dehydration (Shi and Klotz, 2011). Pharmacodynamic changes are not as predictable and clear as pharmacokinetic ones.

Discussion

In humans, isoforms CYP2D6 and 3A4 are responsible for the metabolism of most psychotropics, and may be induced or inhibited by other drugs or substances. Besides co-administered drugs, the patient's physiological status (age, gender, ethnicity, diet, and comorbidity) as well as genetic polymorphisms in CYP enzymes may substantially impact drug-metabolizing enzyme activity (Sandson et al., 2005). It has been estimated that genetic factors may explain 20–95% of the inter-individual variability, therapeutic response, and tolerability of psychiatric drugs. In 2006, the FDA issued updated guidelines for in vitro and in vivo drug interaction studies of drugs in developmental phase. A change of 30% in drug clearance has been proposed as a clinically significant threshold. The time-course of DDIs is often neglected. For example, plasma concentrations of most second-generation antipsychotics may decline rapidly one to two weeks after the addition of carbamazepine and may continue to decrease for up to one month. Conversely, when an inducer is discontinued, plasma drug levels may continue to increase steadily for several weeks. In drug interactions involving either inhibition or induction, a patient's clinical status could remain altered long after changes in therapeutic regimens. Therefore, adverse events and a worsening clinical scenario are often not attributed to an underlying drug interaction. The spectrum of drug interactions with psychotropic medications varies widely in intensity, onset, and duration. Even if the interaction is not severe and life threatening, long-term DDIs can result in poor tolerability and/or reduced efficacy, with possible impact on clinical outcomes and/or treatment compliance. Based on a review of relevant publications (Ereshefsky, 2009; Schellander and Donnerer, 2010; Preskorn and Flockhart, 2006; Kennedy et al., 2013), the following guidelines are recommended to avoid clinically significant DDIs.

Recommendations

1. Most severe DDIs result in cardiovascular complications, and therefore taking a careful medical history is important, including screening for known cardiac risk factors, and regular monitoring of ECG changes from baseline, especially in middle-aged and older adults and in individuals at risk for cardiovascular illnesses.

2. The frequency of adverse reactions occurring as a result of DDIs is proportional to the number of medications a patient takes. Thus, the number of prescribed medications should be kept as low as possible, while the elimination of unnecessary medications, including OTC medications and herbal supplements should be prioritized. The patient should be requested to prepare the list of medications (and doses), including OTC medications, herbal supplements, and dietary patterns. Information regarding the use of alcohol, recreational drugs, and tobacco products should also be collected. The physician should then revise the list of medications, and, if possible, change therapeutic regimens to avoid the occurrence of clinically significant DDIs.

3. Ascertain if drugs involved in DDIs could be substituted by another drug with similar spectrum of efficacy but with lower potential for interactions. Among

antipsychotics, *ziprasidone* and *paliperidone* have the least potential for DDIs via the CYP system. Ziprasidone metabolism is largely mediated by a non-CYP mechanism involving the aldehyde oxidase system, while a CYP3A4 pathway is less relevant. Paliperidone, the active metabolite of risperidone, is largely devoid of phase I metabolism, and undergoes primarily phase II conjugation reactions.

The majority of SSRIs undergo extensive hepatic oxidative metabolism mediated by CYP isoenzymes. Unlike TCAs, newer antidepressants have a relatively wider therapeutic index, limiting the severity of adverse effects when concomitantly administered with enzyme inhibitors or inducers. However, SSRIs, which are potent inhibitors of CYP450, are likely to cause significant DDIs. Examples include fluoxetine and paroxetine, which are potent inhibitors of CYP2D6, and fluvoxamine, a potent inhibitor of CYP1A2 and CYP2C19. Antidepressants like sertraline, citalopram, escitalopram, venlafaxine, mirtazapine, and reboxetine are generally less likely to be potential sources of interactions involving CYP isoenzymes (Spina et al., 2008; Spina et al., 2012).

Among anti-epileptic drugs used as mood stabilizers, a number of DDIs have been reported for valproic acid, which acts as an inhibitor of CYP2C9 and for carbamazepine, which is a potent inducer of CYP3A4, 2B6, 2C9 and 2C19 isoenzymes. Other anti-epileptics like lamotrigine, gabapentin, and topiramate, which are used as mood stabilizers, have been reported to have minimal clinically significant drug-drug interactions.

4. New medications being added to existing pharmacotherapy regimens should be started at low doses and titrated slowly. This is particularly important in special patient populations that are more likely to experience DDIs, including elderly patients, patients with renal or hepatic impairment, as well as those with chronic somatic illnesses requiring long-term pharmacotherapy.

5. When a medication is prescribed concomitantly with either an inhibitor or an inducer of its metabolism, or otherwise if the inhibitor or inducer is discontinued, careful monitoring of clinical response and possible monitoring of plasma concentrations of the medication for several weeks are recommended, since DDIs often occur within one to two weeks following changes in a patient's medication regimen. Continuous monitoring of newly developed side effects and changes in clinical response are also warranted.

6. A detailed explanation of the symptoms that patients might experience helps the physicians build a therapeutic rapport and encourages patients to actively participate in their treatment plan and be aware of the potential side effects and changes in clinical response.

7. Data on potential DDIs involving newly developed medications for treatment of psychiatric conditions, infections, cancer, and other diseases have been growing in a rapid pace. Therefore, clinicians should explore available resources to learn about DDIs, such as updated textbooks, electronic databases (e.g. PubMed and UptoDate), reviews, and updated drug interactions websites (e.g. Lexicomp, Epocrates, Medscape, FDA, Drugs.com, and CDC websites). Furthermore, the use of pharmacogenetic tests should be considered in selected clinical situations.

Conclusion

Drug interactions are an often neglected cause of increased morbidity and mortality. This may significantly increase the expenditure of health care in primary care and other treatment settings. Since most drug interactions are predictable, physicians should be continuously educated about the various mechanisms of drug interactions and follow the appropriate recommendations discussed in this chapter. With the advent of several websites and catalogues documenting potential drug interactions as well as pharmacogenetic testing, most DDIs could be preventable.

References

Adults and Older Adult Adverse Drug Events. Centers for Disease Control and Prevention website. October 2, 2012. Retrieved April 25, 2015, from http://www.cdc.gov/MedicationSafety/Adult_AdverseDrugEvents.html

Akamine, Y, Yasui-Furukori, N, Ieiri, I, and Uno, T. (2012). Psychotropic Drug-Drug Interactions Involving P-Glycoprotein. CNS Drugs, 26: 959–73.

American Psychiatric Association. (1997). Practice guideline for the treatment of patients with schizophrenia. Am J Psychiatry, 154/4: 1–63.

Budnitz, DS, Lovegrove, MC, Shehab, N, and Richards, CL. (2011). Emergency hospitalizations for adverse drug events in older Americans. N Engl J Med, 365/21: 2002–12.

Burger D, Back D, Buggisch P, Buti M, Craxí A, Foster G, Klinker H, Larrey D, Nikitin I, Pol S, Puoti M, Romero-Gómez M, Wedemeyer H, and Zeuzem S. (2013). Clinical management of drug-drug interactions in HCV therapy: Challenges and solutions, J Hepatol, 58: 792–800.

Caraci, F, Crupi, R, Drago, F, and Spina, E. (2011). Metabolic Drug Interactions Between Antidepressants and Anticancer Drugs: Focus on Selective Serotonin Reuptake Inhibitors and Hypericum Extract. Curr Drug Metab, 12: 570–577.

Castberg, I, Skogvoll, E, and Spigset, O. (2007). Quetiapine and drug interactions: evidence from a routine therapeutic drug monitoring service. J Clin Psychiatry, 68: 1540–45.

Ciraulo, DA, Shader, RI, Greenblatt, DJ, and Creelman, W. (2006). Drug interactions in psychiatry, 3rd edn. New York: Lippincott Williams & Wilkins.

Devane CL. (1998). Principles of pharmacokinetics and pharmacodynamics. In: The American Psychiatric Press Textbook of Psychopharmacology, AF Schatzberg and CB Nemeroff, eds., 2nd edn. Washington, DC: American Psychiatric Press Inc.

Dunnill MS and Halley W. (1973). Some observations on the quantitative anatomy of the kidney. J Pathol, 110: 113–21.

English, B, Dortch, M, Ereshefsky, L, and Jhee, S. (2012). Clinically significant psychotropic drug-drug interactions in the primary care settings. Curr Psychiatry Rep, 14/4: 376–90.

Ereshefsky, L, Jhee, S, and Grothe, D. (2005). Antidepressant drug-drug interaction profile ppdate. Drugs R D, 6/6: 323–6.

Ereshefsky, L. (2009). Drug-drug interactions with the use of psychotropic medications: questions and answers. CNS Spectr, 14/8: 1–8.

Fleeman N, Dundar Y, Dickson R, Jorgensen A, Pushpakom S, McLeod C, Pirmohamed M, and Walley T. (2011). Cytochrome P450 testing for prescribing antipsychotics in adults with schizophrenia: systematic review and meta-analyses. Pharmacogenomics J, 11: 1–14.

Gardiner, P, Phillips, R, and Shaughnessy, AF. (2008). Herbal and dietary supplement–drug interactions in patients with chronic illnesses. *Am Fam Physician,* 77/1: 73–78.

Hewick DS, Newbury P, Hopwood S, Naylor G, and Moody J. (1977). Age as a factor affecting lithium therapy. *Br J Clin Pharmacol,* 4: 201–5.

Huang, SM. (2011). *Drug Development and Drug Interactions: Tables of Substrates, Inhibitors, and Inducers.* US Food and Drug Administration website. Retrieved March 23, 2015, from http://www.fda.gov/Drugs/DevelopmentApprovalProcess/DevelopmentResources/DrugInteractionsLabeling/ucm093664.htm#classInhibit

Hussar, DA. (2013). Drug Interactions: Factors Affecting Response to Drugs. Merck Manuals website. Retrieved April 08, 2015. http://www.merckmanuals.com/home/drugs/factors_affecting_response_to_drugs/drug_interactions.html

Ingelman-Sundberg, M. (2005). Genetic polymorphisms of cytochrome P450 2D6 (CYP2D6): clinical consequences, evolutionary aspects and functional diversity. *Pharmacogenomics J,* 5/1:6–13.

Kalgutkar, AS, Obach, RS, and Mauer, TS. (2007). Mechanism-based inactivation of cytochrome p450 enzymes: Chemical mechanisms, structure-activity relationships and relationship to clinical drug-drug interactions and idiosyncratic adverse drug reactions. *Curr Drug Metab,* 8: 407–47.

Kelly, CM, Juurlink, DN, Gomes, T, Duong-Hua, M, Pritchard, KL, Austin, PC, and Paszat, LF. (2010). Selective serotonin reuptake inhibitors and breast cancer mortality in women receiving tamoxifen: a population-based cohort study. *BMJ,* Feb 8;**340**:c693, doi: 10.1136/bmj.c693.

Kennedy, WK, Jann, MW and Kutscher, EC. (2013). Clinically significant drug interactions with atypical antipsychotics. *CNS Drugs,* 27: 1021–48.

Klotz, U, Avant, GR, Hoyumpa, A, Schenker, S, and Wilkinson, GR. (1975). The effects of age and liver disease on the disposition and elimination of diazepam in adult man. *J. Clin. Invest,* 55/2: 347–59.

Labos, C, Dasgupta, K, and Nedjar, H. (2011). Risk of bleeding associated with combined use of selective serotonin reuptake inhibitors and antiplatelet therapy following acute myocardial infarction. *Can Med Assoc J,* **183**/16: 1835–43.

Lexicomp Online. (2015). https://online.lexi.com/lco/action/interact

Liston, H, Markowitz, J, and DeVane C. (2001). Drug glucuronidation in clinical psychopharmacology. *J Clin Psychopharmacol,* 21: 500–15.

Madhusoodanan, S, Velama, M, Parmar, J, Goia, D, and Brenner, R. (2014). A current review of cytochrome P450 interactions of psychotropic drugs. *Ann Clin Psychiatry,* 26/2: 120–38.

Mangoni, AA and Jackson, SH. (2004). Age-related changes in pharmacokinetics and pharmacodynamics: basic principles and practical applications. *Br J Clin Pharmacol,* 57/1: 6–14.

Muscatello, MR, Spina, E, Bandelow, B,and Baldwin, D. (2012). Clinically relevant drug interactions in anxiety disorders. *Hum Psychopharmacol Clin,* 27: 239–53.

Nadkarni, A, Oldham, M, Howard, M, and Berenhaum, I. (2012). Drug-drug interactions between warfarin and psychotropics: updated review of the literature. *Pharmacotherapy,* 32/10: 932–42.

Nebert DW, Adensik M, Coon MJ, Estabrook RW, Gonzalez FJ, Guengerich FP, Gunsalus IC, Johnson EF, Kemper B, Levin W, Phillips, IR, Sato R, and Waterman MR. (1987). The P450 gene superfamily: recommended nomenclature. *DNA,* 6/1: 1–11.

Preskorn, S Hand Flockhart, D. (2006). 2006 Guide to Psychiatric Drug Interactions. *Prim psychiatry*, 13/4: 35–64.

Rasmussen-Torvik, LJ and McAlpine, DD. (2007). Genetic screening for SSRI drug response among those with major depression: greatpromise and unseen perils. *Depress Anxiety*, 24/5:350–7.

Sajatovic, M, Madhusoodanan, S, and Buckley, P. (2000). Schizophrenia in the Elderly. *CNS drugs*, 13/2: 103–15.

Sandson, N, Armstrong, S, and Cozza, K. (2005). An Overview of Psychotropic Drug-Drug Interactions. *Psychosomatics*, 46: 464–94.

Schellander, R and Donnerer, J. (2010). Antidepressants: Clinically Relevant Drug Interactions to Be Considered. *Pharmacology*, 86: 203–15.

Shi, S and Klotz, U. (2011). Age-related changes in pharmacokinetics. *Curr Drug Metab* 12/7: 601–10.

Short, DD, Hawley, JM, and McCarthy, MF. 2009. Management of schizophrenia with medical disorders: cardiovascular, pulmonary, and gastrointestinal. *Psychiatr Clin North Am*, 32/4: 759–73.

Sockalingam, S, Tseng, A, Giguere, P, and Wong, D. (2013). Psychiatric treatment considerations with direct acting antivirals in hepatitis C. *BMC Gastroenterol*, 13: 86.

Spina, E and de Leon, J. (2007). Metabolic drug interactions with newer antipsychotics: a comparative review. *Basic Clin Pharmacol Toxicol*, 100: 4–22.

Spina, E, Santoro, V, and D'Arrigo, C. (2008). Clinically relevant pharmacokinetic drug interactions with second-generation antidepressants: an update. *Clin Ther*, 30/7: 1206–27.

Spina, E, Trifiro, G, and Caraci, F. (2012). Clinically significant drug interactions with newer antidepressants. *CNS Drugs*, 26: 39–67.

Stahl, SM. (2013). *Stahl's Essential Psychopharmacology: Neuroscientific Basis and Practical Applications*, 4th edN. Cambridge: Cambridge University Press.

Sternbach, H. (1991). The serotonin syndrome. *Am J Psychiatry*, 148/6: 705–13.

Thompson, A, Silverman, B, Dzeng, L, and Treisman, G. (2006). Psychotropic medications and HIV. *Clin Infect Dis*, 42: 1305–10.

Turnheim, K. (2003). When drug therapy gets old: pharmacokinetics and pharmacodynamics in the elderly. *Exp Gerontol*, 38/8: 843–53.

Wilkinson, G. (2001). Pharmacokinetics: the dynamics of drug absorption, distribution, and elimination. In *Goodman and Gilman's: The Pharmacological Basis of Therapeutics*, JG Hardman, LE Limbird, and AG Gilman AG, eds, (10th edn. New York: McGraw-Hill.

Index

3-methoxy-4-hydroxyphenylglycol (MHPG) 61
5-hydroxyindoleacetic acid (5-HIAA) 61